Diabetes Mellitus in Cats and Dogs

Editors

CHEN GILOR
THOMAS K. GRAVES

VETERINARY CLINICS OF NORTH AMERICA: SMALL ANIMAL PRACTICE

www.vetsmall.theclinics.com

May 2023 • Volume 53 • Number 3

ELSEVIER

1600 John F. Kennedy Boulevard • Suite 1800 • Philadelphia, Pennsylvania, 19103-2899
http://www.vetsmall.theclinics.com

VETERINARY CLINICS OF NORTH AMERICA: SMALL ANIMAL PRACTICE Volume 53, Number 3
May 2023 ISSN 0195-5616, ISBN-13: 978-0-323-94023-8

Editor: Stacy Eastman
Developmental Editor: Axell Ivan Jade Purificacion

Veterinary Clinics of North America: Small Animal Practice (ISSN 0195-5616) is published bimonthly by Elsevier Inc., 360 Park Avenue South, New York, NY 10010-1710. Months of issue are January, March, May, July, September, and November. Business and Editorial Offices: 1600 John F. Kennedy Blvd., Ste. 1800, Philadelphia, PA 19103-2899. Customer Service Office: 3251 Riverport Lane, Maryland Heights, MO 63043. Periodicals postage paid at New York, NY and additional mailing offices. Subscription prices are $387.00 per year (domestic individuals), $844.00 per year (domestic institutions), $100.00 per year (domestic students/residents), $488.00 per year (Canadian individuals), $1049.00 per year (Canadian institutions), $528.00 per year (international individuals), $1049.00 per year (international institutions), $100.00 per year (Canadian students/residents), and $220.00 per year (international students/residents). To receive student/resident rate, orders must be accompanied by name of affiliated institution, date of term, and the *signature* of program/residency coordinator on institution letterhead. Orders will be billed at individual rate until proof of status is received. Foreign air speed delivery is included in all *Clinics* subscription prices. All prices are subject to change without notice. **POSTMASTER:** Send address changes to *Veterinary Clinics of North America: Small Animal Practice*, Elsevier Health Sciences Division, Subscription Customer Service, 3251 Riverport Lane, Maryland Heights, MO 63043. Customer Service (orders, claims, online, change of address): Elsevier Periodicals Customer Service, Elsevier Health Sciences Division Subscription **Customer Service 3251 Riverport Lane Maryland Heights, MO 63043. Tel: 1-800-654-2452 (U.S. and Canada); 314-447-8871 (outside U.S. and Canada). Fax: 314-447-8029. E-mail: journalscustomerservice-usa@elsevier.com (for print support); journalsonlinesupport-usa@elsevier.com (for online support).**

Reprints. For copies of 100 or more of articles in this publication, please contact the Commercial Reprints Department, Elsevier Inc., 360 Park Avenue South, New York, NY 10010-1710. Tel.: 212-633-3874; Fax: 212-633-3820; E-mail: reprints@elsevier.com.

Veterinary Clinics of North America: Small Animal Practice is also published in Japanese by Inter Zoo Publishing Co., Ltd., Aoyama Crystal-Bldg 5F, 3-5-12 Kitaaoyama, Minato-ku, Tokyo 107-0061, Japan.

Veterinary Clinics of North America: Small Animal Practice is covered in *Current Contents/Agriculture, Biology and Environmental Sciences, Science Citation Index, ASCA, MEDLINE/PubMed (Index Medicus), Excerpta Medica, and BIOSIS.*

Contributors

EDITORS

CHEN GILOR, DVM, PhD
Diplomate, American College of Veterinary Internal Medicine; Associate Professor, Small Animal Internal Medicine, Department of Small Animal Clinical Sciences, College of Veterinary Medicine, University of Florida, Gainesville, Florida, USA

THOMAS K. GRAVES, DVM, MS, PhD
Diplomate, American College of Veterinary Internal Medicine; College of Veterinary Medicine, Midwestern University, Glendale, Arizona, USA

AUTHORS

RENEA BARRETT, BSc, DVM, MANZCVS
Animal Diabetes Australia, Melbourne, Victoria, Australia

RICHARD K. BURCHELL, BSc, BVSc, MMedVet
Diplomate, European College of Veterinary Internal Medicine - Companion Animal; North Coast Veterinary Specialist and Referral Centre, Sippy Downs, Sunshine Coast, Australia

RENATA S. COSTA, DVM, MPhil, GradDipEd, MANZCVS
Diplomate, American College of Veterinary Anesthesia and Analgesia; Assistant Professor of Anesthesiology and Service Chief, Specialty Medicine, Midwestern University, Glendale, Arizona, USA

LUCY J. DAVISON, MA, VetMB, MRVCS
Diplomate, Small Animal Medicine; Diplomate, European College of Veterinary Internal Medicine - Companion Animal; Royal Veterinary College, Clinical Sciences and Services, Hertfordshire, United Kingdom

FRANCESCA DEL BALDO, DVM, MRCVS, PhD
Diplomate, European College of Veterinary Internal Medicine - Companion Animal (Internal Medicine); Department of Veterinary Medical Science, University of Bologna, Bologna, Italy

LINDA FLEEMAN, BVSc, PhD, MANZCVS
Director, Animal Diabetes Australia, Melbourne, Victoria, Australia

FEDERICO FRACASSI, DVM, PhD
Diplomate, European College of Veterinary Internal Medicine - Companion Animal; Department of Veterinary Medical Science, University of Bologna, Bologna, Italy

ARNON GAL, DVM, PhD
Diplomate, American College of Veterinary Internal Medicine (Small Animal Internal Medicine); Diplomate, American College of Veterinary Pathologists (Anatomic Pathology); Assistant Professor in Small Animal Internal Medicine, Department of Veterinary Clinical

Medicine, College of Veterinary Medicine, University of Illinois at Urbana-Champaign, Urbana, Illinois, USA

CHEN GILOR, DVM, PhD
Diplomate, American College of Veterinary Internal Medicine; Associate Professor, Small Animal Internal Medicine, Department of Small Animal Clinical Sciences, College of Veterinary Medicine, University of Florida, Gainesville, Florida, USA

RUTH GOSTELOW, BVetMed(Hons), PhD, FHEA
Diplomate, European College of Veterinary Internal Medicine (Companion Animal); Diplomate, American College of Veterinary Internal Medicine (Companion Animal); MRCVS, Senior Lecturer in Small Animal Internal Medicine, RCVS Recognised Specialist in Small Animal Medicine, The Royal Veterinary College, North Mymms, Hertfordshire, United Kingdom

THOMAS K. GRAVES, DVM, MS, PhD
Diplomate, American College of Veterinary Internal Medicine; College of Veterinary Medicine, Midwestern University, Glendale, Arizona, USA

KATARINA HAZUCHOVA, MVDr, PhD, MRCVS
Diplomate, European College of Veterinary Internal Medicine (Companion Animal); Senior Clinician and Lecturer in Small Animal Internal Medicine, Small Animal Clinic (Internal Medicine), Justus-Liebig-Universität Gießen, Gießen, Germany

RICHARD C. HILL, MA, VetMB, PhD, MRCVS
Diplomate, American College of Veterinary Internal Medicine (Small Animal Internal Medicine, Nutrition); University of Florida College of Veterinary Medicine, Gainesville, Florida, USA

TEELA JONES, DVM, MVetSc
Diplomate, American College of Veterinary Anesthesia and Analgesia; Anesthesiologist, Summit Veterinary Referral Center, Tacoma, Washington, USA

JOCELYN MOTT, DVM
Diplomate, American College of Veterinary Internal Medicine (Small Animal Internal Medicine); Post-Doctoral Associate in Diabetes, College of Veterinary Medicine, University of Florida, Gainesville, Florida, USA

STIJN J.M. NIESSEN, DVM, PhD, PGCertVetEd, FHEA
Diplomate, European College of Veterinary Internal Medicine; MRCVS, Professor, Royal Veterinary College London, United Kingdom; Co-Founder, Veterinary Specialist Consultations and VIN Europe, Hilversum, the Netherlands

ALLISON L. O'KELL, DVM, MS
Diplomate, American College of Veterinary Internal Medicine (Small Animal Internal Medicine); Department of Small Animal Clinical Sciences, University of Florida, Gainesville, Florida, USA

ADESOLA ODUNAYO, DVM, MS
Diplomate, American College of Veterinary Emergency and Critical Care; Clinical Associate Professor of Emergency and Critical Care, Department of Small Animal Clinical Sciences, College of Veterinary Medicine, University of Florida, Gainesville, Florida, USA

VALERIE J. PARKER, DVM
Diplomate, American College of Veterinary Internal Medicine (Small Animal Internal Medicine and Nutrition); The Ohio State University Veterinary Medical Center, Columbus, Ohio, USA

JENNIFER M. REINHART, DVM, PhD
Department of Veterinary Clinical Medicine, College of Veterinary Medicine, University of Illinois Urbana-Champaign, Urbana, Illinois, USA

Contents

Preface: Diabetes Mellitus in Cats and Dogs   xiii

Chen Gilor and Thomas K. Graves

Etiology and Pathophysiology of Diabetes Mellitus in Dogs   493

Allison L. O'Kell and Lucy J. Davison

Canine diabetes results from a wide spectrum of clinical pathophysiological processes that cause a similar set of clinical signs. Various causes of
insulin deficiency and beta cell loss, insulin resistance, or both charac-
terize the disease, with genetics and environment playing a role. Understanding the genetic and molecular causes of beta cell loss will provide
future opportunities for precision medicine, both from a therapeutic and
preventative perspective. This review presents current knowledge of the
etiology and pathophysiology of canine diabetes, including the importance
of disease classification. Examples of potential targets for future precision
medicine–based approaches to therapy are discussed.

Pathophysiology of Prediabetes, Diabetes, and Diabetic Remission in Cats   511

Ruth Gostelow and Katarina Hazuchova

 Video content accompanies this article at http://www.vetsmall.
theclinics.com.

Diabetes mellitus (DM) has a heterogenous cause, and the exact pathogenesis differs between patients. Most diabetic cats have a cause similar
to human type 2 DM but, in some, DM is associated with underlying conditions, such as hypersomatotropism, hyperadrenocorticism, or administration of diabetogenic drugs. Predisposing factors for feline DM include
obesity, reduced physical activity, male sex, and increasing age. Gluco(-
lipo)toxicity and genetic predisposition also likely play roles in pathogenesis. Prediabetes cannot be accurately diagnosed in cats at the current
time. Diabetic cats can enter remission, but relapses are common, as
these cats might have ongoing, abnormal glucose homeostasis.

**Diabetes Ketoacidosis and Hyperosmolar Hyperglycemic Syndrome in Companion
Animals**   531

Arnon Gal and Adesola Odunayo

Diabetes mellitus is a common endocrinopathy in dogs and cats. Diabetes
ketoacidosis (DKA) and hyperosmolar hyperglycemic state (HHS) are life-
threatening complications of diabetes resulting from an imbalance between insulin and the glucose counter-regulatory hormones. The first
part of this review focuses on the pathophysiology of DKA and HHS,
and rarer complications such as euglycemic DKA and hyperosmolar
DKA. The second part of this review focuses on the diagnosis and treatment of these complications.

Glucose Counterregulation: Clinical Consequences of Impaired Sympathetic
Responses in Diabetic Dogs and Cats   551

Jocelyn Mott and Chen Gilor

> Insulin induced hypoglycemia (IIH) is common in veterinary patients and
> limits the clinician's ability to obtain adequate glycemic control with insulin
> therapy. Not all diabetic dogs and cats with IIH exhibit clinical signs and
> hypoglycemia might be missed by routine blood glucose curve monitoring.
> In diabetic patients, counterregulatory responses to hypoglycemia are
> impaired (lack of decrease in insulin levels, lack of increase in glucagon,
> and attenuation of the parasympathetic and sympathoadrenal autonomic
> nervous systems) and have been documented in people and in dogs but
> not yet in cats. Antecedent hypoglycemic episodes increase the patient's
> risk for future severe hypoglycemia.

Diabetes Mellitus and the Kidneys   565

Arnon Gal and Richard K. Burchell

> The pathomechanisms implicated in diabetic kidney disease in people are
> present in dogs and cats and, in theory, could lead to renal complications
> in companion animals with long-standing diabetes mellitus. However,
> these renal complications develop during a long period, and there is little
> to no clinical evidence that they could lead to chronic kidney disease in
> companion animals.

Anesthetic Considerations in Dogs and Cats with Diabetes Mellitus   581

Renata S. Costa and Teela Jones

> Understanding the effects of diabetes and hyperglycemia on hydration,
> acid–base status, and immune function is paramount to safely anesthetiz-
> ing diabetic cats and dogs. Preoperative stabilization of glucose concen-
> trations, hydration, and electrolyte imbalances is key to minimizing
> morbidity and mortality. Blood glucose monitoring perioperatively will
> help guide insulin and dextrose administration. Specific anesthetic consid-
> erations, and peri-anesthetic management of animals with diabetes melli-
> tus, including anesthetic drugs and recommended insulin protocols are
> discussed.

Continuous Glucose Monitoring in Dogs and Cats: Application of New Technology
to an Old Problem   591

 Video content accompanies this article at http://www.vetsmall.
theclinics.com.

Francesca Del Baldo and Federico Fracassi

> In recent years, glucose monitoring has been revolutionized by the devel-
> opment of continuous glucose monitoring systems (CGMS), which are
> wearable non/minimally invasive devices that measure glucose concentra-
> tion almost continuously for several consecutive d/wk. The Abbott Free-
> Style Libre is the CGMS used most commonly. It has adequate clinical
> accuracy both in dogs and cats, even though the accuracy is lower in
> the hypoglycemic range. It allows an accurate identification of glycemic
> excursions occurring throughout the day as well as of glucose variations

during consecutive days, enabling the clinician to make a more informed decision about the insulin dose and frequency of administration.

Insulin Therapy in Small Animals, Part 1: General Principles   615

Linda Fleeman and Chen Gilor

Understanding the pharmacology of insulin and how it relates to the pathophysiology of diabetes can lead to better clinical outcomes. No insulin formulation should be considered "best" by default. Insulin suspensions (NPH, NPH/regular mixes, lente, and PZI) as well as insulin glargine U100 and detemir are intermediate-acting formulations that are administered twice daily. For a formulation to be an effective and safe basal insulin, its action should be roughly the same every hour of the day. Currently, only insulin glargine U300 and insulin degludec meet this standard in dogs, whereas in cats, insulin glargine U300 is the closest option.

Insulin Therapy in Small Animals, Part 2: Cats   635

Linda Fleeman and Chen Gilor

No insulin formulation should be considered best by default for management of feline diabetes. Rather, the choice of insulin formulation should be tailored to the specific clinical situation. In most cats that have some residual beta cell function, administering only a basal insulin might lead to complete normalization of blood glucose concentrations. Basal insulin requirements are constant throughout the day. Therefore, for an insulin formulation to be effective and safe as a basal insulin, its action should be roughly the same every hour of the day. At present, only insulin glargine U300 approaches this definition in cats.

Insulin Therapy in Small Animals, Part 3: Dogs   645

Linda Fleeman and Chen Gilor

Insulin therapy should ideally mimic a basal-bolus pattern. Lente, NPH, NPH/regular mixes, PZI, glargine U100, and detemir are intermediate-acting formulations that are administered twice daily in dogs. To minimize hypoglycemia, intermediate-acting insulin protocols are usually geared towards alleviating (but not eliminating) clinical signs. Insulin glargine U300 and insulin degludec meet the criterla for an effective and safe basal insulin in dogs. In most dogs, good control of clinical signs is achieved when using a basal insulin alone. In a small minority, bolus insulin at the time of at least one meal per day may be added to optimize glycemic control.

Nutritional Management of Cats and Dogs with Diabetes Mellitus   657

Valerie J. Parker and Richard C. Hill

This article reviews the nutritional assessment and management of diabetic dogs and cats. It discusses how to determine appropriate nutritional goals for individual patients, including comorbid patients with diabetes. Considerations for macronutrient and micronutrient modifications will be reviewed.

The Future of Diabetes Therapies: New Insulins and Insulin Delivery Systems, Glucagon-Like Peptide 1 Analogs, Sodium-Glucose Cotransporter Type 2 Inhibitors, and Beta Cell Replacement Therapy   675

Jennifer M. Reinhart and Thomas K. Graves

As the prevalence of diabetes mellitus increases, so too does the number of available treatment modalities. Many diabetic therapies available in human medicine or on the horizon could hold promise in the management of small animal diabetes. However, it is important to consider how species differences in pathophysiology, management practices and goals, and lifestyle may affect the translation of such treatment modalities for veterinary use. This review article aimed to familiarize veterinarians with the more promising novel diabetic therapies and explore their possible applications in the treatment of canine and feline diabetes mellitus.

Hypersomatotropism and Other Causes of Insulin Resistance in Cats   691

Stijn J.M. Niessen

True insulin resistance should be differentiated from management-related difficulties (eg, short insulin duration, inappropriate insulin injection, inappropriate storage). Hypersomatotropism (HST) is the number one cause of insulin resistance in cats, with hypercortisolism (HC) occupying a more distant second place. Serum insulinlike growth factor-1 is adequate for screening for HST, and screening at the time of diagnosis, regardless of presence of insulin resistance, is advocated. Treatment of either disease centers on removal of the overactive endocrine gland (hypophysectomy, adrenalectomy) or inhibition of the pituitary or adrenal glands by using drugs such as trilostane (HC), pasireotide (HST, HC) or cabergoline (HST, HC).

Cushing's Syndrome and Other Causes of Insulin Resistance in Dogs   711

Linda Fleeman and Renea Barrett

The most common causes of insulin resistance in diabetic dogs are Cushing syndrome, diestrus, and obesity. Cushing-associated effects include insulin resistance, excessive postprandial hyperglycemia, perceived short duration of insulin action, and/or substantial within-day and/or day-to-day glycemic variability. Successful strategies to manage excessive glycemic variability include basal insulin monotherapy and combined basal-bolus insulin treatment. Ovariohysterectomy and insulin treatment can achieve diabetic remission in about 10% of cases of diestrus diabetes. Different causes of insulin resistance have an additive effect on insulin requirements and the risk of progression to clinical diabetes in dogs.

VETERINARY CLINICS OF NORTH AMERICA: SMALL ANIMAL PRACTICE

FORTHCOMING ISSUES

July 2023
Rehabilitation Therapy
Molly J. Flaherty, *Editor*

September 2023
Small Animal Theriogenology
Bruce W. Christensen, *Editor*

November 2023
Advancements in Companion Animal Cardiology
Joshua Stern, *Editor*

RECENT ISSUES

March 2023
Ophthalmology in Small Animal Care
Bruce Grahn, *Editor*

January 2023
Clinical Pathology
Maxey L. Wellman, M. Judith Radin, *Editors*

November 2022
Vector-Borne Diseases
Linda Kidd, *Editor*

SERIES OF RELATED INTEREST

Veterinary Clinics: Exotic Animal Practice
https://www.vetexotic.theclinics.com/
Advances in Small Animal Care
https://www.advancesinsmallanimalcare.com/

THE CLINICS ARE NOW AVAILABLE ONLINE!
Access your subscription at:
www.theclinics.com

Preface

Diabetes Mellitus in Cats and Dogs

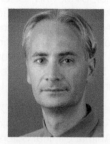 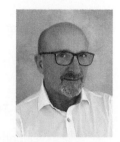

Chen Gilor, DVM, PhD, DACVIM   Thomas K. Graves, DVM, PhD, DACVIM
Editors

If we could have three wishes for the management of diabetes in dogs and cats, they would probably be these:

1. That diabetes mellitus be viewed not as two specific diseases, type 1 and type 2, but as a syndrome of glucose dysregulation of myriad causes and mechanisms.
2. That the frustrations suffered by veterinarians and their clients over the treatment of diabetes in animals be quelled by understanding of the pathophysiologic basis of modern insulin therapy, and by setting clear and reasonable expectations for treatment outcomes.
3. That traditional blood glucose curves, misleading as they are when performed by intermittent sampling of blood glucose throughout the day, would cease to exist.

Prefaces, in general, tend to be full of hyperbole, and we won't disappoint. Diabetes is the largest, deadliest, most tenacious, and most expensive pandemic facing humankind, and it continues to threaten dogs and cats as well. Veterinary patients can benefit from the oceans of research aimed at diagnosis, treatment, and prevention of diabetes in people, but this requires that veterinarians possess constantly updated knowledge of diabetes trends on all fronts. Our aim is to present the most current and evidence-based ideas on the treatment of diabetes, and also to provide veterinarians with updated information on the pathobiology of the disease. It is our hope that having a better understanding of disease mechanisms and the intricacies of insulin pharmacology will not only satisfy the intellectual curiosity of readers but also position them to provide the best care for their patients. We have tried to include much practical information in this issue, and our hope is that even the more esoteric aspects of diabetes presented herein might prove useful, or at the very least, of interest.

Vet Clin Small Anim 53 (2023) xiii–xiv
https://doi.org/10.1016/j.cvsm.2023.02.018
0195-5616/23/© 2023 Published by Elsevier Inc.

vetsmall.theclinics.com

We are grateful for the expert contributions made by a list of authors that includes some of the world's top experts in animal diabetes, as well as some up-and-coming future leaders in the field. Working with them has taught us many new things and has made us better veterinarians. We hope the readers of this issue are similarly enriched. It might be asking a lot, but we also hope that at least two of our wishes come true (we are not holding out for the glucose curve moratorium).

Chen Gilor, DVM, PhD, DACVIM
Small Animal Internal Medicine
Department of Small Animal Clinical Sciences
College of Veterinary Medicine
University of Florida
2015 Southwest 16th Avenue
Gainesville, FL 32608, USA

Thomas K. Graves, DVM, PhD, DACVIM
Small Animal Internal Medicine
Department of Small Animal Clinical Sciences
College of Veterinary Medicine
Midwestern University
19555 N 59th Avenue
Glendale, AZ 85308, USA

E-mail addresses:
cgilor@ufl.edu (C. Gilor)
t.graves@midwestern.edu (T.K. Graves)

Etiology and Pathophysiology of Diabetes Mellitus in Dogs

Allison L. O'Kell, DVM, MS, DACVIM (SAIM)[a],*,
Lucy J. Davison, MA, PhD, VetMB, DipECVIM-CA, MRVCS[b]

KEYWORDS

- Canine diabetes • Pathogenesis • Beta cell • Insulin deficiency • Insulin resistance

KEY POINTS

- Diabetes mellitus in dogs results from one or more underlying mechanisms related to insulin deficiency/β-cell loss, insulin resistance, or both.
- Autoimmunity seems to be a less important aspect of pathophysiology than was previously believed, with focus shifting toward β-cell health.
- Genetics and the environment likely play a role, but require further study to better define these as underlying risk factors.
- Underlying disease mechanisms may in part be breed dependent, and optimal management from a precision medicine standpoint will likely rely on uncovering the genetic and molecular basis for the disease among breeds.

INTRODUCTION

Diabetes mellitus (DM) has been defined[a] by the European Society for Veterinary Endocrinology and Society for Comparative Endocrinology as a heterogeneous group of diseases with multiple causes, characterized by hyperglycemia resulting from inadequate insulin secretion, inadequate insulin action, or both.[1]

In veterinary practice, it is well established that all dogs with diabetes, almost without exception, require lifelong daily insulin injections. This implies a state of permanent insulin deficiency, and is typically associated with pancreatic β-cell loss. There are, however, many and varied routes by which this β-cell loss may occur. Some routes have a more direct impact on the β-cell, whereas others may result in β-cell death more indirectly.

---

[a]Note: Current affiliation is with PetDx, but affiliation was the University of Florida at the time of writing.
[a] Department of Small Animal Clinical Sciences, University of Florida, 2015 Southwest 16th Avenue, Gainesville, FL 32610, USA; [b] Royal Veterinary College, Clinical Sciences and Services, Hawkshead Lane, Hertfordshire AL9 7TA, UK
* Corresponding author.
E-mail address: aokelldvm@gmail.com

Vet Clin Small Anim 53 (2023) 493–510
https://doi.org/10.1016/j.cvsm.2023.01.004
0195-5616/23/© 2023 Elsevier Inc. All rights reserved.

In the developing era of precision medicine, in which management of human DM has been at the forefront, it has become increasingly important to understand the molecular basis of disease, and disease risk, in every individual patient. Precision medicine has been defined as "providing the right therapy for the right patient at the right time,"[2] a concept also described as "precision care" or "personalized medicine." This principle of individualized care is underpinned by the ability to distinguish between different subtypes of a particular condition, each requiring a different approach. In human DM precision medicine, such tools as genome sequencing, autoantibody evaluation, and measurement of insulin C-peptide are important in informing the most effective strategy for management, and potentially even prevention, of DM. Although the understanding of the molecular basis of canine DM is still in its infancy, it is anticipated that with improved knowledge, the ability of the veterinary profession to deliver diabetes care with greater precision to canine patients will improve.

This review presents what is currently known about the cause and pathophysiology of DM in dogs, including the importance of disease classification. Examples of potential targets for future precision medicine–based approaches to therapy are also discussed.

CLASSIFICATION AND DESCRIPTION

Although dogs with DM all present with similar clinical signs of polydipsia, polyuria, polyphagia, and persistent hyperglycemia, classification of the underlying mechanism of their disease is vitally important for optimal management.[3] In human medicine, the type 1/type 2 diabetes classification has been described as inadequately capturing the heterogeneity of the condition, and there is currently a clear focus on defining different diabetes subtypes more effectively.[4] **Box 1** represents the Project ALIVE (Agreeing Language in Veterinary Endocrinology) etiologic classification of DM in dogs (and cats). Importantly, however, it is not yet clear what proportion of dogs with diabetes fall into each category, and also whether certain categories are overrepresented in DM within particular breeds. There are also some categories that are purely theoretical at present, and not reported in the veterinary literature, such as diabetes induced by thiazide diuretics. These are included on the list because they are known to exist in people.[5,6] Although some more unusual and rare forms of DM do exist, such as juvenile diabetes in the Labrador retriever and other breeds,[7,8] diabetes following partial pancreatectomy for insulinoma,[9] and diabetes associated with drug treatment (eg, streptozotocin),[10] this review focuses on the more commonly presented forms of canine DM.

Insulin-Deficient Diabetes Mellitus

Pancreatic pathology and β-cell loss
Unfortunately, large studies of the histopathologic appearance of the canine diabetic pancreas at the time of diagnosis are lacking, making it more challenging to dissect the mechanisms leading up to and causing β-cell damage in this species. Mechanisms involved in β-cell death or survival in human diabetic patients include apoptosis, necroptosis, autophagy, and pyroptosis,[11] and these can reasonably be assumed to play a role in canine DM. Although apoptosis is a shared and common form of β-cell death in type 1 and type 2 human diabetes, the two conditions are notably distinct in histopathologic appearance. Autoimmune type 1 DM is characterized by an islet infiltrate of lymphocytes, known as insulitis, which is absent in type 2 diabetes.[12] The presence of autoimmune insulitis in canine DM has only rarely

---

Box 1
Etiologic classification of diabetes mellitus in dogs and cats as defined by the ALIVE project

Insulin-deficient DM (β-cell-related disorders)
- Reduced insulin secretion
  - β-cell dysfunction
  - β-cell destruction
    - *Immune mediated*
    - *β-cell loss associated with exocrine pancreatic disease*
      - *Pancreatitis*
      - *Neoplasia*
      - *Idiopathic*
    - Toxicity (diazoxide)
    - Infection
    - Idiopathic
  - β-cell death
    - Glucotoxicity
    - Lipotoxicity
    - Idiopathic
  - *β-cell aplasia/abiotrophy/hypoplasia*
- Production of defective insulin

Insulin-resistant DM (target-organ disorders)
- Endocrine influence
  - *Growth hormone*
    - Endogenous hypersecretion
      - Pituitary origin
      - *Mammary origin*
    - Exogenous growth hormone
  - Steroids
    - *Glucocorticoids*
      - *Endogenous hypersecretion*
      - *Exogenous glucocorticoids*
    - *Progesterone/progestines*
      - *Luteal phase*
        - *Pregnancy*
        - *Diestrus (dog)*
      - *Exogenous progestins*
    - Other
  - Catecholamines
  - Thyroid hormone
    - Hyperthyroidism
- Obesity
- Drugs
  - Thiazide diuretics
  - β-adrenergic agonists
- Inflammatory mediators
- Disorders of receptor and intracellular signaling

Annotated to highlight in *bold/italic* those conditions that are most commonly recognized in canine diabetes mellitus. Note that an individual can concurrently have more than one underlying cause.

European Society for Veterinary Endocrinology, Project ALIVE..[1]

---

been reported, with acute or chronic inflammation of the exocrine pancreas appearing more commonly.[13] Overall, most published pathology studies in canine DM describe a complete absence of pancreatic β-cells in the diabetic pancreas[14,15] because samples have usually been collected from patients with long-standing disease.

Autoimmunity

In addition to insulitis, the hallmark of human type 1 DM is the presence of circulating antibodies to pancreatic autoantigens, such as insulin, proinsulin, glutamic acid decarboxylase (GAD65), and insulinoma antigen 2 (IA-2).[16] These autoantibodies are considered to be a consequence of β-cell destruction rather than a cause, with the infiltrating cytotoxic CD8 T lymphocytes being primarily responsible for islet destruction. Because affected dogs are insulin-dependent, canine DM has often been aligned with human type 1 DM, and in some dogs, similar pancreatic autoimmunity may be present.[17] Several studies have examined sera from dogs with diabetes for autoantibodies to insulin, proinsulin, GAD65, IA-2, and other pancreatic proteins.[18–23] Results have been highly variable, and although a small number of individual autoantibody-positive dogs with diabetes have been identified, serologic evidence for autoimmunity as a common primary underlying mechanism in canine DM is limited. Despite this, the association of particular haplotypes of the canine major histocompatibility complex with diabetes risk (encoded by the Dog Leukocyte Antigen [DLA] genes) does point to a role for the adaptive immune system in the pathogenesis of canine DM, at least in some breeds.[24]

Exocrine pancreatic disease

The relationship between canine DM and pancreatitis is well recognized but still not fully understood.[25] Pancreatogenic DM in humans is DM caused by any disease associated with the exocrine pancreas, including pancreatitis (acute or chronic), pancreatic cancer, and pancreatectomy. Similar to dogs, it represents a heterogeneous spectrum of clinical presentations.[26]

One of the challenges of evaluating the relationship between canine pancreatitis and DM is the poor specificity and sensitivity of diagnostic tests for pancreatitis, including pancreatic lipase assays and diagnostic imaging.[27,28] It is especially difficult to make a clinical diagnosis of chronic pancreatitis rather than acute pancreatitis,[29,30] and it is therefore possible that the DM diagnosis could precede recognition of exocrine pancreatic inflammation, even if the pancreatitis was present first.

Although there is published evidence that "bystander" damage to islets in pancreatitis can impact on β-cell function and lead to DM with or without exocrine pancreatic insufficiency,[31] in other studies, it seems that the hyperglycemic[32] and hyperlipidemic[33] diabetic state itself can contribute to the development of secondary pancreatitis. Therefore pancreatitis, which has been estimated to be present in 28% to 40% of canine DM patients,[13,34] may be causal or consequential in canine DM.

In addition, given that pancreatitis is more prevalent in certain breeds, and may have different mechanisms depending on the breed,[35–37] it is also possible that the causal association between pancreatitis and DM is more important in some breeds than others. There are shared putative risk factors for the development of DM and pancreatitis, such as obesity and hyperglycemia,[25] therefore it may also be the case that the conditions arise independently in the same individual. However, the close anatomic proximity of β-cells and pancreatic exocrine tissue supports the hypothesis that one condition becomes more likely once the other is present.

Insulin-Resistant Diabetes Mellitus

In some cases, canine DM may arise as the result of insulin resistance. This may be associated, at least initially, with hyperinsulinemia,[38] and persistent and often progressive glucose intolerance. The detrimental impact of persistent hyperglycemia (glucotoxicity) and/or hyperlipidemia (lipotoxicity) on human β-cell function is well documented,[39] but it is considerably less well understood in dogs. Additional discussion of insulin resistance in dogs is found elsewhere in this issue.

Glucocorticoids

Endogenous and exogenous glucocorticoids cause insulin resistance.[40] There are reports of the development of transient or permanent DM after glucocorticoid therapy in dogs[41,42]; however, this seems to be much less common than in cats. Healthy dogs given anti-inflammatory (prednisone for 4 weeks[43]) and immunosuppressive (prednisolone for 3 weeks[44]) doses of glucocorticoids did not have evidence of glucose intolerance or hyperinsulinemia. Given that the use of glucocorticoids in clinical practice is extremely common, many experts hypothesize that pre-existing abnormalities of the endocrine pancreas are likely present in dogs that develop DM after exogenous glucocorticoid administration.[45]

Naturally occurring hypercortisolism causes insulin resistance and glucose intolerance.[46] Recent studies have found that 10.5% to 13.6% of dogs with hyperadrenocorticism had concurrent DM[47,48]; conversely, 23% of dogs with DM had concurrent hypercortisolism.[34] It is difficult to determine which disease developed first in many cases reported in these studies. Additionally, in dogs treated for hypercortisolism with retinoic acid and cabergoline[48] or 9-cis isotreinoin,[49] those with blood glucose of greater than 5.6 mmol/L (100 mg/dL) or greater than 5.83 mmol/L (105 mg/dL), respectively, at diagnosis had an increased risk of future development of DM. Dogs with blood glucose greater than 5.83 mmol/L (105 mg/dL) at the time of diagnosis of hypercortisolism and that were treated with low-dose insulin detemir in addition to therapy for hypercortisolism were less likely to develop DM, suggesting a component of β-cell exhaustion in these cases.[49] Given that dogs with hypercortisolism and DM remain insulin dependent even with treatment of hyperadrenocorticism,[46,50,51] additional mechanisms underlying diabetes likely exist, again pointing to the potential fragility of the canine β-cell in the face of hyperglycemia.

Progesterone and growth hormone

Both naturally occurring increases in progesterone and exogenous progesterone administration can lead to increases in growth hormone, insulin resistance, and DM in dogs, sometimes with concurrent clinical signs of acromegaly.[52,53] In dogs, progesterone induces mammary overproduction of growth hormone, which also antagonises insulin.[54] Diabetes has been associated with both diestrus[55,56] and pregnancy.[56–58] Although this has been reported in a variety of breeds, it is suspected that susceptibility to progesterone-controlled growth hormone overproduction DM may be related to breed. Mared and colleagues[59] found that Elkhounds had higher serum C-peptide, increased estimates of β-cell function, and a trend toward lower insulin sensitivity when measured in diestrus compared with anestrus; these differences were not detected among dogs of other breeds. No difference in growth hormone was detected in diestrus versus anestrus in this study; however, this study was limited by reliance on the owner's estimation of timing of sample collection after a heat cycle and measurement at only a single time point.[59] With respect to gestational DM, Nordic Spitz breeds were overrepresented.[57] Ovariohysterectomy or pregnancy termination improves the chances for remission in dogs with progesterone-controlled growth hormone overproduction DM,[52,56,57] further supporting insulin resistance in the pathogenesis.

Primary hypothyroidism also can lead to hypersecretion of growth hormone in dogs[60,61] likely in part as a result of transdifferentiation of pituitary somatotropes into thyrotropes producing growth hormone and thyroid-stimulating hormone.[61] A recent case report described a dog with hypothyroidism and concurrent DM characterized by increased serum insulin along with elevated growth hormone and clinical signs of acromegaly; insulin therapy was eventually discontinued after euthyroid was achieved.[62] This is a rarely reported or clinically recognized form of DM in dogs.

Obesity

Obesity as a cause of insulin hypersecretion and insulin resistance is well documented in dogs.[63–65] Additionally, being overweight has been associated with a diagnosis of DM in dogs.[55,66] A "type 2 DM" model has been developed in dogs that consists of induction of obesity via feeding along with use of β-cell-toxic streptozotocin.[67] However, only after streptozotocin is administered do dogs develop hyperglycemia or overt DM, suggesting that factors other than obesity are important in the development of diabetes in obese dogs.

One way of exploring β-cell function is to examine insulin release in response to intravenous glucose. This test is imperfect because it does not involve responses with oral glucose and the incretin effect. However, in studies of naturally occurring obesity in dogs without diabetes, fasted and first-phase insulin concentrations were higher during an intravenous glucose tolerance test in obese compared with lean dogs, along with peak insulin after glucagon stimulation.[63] Most dogs had normal glucose tolerance, and insulin secretion compensated for insulin resistance.[63] When evaluating insulin secretion and glucose tolerance postprandially, obese dogs had normal glucose at baseline but higher glucose postprandially than lean dogs; however, only four of nine obese dogs were persistently hyperglycemic.[64] Insulin and triglyceride concentrations were also higher at baseline and postprandially.[64] Despite some obese dogs having persistent hyperglycemia for more than two-thirds of the day, none were reported to develop diabetes after a median of 2.6 years of follow-up.[64] In Labrador retrievers, the *pro-opiomelanocortin (POMC)* gene that has been associated with obesity and appetite in this breed does not currently seem to be directly linked with the risk of diabetes.[68] However, it is clear that overweight or obese dogs have insulin resistance and possibly glucose intolerance, and that being overweight has been associated with DM in dogs.[55,66] Based on available evidence, a direct cause and effect relationship remains to be proven.

Other Forms of Diabetes Mellitus

It is likely that within some breeds, distinct forms of DM exist that are unique to the breed and require a specific management approach. The concept of breed-related diabetic phenotypes will be fascinating for future study and delivery of precision medicine. For example, a more intensive approach to management may be required in the diabetic miniature schnauzer with hyperlipidemia, or the Cavalier King Charles spaniel with pancreatitis. Monogenic forms of DM may also exist in some breeds, some forms of which respond better to oral medication than insulin injections. For example, a dog with a mutation disrupting one of the ion channels involved in β-cell glucose sensing and insulin release may demonstrate improved glycemic control with sulphonylureas rather than insulin, as has been seen in humans.[69]

UNDERLYING RISK FACTORS

In many species, DM risk has long been recognized as a combination of genetic and environmental factors, raising the nature or nurture debate.[70] More detailed study of both these elements in canine DM has the potential to reveal new mechanisms for intervention to prevent or manage disease. The study of canine diabetes genetics must be undertaken with great care, because phenocopies, cases with the same clinical signs but different underlying pathogenesis, result in reduced statistical power to find genetic variants associated with disease. Although it is possible that some genetic factors may work in isolation to cause canine DM (monogenic disease), canine DM is likely to be a complex genetic disease, with many associated genetic variants, each of small effect contributing to overall risk. It is also possible that the genetic variants contributing to risk or protection may differ among breeds.

Genetic Diabetes Mellitus Risk Factors

The current status of canine diabetes genetics research has recently been reviewed extensively elsewhere and is only summarized here.[71,72] The hypothesis that there is a genetic basis for some types of canine DM comes from the consistent observation across many studies that certain breeds are highly predisposed to DM (eg, Samoyed, Tibetan terrier, West Highland white terrier, and miniature poodle), whereas others experience relative protection from DM (eg, boxer, golden retriever, German shepherd dog).[8,73–77] This suggests that certain breed-distinct genetic variants exist, which may predispose or protect the whole breed from DM. Work is currently underway to identify these variants by comparison of the whole genome sequence of high-risk and low-risk breeds.[72] Such variants may have a direct effect on β-cell function or health, but they may also have indirect roles in DM risk, such as by predisposing to conditions that may eventually result in DM (eg, hyperlipidemia, hypercortisolism, or pancreatitis).

In addition to genetic variants affecting DM risk in a whole breed, further variants have already been identified within breeds that predispose only some individuals of that breed to DM. These risk-modifying variants are discovered by comparing genetic variation in DM cases and control animals from the same breed. To date most such studies have focused on variants in candidate regions already associated with type 1, type 2, or monogenic human DM.[24,78–81] Many of the variants known to be associated with canine DM are in genes with immune function, including cytokines and the major histocompatibility complex. However, this is more likely to reflect immune bias in the selection of candidate regions for study rather than indicating that canine DM is primarily immune-mediated, because many other genes with different functions (eg, β-cell biology) have not yet been investigated. There are also a notable number of breeds in which DM is common, but no variants in immune genes have been identified.

Environmental Diabetes Mellitus Risk Factors

The role of environmental factors on canine DM risk has not been extensively studied, but is likely to be critically important, at least in some breeds. The role of the environment in type 1 and type 2 DM risk in humans was first highlighted by concordance rates of less than 100% in identical twin studies,[82] indicating that some form of trigger, in addition to genetic susceptibility, was required for DM to develop. This may also be the case in high diabetes risk dog breeds, sharing many genetic variations, but experiencing different environments in terms of diet, exercise, medications, and exposure to infections.

There are some well understood canine DM environmental triggers, such as diestrus and the use of corticosteroids, but there are likely to be others that have not been discovered. There is suggestion in some studies of seasonality in canine DM diagnosis,[8] which could relate to one or more environmental factors, and the reported rising incidence of DM in the canine population[b] would also fit with the emergence of a common environmental trigger.

The diverse mechanisms for canine DM are all likely to be influenced by different environmental factors. For example, pancreatitis has been associated with a high-fat diet and with DM, but it is not clear whether a high-fat diet can act directly as a risk factor for diabetes independent of pancreatitis in dogs. It may also be the case that some environmental risk factors and genes are important in some breeds or some types of DM but not others.

The expanding literature on environmental triggers in human type 1 diabetes has implicated vitamin D status, microbiome diversity, nutritional factors, and viral infections among a wide range of environmental associations with DM risk.[83] Although microbiome disruption has been reported in association with canine DM,[84] there is, as yet, no evidence of causality. There is also increasing evidence of an increased intestinal permeability affecting human DM risk, secondary to a range of factors including inflammation, infection, and diet.[85,86] In human type 2 diabetes, obesity and inactivity are the most important known environmental risk factors, but the microbiome has also been implicated here too, along with a range of other factors including diet and geographic location.[87,88]

Improved knowledge of environmental triggers in canine DM has the potential to lead to preventative or therapeutic breakthroughs, because it may prove more straightforward to avoid such triggers than reduce genetic risk.

PATHOPHYSIOLOGY

Canine DM is a disease of insulin deficiency, whether absolute or relative. At the time of diagnosis, dogs almost invariably require insulin for treatment, leading to the disease often being described as insulin-dependent or consistent with type 1 diabetes in humans.[45,76] The pathogenesis of the disease is much more complicated than this simplified classification. Many dogs with diabetes described in the literature do have insulin deficiency, with inappropriate low insulin (as measured by C-peptide) at baseline for the level of hyperglycemia and a suboptimal response to an insulin secretagogue (glucagon).[89–91] C-peptide is formed from the cleavage of proinsulin and is secreted equimolar with insulin,[91] and is a preferred indicator of β-cell function because endogenous insulin concentrations cannot be measured reliably in dogs treated with insulin, and because a large portion of insulin is degraded in the liver before it can be measured in peripheral blood.[89–91] However, in looking closely at the data in these studies, it is apparent that some dogs do retain C-peptide production and there is overlap between fasting C-peptide concentration in dogs with diabetes and dogs without diabetes.[89,90] There is also variability in response to glucagon, with some individual dogs with diabetes having an increase in C-peptide during the glucagon response test. Two of these dogs were intact females that later reverted to non-insulin-dependent state following ovariohysterectomy, suggestive of an insulin-resistant form of DM.[90]

Montgomery and colleagues[89] found that dogs with diabetes treated with insulin for less than 6 months had a higher basal C-peptide than those treated for greater than 6 months, suggesting that loss of β-cell function may be progressive. The author (ALO) has studied several dogs with diabetes within a month of diagnosis and measured C-peptide at baseline (fasted) and after a glucose-rich liquid meal (Ensure Plus; 15% protein, 28% fat, 57% carbohydrates) (unpublished data). As shown in **Fig. 1**, C-peptide was variable at baseline and after the meal in dogs with diabetes (n = 6) and healthy control (n = 4) dogs, suggesting that there is heterogeneity in the disease in dogs. Given the inconsistent responses in the healthy control dogs it is unclear whether this meal maximally stimulated insulin secretion, however, so these results should be interpreted within that context. Unfortunately, there are currently no commercial laboratories offering canine C-peptide assays and therefore the routine measurement is difficult and not part of a standard clinical work-up for diabetes.

In human type 1 diabetes, measurement of C-peptide has been key to the understanding of residual β-cell function at the time of diagnosis, and in the use of novel therapies. The development of ultrasensitive C-peptide assays has allowed detection

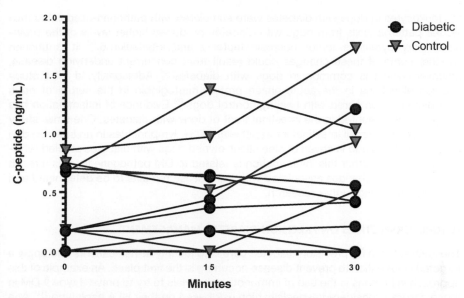

Fig. 1. Serum C peptide at baseline (12-hour fasted sample) and then 15 and 30 minutes following a glucose-rich liquid meal. Samples were taken within 1 month of diagnosis of diabetes in the diabetic group.

of low levels of C-peptide secretion in many patients long after diagnosis, and higher C-peptide has been associated with better metabolic control of the disease.[92] Additionally, assessment of β-cell function with C-peptide is used to assess the effectiveness of immunomodulatory therapies or determine which patients may benefit most from therapies aimed at preserving insulin secretion.[92] To better understand the potential for different subsets of diabetes in dogs, and to provide a knowledge base for the development of individualized and novel therapies, additional study of C-peptide secretion in dogs with diabetes is needed.

Insulin deficiency leads to a decrease in tissue use of glucose, fatty acids, and amino acids and an increase in hepatic gluconeogenesis and glycogenolysis.[93] One study documented increased circulating glucagon concentrations in dogs with diabetes compared with healthy control dogs; however, it is unclear whether samples were collected in a fasted or postprandial state, which could affect glucagon concentrations.[94] These abnormalities lead to hyperglycemia that exceeds the renal threshold for glucose and subsequent glucosuria,[93] and increases in circulating fatty acids and ketone bodies.[94,95] Glucosuria may cause an osmotic diuresis that leads to polyuria and a compensatory polydipsia.[93] Metabolomic analysis has identified abnormalities in serum metabolites in dogs with diabetes compared with control dogs, including increases in branched chain amino acids and γ-aminobutyric acid and decreases in glutamine, tyrosine, and tryptophan pathway metabolites (kynurenine, anthranilic acid).[96] Whether these changes represent a consequence or cause of insulin deficiency remains to be determined, and several of these findings are shared in DM in other species, including rodents and humans.[96]

DM also is associated with a proinflammatory state in dogs, as already mentioned in the case of hyperglycemia-induced pancreatic inflammation.[32] Compared with healthy control animals, dogs with uncomplicated DM had higher serum CXCl8 and monocyte chemoattractant protein-1 (proinflammatory chemokines).[97] When the leukocytes of dogs with diabetes were stimulated with pathogen-associated molecular patterns, cells from dogs with diabetes produced higher levels of the proinflammatory cytokines tumor necrosis factor-α and interleukin-6.[98] It is unclear whether some of these changes could result from concurrent underlying disease, however, which is common in dogs with diabetes.[34] Additionally, a pilot study showed elevations in the acute-phase protein haptoglobin in the serum of dogs with diabetes compared with healthy control dogs.[99] Evidence of inflammation has also been documented in the intestinal tract of dogs with diabetes. One small study found increased small intestinal intraepithelial CD3+ lymphocytes in an induced diabetes dog model and in seven of nine client-owned dogs with diabetes studied retrospectively.[100] Whether this inflammation is related to DM pathogenesis or is a result of the metabolic changes associated with the disease remains to be determined and is an area requiring further research.

FUTURE PERSPECTIVES ON PRECISION DIABETES MANAGEMENT

The ideal solution for precision diabetes care is to identify at-risk patients and apply a targeted intervention to prevent disease occurring in the first place. An example of this approach in humans is the use of immunotherapy trials to try to prevent type 1 DM in those children considered especially high risk based on their HLA haplotype.[101] At a basic level, this is already happening in veterinary medicine, such as the recommendation to neuter entire females of high-risk breeds to limit the risk of diestrus diabetes, or monitoring of patients with diabetes and chronic pancreatitis for the development of exocrine pancreatic insufficiency, and providing exocrine pancreatic supplementation as required. However, for a precision medicine approach at a molecular level, it is first necessary to identify the genes and mechanisms underlying diabetes risk within different breeds. This approach may, for example, allow use of oral hypoglycemic drugs rather than insulin where certain types of monogenic diabetes are known to be present.[69] For example, a DM-associated mutation in Labrador retriever has recently been reported in the KCNJ11 gene, which encodes part of an ATP-sensitive potassium channel in the β-cell involved in insulin release.[102] Mutations in this gene can lead to sulphonylurea-responsive DM in young children.[69] There is therefore a possibility that oral medication may be appropriate for the small number of diabetic Labrador retrievers carrying a homozygous KCNJ11 mutation.

Another future focus area for precision veterinary medicine is likely to be on preservation of β-cell health in response to different types of stress, such as infection, inflammation, autoimmune attack, and hyperglycemia. Even in autoimmune human type 1 diabetes, there has been a recent shift of interest toward β-cell robustness, and the ongoing focus on immune tolerance.[103] One reason for the apparent difference in diabetes risk across different dog breeds may be related to genetically programmed variation in β-cell survival and renewal. It is even possible to hypothesize that selective breeding for particular phenotypic traits (eg, endurance, speed, hunting) has inadvertently led to subtle alterations in glucose homeostasis, metabolism, and β-cell biology in different breeds. Intriguingly, the boxer breed, with the lowest risk of DM,[104] is overrepresented in studies of canine insulinoma,[105] implying that boxer β-cells may have an increased capacity for renewal or survival.

Some potential sites of precision medicine–based DM prevention or management in dogs are summarized in **Fig. 2**. Such interventions may include oral hypoglycemic drugs, small molecules, immunotherapies, or dietary intervention. Some of the β-cell and immunologic elements on this diagram are likely to be under genetic control, such as β-cell survival or renewal capacity, level of hyperglycemia resulting

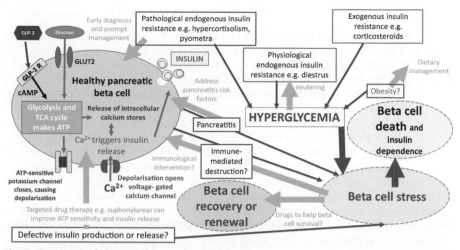

Fig. 2. Summary of the possible mechanisms for development and theoretical management of canine DM from a β-cell perspective. *Red arrows* show factors contributing to hyperglycemia and *green arrows* potential mechanisms by which β-cell health and function may be restored. This diagram represents a simplified version of events and not all biologic mechanisms are represented.

from diestrus, and potential for autoimmunity. Therefore, the future development of canine diabetes polygenic risk scoring, as in human genomic medicine, may also help to inform clinical decisions in diabetes prevention or treatment.[106]

SUMMARY

It is increasingly apparent that canine DM represents a wide spectrum of clinical pathophysiologic processes that converge on a similar set of clinical signs. Autoimmunity is less of a consideration than previously, based on lack of compelling histologic and serologic evidence of autoimmunity, despite genetic studies implicating the immune system in disease risk. β-cell robustness in the face of challenges, such as hyperglycemia, pancreatitis and hormonal antagonism of insulin, is now a focus area. It is only by understanding the molecular basis of DM in each breed and in each individual animal that a future precision approach to this common disease will be feasible. Given the clinical observation that once diagnosed, canine diabetes, unlike feline diabetes, is generally irreversible, any intervention to prevent or reverse diabetes without exogenous insulin must be applied promptly, before all β-cells are lost.

CLINICS CARE POINTS

- Diabetes is not a single disease, but a clinical syndrome that may present as the result of many mechanisms, and understanding the underlying cause can help to inform precision clinical management.

- The paradigm of canine diabetes being most similar to human type 1 (autoimmune) diabetes now seems outdated, and future approaches may focus on assessing and assisting β-cell survival.

- Genetic testing is likely to play a role in future diabetes management.

DISCLOSURES

A.L. O'Kell has no relevant commercial or financial conflicts of interest. Some unpublished data discussed were obtained during support by a grant from the National Institutes of Health (K08DK116735). A.L. O'Kell has previously received research funding from the AKC Canine Health Foundation and Zomedica Inc. She is currently employed by PetDx, which has no relevance to the subject matter of this article. L.J. Davison is supported by a UK MRC Clinician Scientist Fellowship (MR/R007977/1). The UK Canine Diabetes Register and Archive at the RVC has been supported by the Kennel Club Charitable Trust, BSAVA Petsavers, MSD Animal Health, European Commission (FP7-LUPA, GA-201370) and ECVIM-CA Companion Animal Clinical Studies Fund. The Canine Diabetes Genetics Partnership is funded by the Petplan Charitable Trust, with support from Dechra. Additional work, not related to canine diabetes mellitus, is supported by funding from the American Kennel Club Canine Health Foundation, Morris Animal Foundation, UK International Coronavirus Network, Royal Canin, Novo Nordisk Foundation, Evetts-Luff Foundation, BSAVA PetSavers, UK Research and Innovation, Hong Kong Jockey Club. A patent application is in progress associated with canine diabetes genetic data, which may result in a genetic test in future.

REFERENCES

1. Niessen SJM, Bjornvad C, Church DB, et al. Agreeing Language in Veterinary Endocrinology (ALIVE): diabetes mellitus - a modified Delphi-method-based system to create consensus disease definitions. Vet J 2022;289:105910.
2. Chung WK, Erion K, Florez JC, et al. Precision medicine in diabetes: a consensus report from the American Diabetes Association (ADA) and the European Association for the Study of Diabetes (EASD). Diabetes Care 2020;43(7):1617–35.
3. Gilor C, Niessen SJ, Furrow E, et al. What's in a name? Classification of diabetes mellitus in veterinary medicine and why it matters. J Vet Intern Med 2016;30(4):927–40.
4. Deutsch AJ, Ahlqvist E, Udler MS. Phenotypic and genetic classification of diabetes. Diabetologia 2022;65(11):1758–69.
5. ADA Diabetology. Diagnosis and classification of diabetes mellitus. Diabetes Care 2010;33(Suppl 1):S62–9.
6. Zillich AJ, Garg J, Basu S, et al. Thiazide diuretics, potassium, and the development of diabetes. Hypertension 2006;48(2):219–24.
7. Alvarez MS, Herrería-Bustillo V, Utset AF, et al. Juvenile diabetes mellitus and concurrent exocrine pancreatic insufficiency in a Labrador retriever: long-term management. J Am Anim Hosp Assoc 2015;51(6):419–23.
8. Qiu LNY, Cai SV, Chan D, et al. Seasonality and geography of diabetes mellitus in United States of America dogs. PLoS One 2022;17(8):e0272297.
9. Del Busto I, German AJ, Treggiari E, et al. Incidence of postoperative complications and outcome of 48 dogs undergoing surgical management of insulinoma. J Vet Intern Med 2020;34(3):1135–43.
10. Bell R, Mooney CT, Mansfield CS, et al. Treatment of insulinoma in a springer spaniel with streptozotocin. J Small Anim Pract 2005;46(5):247–50.
11. Rojas J, Bermudez V, Palmar J, et al. Pancreatic beta cell death: novel potential mechanisms in diabetes therapy. J Diabetes Res 2018;2018:9601801.
12. Richardson SJ, Pugliese A. 100 years of insulin: pancreas pathology in type 1 diabetes: an evolving story. J Endocrinol 2021;252(2):R41–57.

13. Alejandro R, Feldman EC, Shienvold FL, et al. Advances in canine diabetes mellitus research: etiopathology and results of islet transplantation. J Am Vet Med Assoc 1988;193(9):1050–5.

14. Gilor C, Pires J, Greathouse R, et al. Loss of sympathetic innervation to islets of Langerhans in canine diabetes and pancreatitis is not associated with insulitis. Sci Rep 2020;10(1):19187.

15. Shields EJ, Lam CJ, Cox AR, et al. Extreme beta-cell deficiency in pancreata of dogs with canine diabetes. PLoS One 2015;10(6):e0129809.

16. Ross C, Ward ZJ, Gomber A, et al. The prevalence of islet autoantibodies in children and adolescents with type 1 diabetes mellitus: a global scoping review. Front Endocrinol 2022;13:815703.

17. O'Kell AL, Wasserfall C, Catchpole B, et al. Comparative pathogenesis of autoimmune diabetes in humans, NOD mice, and canines: has a valuable animal model of type 1 diabetes been overlooked? Diabetes 2017;66(6):1443–52.

18. González-Villar F, Pérez-Bravo F. Determination of autoantibodies in dogs with diabetes mellitus. Vet World 2021;14(10):2694–8.

19. O'Kell AL, Wasserfall CH, Henthorn PS, et al. Evaluation for type 1 diabetes associated autoantibodies in diabetic and non-diabetic Australian terriers and Samoyeds. Canine Med Genet 2020;7(1):10.

20. O'Kell AL, Shome M, Qiu J, et al. Exploration of autoantibody responses in canine diabetes using protein arrays. Sci Rep 2022;12(1):2490.

21. Ahlgren KM, Fall T, Landegren N, et al. Lack of evidence for a role of islet autoimmunity in the aetiology of canine diabetes mellitus. PLoS One 2014;9(8):e105473.

22. Davison LJ, Herrtage ME, Catchpole B. Autoantibodies to recombinant canine proinsulin in canine diabetic patients. Res Vet Sci 2011;91(1):58–63.

23. Davison LJ, Weenink SM, Christie MR, et al. Autoantibodies to GAD65 and IA-2 in canine diabetes mellitus. Vet Immunol Immunopathol 2008;126(1–2):83–90.

24. Denyer AL, Massey JP, Davison LJ, et al. Dog leucocyte antigen (DLA) class II haplotypes and risk of canine diabetes mellitus in specific dog breeds. Canine Med Genet 2020;7(1):15.

25. Davison LJ. Diabetes mellitus and pancreatitis: cause or effect? J Small Anim Pract 2015;56(1):50–9.

26. Olesen SS, Toledo FGS, Hart PA. The spectrum of diabetes in acute and chronic pancreatitis. Curr Opin Gastroenterol 2022;38(5):509–15.

27. Lim SY, Steiner JM, Cridge H. Understanding lipase assays in the diagnosis of pancreatitis in veterinary medicine. J Am Vet Med Assoc 2022;260(11):1249–58.

28. Cridge H, Twedt DC, Marolf AJ, et al. Advances in the diagnosis of acute pancreatitis in dogs. J Vet Intern Med 2021;35(6):2572–87.

29. Watson P. Pancreatitis in dogs and cats: definitions and pathophysiology. J Small Anim Pract 2015;56(1):3–12.

30. Watson PJ, Roulois AJ, Scase T, et al. Prevalence and breed distribution of chronic pancreatitis at post-mortem examination in first-opinion dogs. J Small Anim Pract 2007;48(11):609–18.

31. Watson PJ, Herrtage ME. Use of glucagon stimulation tests to assess beta-cell function in dogs with chronic pancreatitis. J Nutr 2004;134(8 Suppl):2081s–3s.

32. Imamura T, Koffler M, Helderman JH, et al. Severe diabetes induced in subtotally depancreatized dogs by sustained hyperglycemia. Diabetes 1988;37(5):600–9.

33. Verkest KR, Fleeman LM, Morton JM, et al. Association of postprandial serum triglyceride concentration and serum canine pancreatic lipase immunoreactivity in overweight and obese dogs. J Vet Intern Med 2012;26(1):46–53.

34. Hess RS, Saunders HM, Van Winkle TJ, et al. Concurrent disorders in dogs with diabetes mellitus: 221 cases (1993-1998). J Am Vet Med Assoc 2000;217(8): 1166–73.

35. Cridge H, Lim SY, Algül H, et al. New insights into the etiology, risk factors, and pathogenesis of pancreatitis in dogs: potential impacts on clinical practice. J Vet Intern Med 2022;36(3):847–64.

36. Coddou MF, Constantino-Casas F, Scase T, et al. Chronic inflammatory disease in the pancreas, kidney and salivary glands of English cocker spaniels and dogs of other breeds shows similar histological features to human IgG4-related disease. J Comp Pathol 2020;177:18–33.

37. Xenoulis PG, Suchodolski JS, Ruaux CG, et al. Association between serum triglyceride and canine pancreatic lipase immunoreactivity concentrations in miniature schnauzers. J Am Anim Hosp Assoc 2010;46(4):229–34.

38. Ader M, Bergman RN. Hyperinsulinemic compensation for insulin resistance occurs independent of elevated glycemia in male dogs. Endocrinology 2021; 162(9):bqab119.

39. Del Prato S. Role of glucotoxicity and lipotoxicity in the pathophysiology of type 2 diabetes mellitus and emerging treatment strategies. Diabet Med 2009; 26(12):1185–92.

40. Reusch CE. Glucocorticoid therapy. In: Feldman ENR, Reusch C, Scott-Moncrief JCR, editors. Canine and feline Endocrinology. 4th edition. St. Louis: Elsevier; 2015. p. 555–77.

41. Jeffers JG, Shanley KJ, Schick RO. Diabetes mellitus induced in a dog after administration of corticosteroids and methylprednisolone pulse therapy. J Am Vet Med Assoc 1991;199(1):77–80.

42. Campbell KL, Latimer KS. Transient diabetes mellitus associated with prednisone therapy in a dog. J Am Vet Med Assoc 1984;185(3):299–301.

43. Moore GE, Hoenig M. Effects of orally administered prednisone on glucose tolerance and insulin secretion in clinically normal dogs. Am J Vet Res 1993; 54(1):126–9.

44. Wolfsheimer KJ, Flory W, Williams MD. Effects of prednisolone on glucose tolerance and insulin secretion in the dog. Am J Vet Res 1986;47(5):1011–4.

45. Nelson RW, Reusch CE. Animal models of disease: classification and etiology of diabetes in dogs and cats. J Endocrinol 2014;222(3):T1–9.

46. Peterson ME, Altszuler N, Nichols CE. Decreased insulin sensitivity and glucose tolerance in spontaneous canine hyperadrenocorticism. Res Vet Sci 1984;36(2): 177–82.

47. Hoffman JM, Lourenço BN, Promislow DEL, et al. Canine hyperadrenocorticism associations with signalment, selected comorbidities and mortality within North American veterinary teaching hospitals. J Small Anim Pract 2018;59(11): 681–90.

48. Miceli DD, Pignataro OP, Castillo VA. Concurrent hyperadrenocorticism and diabetes mellitus in dogs. Res Vet Sci 2017;115:425–31.

49. Miceli DD, Gallelli MF, Cabrera Blatter MF, et al. Low dose of insulin detemir controls glycaemia, insulinemia and prevents diabetes mellitus progression in the dog with pituitary-dependent hyperadrenocorticism. Res Vet Sci 2012;93(1): 114–20.

50. Peterson ME, Nesbitt GH, Schaer M. Diagnosis and management of concurrent diabetes mellitus and hyperadrenocorticism in thirty dogs. J Am Vet Med Assoc 1981;178(1):66–9.

51. McLauchlan G, Knottenbelt C, Augusto M, et al. Retrospective evaluation of the effect of trilostane on insulin requirement and fructosamine concentration in eight diabetic dogs with hyperadrenocorticism. J Small Anim Pract 2010; 51(12):642–8.

52. Eigenmann JE, Eigenmann RY, Rijnberk A, et al. Progesterone-controlled growth hormone overproduction and naturally occurring canine diabetes and acromegaly. Acta Endocrinol 1983;104(2):167–76.

53. Cui Y, Bauer N, Hausmann L, et al. Clinical diabetes mellitus in association with diestrus-induced acromegaly in 2 bitches. Tierarztl Prax Ausg K Kleintiere Heimtiere 2019;47(3):193–201.

54. Selman PJ, Mol JA, Rutteman GR, et al. Progestin-induced growth hormone excess in the dog originates in the mammary gland. Endocrinology 1994; 134(1):287–92.

55. Pöppl AG, de Carvalho GLC, Vivian IF, et al. Canine diabetes mellitus risk factors: a matched case-control study. Res Vet Sci 2017;114:469–73.

56. Fall T, Hedhammar A, Wallberg A, et al. Diabetes mellitus in elkhounds is associated with diestrus and pregnancy. J Vet Intern Med 2010;24(6):1322–8.

57. Fall T, Johansson Kreuger S, Juberget A, et al. Gestational diabetes mellitus in 13 dogs. J Vet Intern Med 2008;22(6):1296–300.

58. Armenise A, Pastorelli G, Palmisano A, et al. Gestational diabetes mellitus with diabetic ketoacidosis in a Yorkshire terrier bitch. J Am Anim Hosp Assoc 2011; 47(4):285–9.

59. Mared M, Catchpole B, Kämpe O, et al. Evaluation of circulating concentrations of glucose homeostasis biomarkers, progesterone, and growth hormone in healthy Elkhounds during anestrus and diestrus. Am J Vet Res 2012;73(2): 242–7.

60. Diaz-Espiñeira MM, Galac S, Mol JA, et al. Thyrotropin-releasing hormone-induced growth hormone secretion in dogs with primary hypothyroidism. Domest Anim Endocrinol 2008;34(2):176–81.

61. Diaz-Espiñeira MM, Mol JA, van den Ingh TS, et al. Functional and morphological changes in the adenohypophysis of dogs with induced primary hypothyroidism: loss of TSH hypersecretion, hypersomatotropism, hypoprolactinemia, and pituitary enlargement with transdifferentiation. Domest Anim Endocrinol 2008;35(1):98–111.

62. Johnstone T, Terzo E, Mooney CT. Hypothyroidism associated with acromegaly and insulin-resistant diabetes mellitus in a Samoyed. Aust Vet J 2014;92(11): 437–42.

63. Verkest KR, Fleeman LM, Rand JS, et al. Evaluation of beta-cell sensitivity to glucose and first-phase insulin secretion in obese dogs. Am J Vet Res 2011; 72(3):357–66.

64. Verkest KR, Rand JS, Fleeman LM, et al. Spontaneously obese dogs exhibit greater postprandial glucose, triglyceride, and insulin concentrations than lean dogs. Domest Anim Endocrinol 2012;42(2):103–12.

65. Brunetto MA, Sá FC, Nogueira SP, et al. The intravenous glucose tolerance and postprandial glucose tests may present different responses in the evaluation of obese dogs. Br J Nutr 2011;106(Suppl 1):S194–7.

66. Mattin M, O'Neill D, Church D, et al. An epidemiological study of diabetes mellitus in dogs attending first opinion practice in the UK. Vet Rec 2014; 174(14):349.

67. Ionut V, Liu H, Mooradian V, et al. Novel canine models of obese prediabetes and mild type 2 diabetes. Am J Physiol Endocrinol Metab 2010;298(1):E38–48.

68. Davison LJ, Holder A, Catchpole B, et al. The Canine POMC Gene, obesity in Labrador retrievers and susceptibility to diabetes mellitus. J Vet Intern Med 2017;31(2):343–8.

69. Bonnefond A, Semple RK. Achievements, prospects and challenges in precision care for monogenic insulin-deficient and insulin-resistant diabetes. Diabetologia 2022;65(11):1782–95.

70. Rand JS, Fleeman LM, Farrow HA, et al. Canine and feline diabetes mellitus: nature or nurture? J Nutr 2004;134(8 Suppl):2072s–80s.

71. Denyer AL, Catchpole B, Davison LJ. Genetics of canine diabetes mellitus part 1: phenotypes of disease. Vet J 2021;270:105611.

72. Denyer AL, Catchpole B, Davison LJ. Genetics of canine diabetes mellitus part 2: current understanding and future directions. Vet J 2021;270:105612.

73. Ringstad NK, Lingaas F, Thoresen SI. Breed distributions for diabetes mellitus and hypothyroidism in Norwegian dogs. Canine Med Genet 2022;9(1):9.

74. Yoon S, Fleeman LM, Wilson BJ, et al. Epidemiological study of dogs with diabetes mellitus attending primary care veterinary clinics in Australia. Vet Rec 2020;187(3):e22.

75. Heeley AM, O'Neill DG, Davison LJ, et al. Diabetes mellitus in dogs attending UK primary-care practices: frequency, risk factors and survival. Canine Medicine and Genetics 2020;7(1):6.

76. Catchpole B, Ristic JM, Fleeman LM, et al. Canine diabetes mellitus: can old dogs teach us new tricks? Diabetologia 2005;48(10):1948–56.

77. Davison LJ, Herrtage ME, Catchpole B. Study of 253 dogs in the United Kingdom with diabetes mellitus. Vet Rec 2005;156(15):467–71.

78. Hess R, Henthorn P, Devoto M, et al. An exploratory association analysis of the insulin gene region with diabetes mellitus in two dog breeds. J Hered 2019; 110(7):793–800.

79. Short AD, Holder A, Rothwell S, et al. Searching for "monogenic diabetes" in dogs using a candidate gene approach. Canine Genet Epidemiol 2014;1:8.

80. Short AD, Catchpole B, Kennedy LJ, et al. Analysis of candidate susceptibility genes in canine diabetes. J Hered 2007;98(5):518–25.

81. Short AD, Catchpole B, Kennedy LJ, et al. T cell cytokine gene polymorphisms in canine diabetes mellitus. Vet Immunol Immunopathol 2009;128(1–3):137–46.

82. Burch PR. Diabetes mellitus: concordance in monozygotic twins. Lancet 1976; 2(7986):632.

83. Houeiss P, Luce S, Boitard C. Environmental triggering of type 1 diabetes autoimmunity. Front Endocrinol 2022;13:933965.

84. Jergens AE, Guard BC, Redfern A, et al. Microbiota-related changes in unconjugated fecal bile acids are associated with naturally occurring, insulin-dependent diabetes mellitus in dogs. Front Vet Sci 2019;6:199.

85. Mønsted M, Falck ND, Pedersen K, et al. Intestinal permeability in type 1 diabetes: an updated comprehensive overview. J Autoimmun 2021;122:102674.

86. Cox AJ, Zhang P, Bowden DW, et al. Increased intestinal permeability as a risk factor for type 2 diabetes. Diabetes Metab 2017;43(2):163–6.

87. Dendup T, Feng X, Clingan S, et al. Environmental risk factors for developing type 2 diabetes mellitus: a systematic review. Int J Environ Res Public Health 2018;15(1):78.
88. Beulens JWJ, Pinho MGM, Abreu TC, et al. Environmental risk factors of type 2 diabetes-an exposome approach. Diabetologia 2022;65(2):263–74.
89. Montgomery TM, Nelson RW, Feldman EC, et al. Basal and glucagon-stimulated plasma C-peptide concentrations in healthy dogs, dogs with diabetes mellitus, and dogs with hyperadrenocorticism. J Vet Intern Med 1996;10(3):116–22.
90. Fall T, Holm B, Karlsson A, et al. Glucagon stimulation test for estimating endogenous insulin secretion in dogs. Vet Rec 2008;163(9):266–70.
91. Fleeman LM, Rand JS, Morton JM. Pharmacokinetics and pharmacodynamics of porcine insulin zinc suspension in eight diabetic dogs. Vet Rec 2009; 164(8):232–7.
92. Jamiołkowska-Sztabkowska M, Głowińska-Olszewska B, Bossowski A. C-peptide and residual β-cell function in pediatric diabetes: state of the art. Pediatr Endocrinol Diabetes Metab 2021;27(2):123–33.
93. Nelson R. Canine diabetes mellitus. In: Feldman E, Nelson R, Reusch C, et al, editors. Canine and feline Endocrinology. 4 edition. St. Louis: Elsevier; 2015. p. 213–57.
94. Durocher LL, Hinchcliff KW, DiBartola SP, et al. Acid-base and hormonal abnormalities in dogs with naturally occurring diabetes mellitus. J Am Vet Med Assoc 2008;232(9):1310–20.
95. Fracassi F. Canine diabetes mellitus. In: Ettinger S, Feldman E, Cote E, editors. Textbook of veterinary internal medicine: diseases of the dog and cat. Vol 2. 8th edition. St. Louis, MO: Elsevier; 2017. p. 1767–81.
96. O'Kell AL, Wasserfall C, Guingab-Cagmat J, et al. Targeted metabolomic analysis identifies increased serum levels of GABA and branched chain amino acids in canine diabetes. Metabolomics 2021;17(11):100.
97. O'Neill S, Drobatz K, Satyaraj E, et al. Evaluation of cytokines and hormones in dogs before and after treatment of diabetic ketoacidosis and in uncomplicated diabetes mellitus. Vet Immunol Immunopathol 2012;148(3–4):276–83.
98. DeClue AE, Nickell J, Chang CH, et al. Upregulation of proinflammatory cytokine production in response to bacterial pathogen-associated molecular patterns in dogs with diabetes mellitus undergoing insulin therapy. J Diabetes Sci Technol 2012;6(3):496–502.
99. Franco-Martínez L, Gelemanović A, Horvatić A, et al. The serum and saliva proteome of dogs with diabetes mellitus. Animals (Basel) 2020;10(12):2261.
100. Crakes KR, Pires J, Quach N, et al. Fenofibrate promotes PPARα-targeted recovery of the intestinal epithelial barrier at the host-microbe interface in dogs with diabetes mellitus. Sci Rep 2021;11(1):13454.
101. Warshauer JT, Bluestone JA, Anderson MS. New frontiers in the treatment of type 1 diabetes. Cell Metab 2020;31(1):46–61.
102. Falcone S., Wallace M., Denyer A., et al., A mutation in the KCNJ11 gene and diabetes mellitus in the Labrador retriever (abstract), J Vet Intern Med, 36 (6), 2022, 2512.
103. Roep BO, Thomaidou S, van Tienhoven R, et al. Type 1 diabetes mellitus as a disease of the β-cell (do not blame the immune system?). Nat Rev Endocrinol 2021;17(3):150–61.
104. Catchpole B, Adams JP, Holder AL, et al. Genetics of canine diabetes mellitus: are the diabetes susceptibility genes identified in humans involved in breed susceptibility to diabetes mellitus in dogs? Vet J 2013;195(2):139–47.

105. Ryan D, Pérez-Accino J, Gonçalves R, et al. Clinical findings, neurological manifestations and survival of dogs with insulinoma: 116 cases (2009-2020). J Small Anim Pract 2021;62(7):531–9.

106. Kumuthini J, Zick B, Balasopoulou A, et al. The clinical utility of polygenic risk scores in genomic medicine practices: a systematic review. Hum Genet 2022; 30:1–8.

Pathophysiology of Prediabetes, Diabetes, and Diabetic Remission in Cats

Ruth Gostelow, BVetMed(Hons), DipACVIM-CA, DipECVIM-CA, PhD, FHEA, MRCVS[a],*, Katarina Hazuchova, MVDr, PhD, DipECVIM-CA, MRCVS[b]

KEYWORDS

• Feline • Diabetes mellitus • β-cell • Insulin resistance • Glucose intolerance

KEY POINTS

• Feline diabetes mellitus (DM) can result from a wide variety of underlying etiologic factors, and the underlying pathogenesis therefore varies between individual patients.

• Prediabetes in cats remains extremely challenging to diagnose in clinical veterinary practice, and identifying ideal screening methods, and how well these might predict future DM, requires substantial further research.

• Diabetic remission can occur in a proportion of diabetic cats, but these cats often have decreased glucose tolerance, and relapses are not uncommon.

 Video content accompanies this article at http://www.vetsmall.theclinics.com.

INTRODUCTION

Diabetes mellitus (DM) is a metabolic disorder characterized by persistent hyperglycemia, resulting from impaired insulin secretion from pancreatic β-cells, defective insulin action (termed "insulin resistance" [IR]), or both.[1,2] In people, a diagnosis of DM is made based on clearly defined cutoffs for fasting plasma glucose (FPG), 2-hour plasma glucose during a 75-g oral glucose tolerance test (OGTT), or elevation in hemoglobin A1c (HbA$_{1c}$) concentration. An HbA$_{1c}$ concentration of $\geq$48 mmol/mol ($\geq$6.5%) is widely used as supportive of DM in people, although this cutoff can have low sensitivity for DM diagnosis when used alone.[3]

People who do not meet criteria for DM, but who have FPG, OGTT, or HbA$_{1c}$ results that exceed normal limits, are termed to have "prediabetes." These patients have impaired fasting glucose (IFG) or impaired glucose tolerance (IGT) and an increased

[a] The Royal Veterinary College, Hawkshead Lane, North Mymms, Hertfordshire AL9 7TA, UK;
[b] Small Animal Clinic (Internal Medicine), Justus-Liebig-Universität Gießen, Frankfurter Strasse 114, Gießen, Germany
* Corresponding author.
E-mail address: rgostelow@rvc.ac.uk

Vet Clin Small Anim 53 (2023) 511–529
https://doi.org/10.1016/j.cvsm.2023.02.001
0195-5616/23/© 2023 Elsevier Inc. All rights reserved.

risk of progressing to overt DM.[4] Throughout the rest of this article, IGT will be used to refer to human patients who have been assigned this diagnosis based on OGTT.

Remission of DM can be seen in both cats and people. A recent consensus statement recommended the following as a reliable, simple criteria for diabetic remission in people: "Maintenance of an HbA1c below the concentration currently used for diagnosis of DM, for at least 3 months after [stopping] antihyperglycemic agents."[5] In contrast, feline diabetic remission is most often defined as maintenance of normoglycemia for at least 4 weeks without the need for antihyperglycemic medications. A carbohydrate-reduced diet is not typically considered an antihyperglycemic medication for this definition.[6] This article discusses the pathophysiology of DM, prediabetes, and diabetic remission in cats.

DIABETES MELLITUS IN CATS

DM has a heterogenous cause, and the exact pathogenesis by which DM develops differs between individual patients (**Fig. 1**). **Fig. 2** provides a simplified depiction of the major etiologic factors that might contribute to DM development in cats. Although these diabetogenic factors vary between individuals, the final stage in the development of prediabetes and DM is failure of pancreatic β-cells to secrete adequate insulin to maintain normoglycemia. This β-cell failure might result from β-cell destruction, abnormal β-cell function, or failure of β-cell production to compensate for peripheral IR.[7] The deciding role of β-cell function accounts for why not all cats with risk factors for DM, such as obesity or glucocorticoid treatment, develop DM because patients

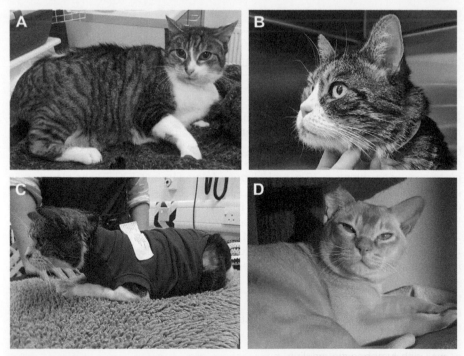

Fig. 1. Four diabetic cats with likely differing cause for their DM: (*A*) An obese DSH cat. (*B*) A DSH cat with HS-associated DM, showing phenotypic changes of acromegaly (prognathism inferior and wide facial features). (*C*) A DSH cat with HA-associated DM. This cat is wearing a protective vest owing to skin fragility and alopecia secondary to HA. (*D*) A Burmese.

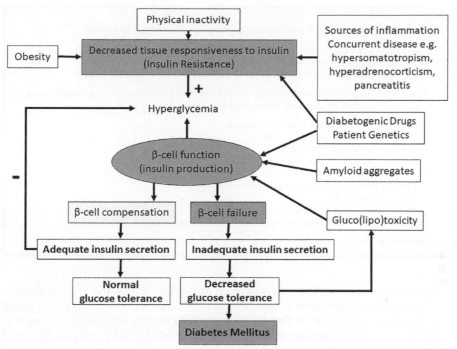

Fig. 2. Major contributing factors that might lead to the development of DM in cats. Although underlying cause can differ between patients, β-cell failure is the common final step in the development of DM.

with sufficient β-cell function can maintain normal glucose tolerance despite these diabetogenic influences.[8]

It is increasingly recommended to clarify the cause of DM in small animal patients as soon as possible following diagnosis, especially as this has important implications for optimizing patient treatment.[9] For example, an overweight diabetic cat is likely to benefit from undergoing planned weight loss as part of their management to improve obesity-associated IR (see **Fig. 1**A). Also, cats with hypersomatotropism (HS)- or hyperadrenocorticism (HA)-associated DM typically experience poor DM control until their underlying endocrinopathy is identified and adequately managed (see article on "Hypersomatotropism and other causes of insulin resistance in cats").[10]

Classifying a patient's DM type according to cause is routinely performed in human medicine. The 4 major categories used in people are shown in **Box 1**, and the causes of DM seen in veterinary medicine are often compared with these groups.[9,11,12] Based on similar risk factors, such as obesity and physical inactivity, most diabetic cats have a form of DM likened to type 2 DM in people.[9] However, many feline DM cases are due to causes classified as "Specific types of DM, due to other causes" in people (see **Box 1**). This includes cats with HS-associated DM,[13] HA-associated DM,[14] or those that have received diabetogenic drugs.[15] There is little evidence for type 1 DM, associated with immune-mediated islet inflammation, in cats. Only a couple of suspected cases, with lymphocytic insulitis, have been reported.[16,17] Gestational DM has not been reported in cats.

Factors from **Fig. 2**, which might contribute to the development of DM in cats, are discussed later. It is highly likely that an individual cat might have more than one of

Box 1
Etiologic classification system used to categorize diabetes mellitus in people[1]

i. *Type 1 DM* (β-cell destruction, usually leading to absolute insulin deficiency)
  a. Immune-mediated (serologic evidence of β-cell autoimmunity)
  b. Idiopathic (permanent insulinopenia without evidence of autoimmunity)

ii. *Type 2 DM* (ranging from predominant insulin resistance with relative insulin deficiency, to a predominant insulin secretion deficit alongside insulin resistance)

iii. Specific types of DM, owing to other causes
  a. Genetic defects of β-cell function
  b. Genetic defects of insulin action
  c. Exocrine pancreatic diseases (eg, *pancreatitis, neoplasia*)
  d. Endocrinopathies (eg, *hypersomatotropism, hyperadrenocorticism*)
  e. Drug or chemical induced (eg, *glucocorticoids*)
  f. Infection-induced
  g. Uncommon forms of immune-mediated DM
  h. Other genetic syndromes occasionally associated with DM

iv. Gestational DM

these factors contributing to the development of their DM. Furthermore, some diabetic people are recognized to have a "mixed" type of DM with features of more than one of the etiologic groups shown in **Box 1**.[18] It is possible for this scenario to also exist in some diabetic cats (eg, an overweight cat diagnosed with DM following glucocorticoid administration).

FACTORS CONTRIBUTING TO DIABETES MELLITUS DEVELOPMENT IN CATS
Obesity

Obesity is a major risk factor for DM in both cats and people, and,[19,20] similar to people, insulin sensitivity is reduced in obese cats compared with those that are lean.[8,21] One study using euglycemic hyperinsulinemic clamps estimated ∼30% loss in insulin sensitivity for each kilogram increase in body weight. However, when obese cats lost weight and became lean, insulin sensitivity returned and was no different from lean cats without a history of obesity.[21] Obesity could therefore represent a reversible cause of IR in cats if weight loss can be achieved. However, it is also possible that the IR documented in obese cats might occur because of factors associated with an overweight state. For example, IR might develop as a result of feeding certain diets, leading to intestinal inflammation and increased intestinal permeability, which has been shown in mouse models fed high-fat diets.[22] Consequently, microbiome modulation or inhibition of intestinal inflammation might have the potential to improve glucose tolerance.[22,23] It has yet to be shown whether these factors are applicable in cats.. Furthermore, it has been discussed that, in people, hyperinsulinemia might be the primary abnormality, leading to weight gain and obesity, which is in contrast with the classical concept of obesity leading to IR and hyperinsulinemia.[24] Studies in mouse models are in support of the primary role of hyperinsulinemia.[25] Furthermore, studies of first-degree relatives of people with type 2 DM have revealed these individuals to have significant IR in muscle and liver as well as hyperinsulinemia at the time when they are neither obese nor glucose intolerant.[26]

As mentioned above, not all cats develop glucose intolerance following the development of obesity. One study suggested that cats who became glucose intolerant after becoming obese typically had several intravenous (IV) glucose tolerance test

(IVGTT) findings suggestive of abnormal glucose homeostasis even when in a lean state. However, this did not reach statistical significance.[8] When cats become obese, both subcutaneous and visceral fat mass increase to a similar extent and correlate with decreased insulin sensitivity.[21] This contrasts to people, where visceral adiposity appears to be more important for the development of IR than subcutaneous fat. Visceral adiposity also seems to be linked to metabolic syndrome in humans, which is defined as concurrent occurrence of obesity, hypertension, dyslipidemia, and IR.[27] Although cats exhibit some of the features of dyslipidemia present in people with this condition, they do not experience the typical cardiovascular complications, such as atherosclerosis, coronary artery disease, and stroke or clinical hypertension.[28] In people, increasing attention is being paid to the role of ectopic lipid accumulation in the muscle and liver, alongside the decreased capacity of adipocytes to store triglycerides, in the pathogenesis of IR.[29] Increased intramyocellular lipid accumulation was also detected in cats following weight gain and was correlated with the presence of IR, based on IVGTT.[30] However, further research is needed to clarify its role in the pathogenesis of DM in cats.

The molecular mechanisms by which obesity might be linked to IR in cats have not been fully elucidated, and it is also possible, as discussed above, that obesity is a consequence of IR rather than being its cause.[31] The glucose transporter GLUT4 is responsible for insulin-mediated glucose uptake in the muscle and adipose tissue, and reduced expression of GLUT4 was demonstrated in people with type 2 DM and severe IR.[32] In cats, the expression of GLUT4 in both muscle and adipose tissue decreased as cats became overweight and was shown to correlate with a decrease in glucose tolerance judged by IVGTT.[33] Obesity in cats and people is also associated with altered production of adipose tissue–derived hormones (adipokines), particularly a decrease in the insulin-sensitizing adipokine, adiponectin and increased concentrations of leptin (hyperleptinemia). Decreased serum total adiponectin concentrations are associated with increased likelihood of DM in people,[34] and overweight cats have been shown to have both decreased concentrations of total adiponectin[35] and a relative decrease in high-molecular-weight adiponectin, which is thought to be the most biologically active form.[36] This decrease in the proportion of high-molecular-weight adiponectin also correlated with decreased insulin sensitivity. Increasing adiposity is associated with the development of hyperleptinemia in both cats and people.[21,37] Leptin also acts on the central nervous system to decrease food intake and promote energy utilization. Obese people show a decreased response to these properties, which is described as leptin-resistance.[38,39] In overweight cats, weight loss is associated with an increase in total adiponectin concentration and a reduction in leptin concentration to levels similar to those of lean cats.[21]

Overweight people develop low-grade adipose tissue inflammation, which includes infiltration of fat deposits by macrophages, and increased production of inflammatory cytokines, such as tumor necrosis factor-α (TNF-α) and interleukin-6 (IL-6). These inflammatory mediators are proposed to cause IR by disrupting normal insulin signaling.[40] In contrast, adipose tissue inflammation might not contribute to IR in overweight cats. Although increased TNF-α concentrations have been documented in the adipose tissue of obese cats,[41] there is little evidence for systemic inflammation. Blood concentration of IL-1, IL-6, and TNF-α do not alter when lean cats become obese,[42] and blood concentrations of the acute phase proteins, serum amyloid A and haptoglobin, do not change in overweight cats that undergo weight loss.[43] This lack of systemic inflammation is a proposed reason overweight cats do not develop the cardiovascular complications of metabolic syndrome in people.[28]

Glucotoxicity/Glucolipotoxicity

Glucotoxicity is the term used to describe the β-cell destruction and dysfunction, which is proposed to result from chronic exposure to supraphysiologic glucose concentrations. By affecting both β-cell function and survival, glucotoxicity is proposed to have both reversible and irreversible components.[44] Iatrogenic hyperglycemia causes a rapid decline in serum insulin concentrations, and β-cell apoptosis, in healthy cats, suggesting that glucotoxicity might play a role in the development of feline DM.[45] Furthermore, human studies imply that insulin secretion is decreased even in the presence of mild hyperglycemia.[46] It is therefore likely that mild, intermittent hyperglycemia contributes to β-cell failure in prediabetic people, even before patients develop overt DM, and the same could occur in cats during the development of DM (**Fig. 2**). Proposed mechanisms of glucotoxicity, based on in vitro studies, include depletion of intracellular insulin stores, which can be replenished by β-cell rest,[47] and endoplasmic reticulum stress, which might lead to β-cell apoptosis and impaired insulin signaling.[48]

Lipotoxicity refers to the potential deleterious effects on β-cell function and mass that might result from excessive fatty acid exposure.[49] In human diabetology, it is increasingly accepted that these deleterious effects only occur in the presence of concurrent hyperglycemia, leading diabetologists to propose "glucolipotoxicity" as a more appropriate name for this effect.[50] This synergistic, deleterious effect is attributed to hyperglycemia directing cellular metabolism away from fatty acid oxidation, leading to a cytosolic accumulation of fatty acid derivatives, which can contribute to β-cell dysfunction.[51] In cats, infusion of fatty acids failed to cause glucose intolerance based on the results of IVGTT performed after 10 days of lipid infusion.[45] However, cats receiving lipid infusion had higher glucose concentrations when compared with saline-infused cats, whereas insulin concentrations did not differ in these 2 groups, suggesting that some impairment of β-cell function might have been present. Nevertheless, the insulin-positive area on pancreatic islet immunostaining did not differ between lipid- and saline-infused cats, and β-cell apoptosis was not documented after 10 days of lipid infusion, indicating that hyperlipidemia alone might not play a major role in the development of DM.[45] However, as this was a short-term exposure (10 days) in previously healthy research cats, it is unknown whether glucolipotoxicity is a pathogenic mechanism in the development of feline DM if present over longer time periods.

Islet Amyloidosis

Islet amyloidosis refers to extracellular amyloid deposition within the islets of Langerhans, which is a common histologic change in diabetic cats.[16] Islet amyloid is formed from insoluble, polymerized fibrils of the β-cell secretory product, amylin, which is cosecreted with insulin.[52] However, the role that amyloid deposits play in the development of feline DM is controversial because the pancreata of nondiabetic cats can show a similar degree of amyloidosis.[16] In vitro research suggests that amyloid-related β-cell death during the development of DM might be caused by toxic amylin oligomers, which form secondary to ER stress and abnormal protein folding, rather than by mature amyloid deposits.[53] Islet amyloid deposition is therefore not considered to be a primary cause of DM in cats, but could contribute to islet damage.[16]

Diabetogenic Drug Treatment

Drug-induced DM is classified as a "Specific type of DM, due to other causes" in people (see **Box 1**). Glucocorticoids are the most commonly used diabetogenic drug in veterinary medicine and could contribute to DM development by decreasing peripheral insulin sensitivity, and promoting endogenous glucose production in the liver.[54] Glucocorticoid therapy is a well-recognized risk factor for feline DM (**Box 2**).[15] The fact that spontaneous HA is usually associated with DM in cats (see later discussion), but only occasionally in dogs, suggests that cats could be particularly susceptible to the diabetogenic effects of glucocorticoids.[55]

Other Endocrinopathies

HS and HA typically lead to secondary DM in affected cats. The cause, diagnosis, and management of these conditions are covered in a separate article in this issue. HS has been estimated to be the underlying cause in up to 25% of feline DM cases in the United Kingdom, although geographic differences in this prevalence might exist.[13,56] The mitogenic effects of growth hormone can result in affected cats also showing phenotypic changes of acromegaly (see **Fig. 1**B). Spontaneous HA is uncommon in cats, although glucocorticoids' diabetogenic effects cause approximately 90% of cats with HA to be diabetic. Most cats with spontaneous HA have concurrent dermatologic lesions, including fragile skin and alopecia (see **Fig. 1**C).[14]

Pancreatitis

Whether pancreatitis is the cause, or the consequence, of DM in cats is debatable, and their role likely differs between individual diabetic patients. Furthermore, in an individual cat with DM and pancreatitis, a third condition might be the trigger for both diseases. Diabetic cats commonly have laboratory or ultrasonographic evidence of pancreatitis, although clinical signs of pancreatitis are often lacking in these cases.[57] Experimental hyperglycemia is shown to increase pancreatic neutrophil count,[45] so it is possible that chronic hyperglycemia in cats with DM contributes to pancreatic inflammation, rather than pancreatitis being a major cause of DM in cats.

Genetics

In human medicine, patient genetics is known to influence an individual's susceptibility to both type 1 and type 2 DM, and the same is likely for type 2–like DM in cats. In people, predisposition for type 2 DM has a polygenic susceptibility pattern, and the disease is observed to run in families, with heritability (h^2) estimates between 0.31 and 0.69.[58]

Similar to people, where certain ethnicities are more susceptible to DM, a predisposition for type 2–like DM is recognized in some cat breeds. Burmese cats in the United Kingdom,[59] Europe,[60] and Australia[61] are predisposed to the development of DM (see **Fig. 1**D, **Box 2**). In contrast, no predisposition has been identified in Burmese cats

---

Box 2
Clinics care points

- Cats receiving prolonged, or high-dose, glucocorticoid therapy should be monitored for diabetes mellitus development, especially if they have other risk factors for diabetes mellitus (eg, obesity). A recent study found that diabetes mellitus developed in nearly 10% of cats that received high-dose prednisolone therapy for at least 3 weeks.[109]

- European/Australian Burmese cats show metabolic derangements typically associated with obesity, even when lean. These include reduced adiponectin concentrations and dyslipidemia and might contribute to their predisposition for diabetes mellitus.[110]

- Management strategies to reduce the risk of diabetes mellitus relapse in cats in remission include ongoing avoidance of diabetogenic influences (eg, weight gain or glucocorticoid therapy), and continued, long-term feeding of a carbohydrate-reduced diet.

bred in the United States,[62] which likely results from the separate breeding history of American and European/Australian Burmese.[63,64] Other cat breeds with increased risk of DM include Tonkinese, which share a genetic similarity with Burmese,[65] as well as Norwegian Forest, Russian Blue, and Abyssinian breeds.[59,60]

Techniques used to study the heritability of DM in people, including genome-wide association studies (GWAS) and whole-genome sequencing (WGS), have recently been applied to feline DM. A single candidate gene study in diabetic cats has been published, which identified a nonsynonymous single nucleotide polymorphism (SNP) in the coding sequence of feline melanocortin-4 receptor gene (MC4R:c.92C>T) to be associated with type 2–like DM in overweight domestic shorthair (DSH) cats.[66] Variants of this gene are also associated with obesity and type 2 DM in people.[67] Three GWAS of DM in cats have been published to date, including 1 in DSH cats[68] and 2 studying DM in Burmese cats.[69,70] These have identified a variety of candidate susceptibility genes, which have also been associated with DM, obesity, and lipid dysregulation in people. Studies assessing the functional impact of SNPs identified in these GWAS are yet to follow, and research using WGS technologies is also ongoing.

Epidemiologic Risk Factors

Reduced physical activity/indoor confinement is a risk factor for DM in cats.[15,19] Exercise increases insulin sensitivity, and sedentary lifestyle is also a risk factor for obesity in people,[71] explaining the link between DM and reduced physical activity. Increasing age is another shared risk factor between human and feline DM.[72] Older cats might suffer from conditions such as obesity, HS, or HA, predisposing them to DM. Declining β-cell function has been described in aging people,[73] but it is unknown whether this also occurs in cats.

Some discrepancies exist regarding the role of diet. One study found feeding dry food was a risk factor for DM,[19] whereas another did not find such an association.[15] The former study identified dry food as a risk factor for DM in normal weight cats only, whereas overweight cats were predisposed irrespective of diet type.[19] Interestingly, male cats have frequently been found to be at greater risk of DM compared with female cats, although this does not seem to apply to Burmese cats.[60,62,72,74] This might be due to male cats' tendency to have lower insulin sensitivity when lean, and a greater increase in body weight when fed ad libitum, compared with female cats.[8]

PREDIABETES IN CATS

Prediabetes is a state of abnormal glucose homeostasis, typically diagnosed following identification of IFG and/or IGT and/or an elevated HbA$_{1c}$ concentration in people. In human medicine, a diagnosis of prediabetes implies an increased risk of developing DM and cardiovascular disease.[3] Although various tests of glucose tolerance have been proposed to identify prediabetes in cats (see later discussion), a diagnosis of prediabetes cannot be applied to feline patients without prognostic information on whether such tests are associated with an increased future risk of DM. The European Society of Veterinary Endocrinology ALIVE Project working group recently commented that there is currently insufficient evidence on prediabetes in cats (and dogs) to draw conclusions on its clinical relevance. However, their guidelines recognize the possibility of subclinical DM.[2] Because of inability to accurately apply a diagnosis of prediabetes in cats, much of this section refers to subclinical DM in cats.

As discussed above, cats can develop reduced insulin sensitivity when exposed to DM risk factors commonly seen in veterinary practice, such as weight gain[21] and glucocorticoid therapy.[75] These findings, combined with the likely rising incidence of feline DM,[62] mean that cats with subclinical DM will almost certainly form part of a typical feline patient population.

Identifying cats with subclinical DM is challenging for several reasons. Although older cats often have blood glucose (BG) checked in routine bloodwork, mild elevations are challenging to interpret and often attributed to stress hyperglycemia.[76] In most cases, the diagnosis of DM is only made when a cat is presented to a veterinarian for clinical signs referable to DM.[77] Recognizing cats with subclinical DM, in which these signs might be absent, is therefore difficult.[2]

The presence of predisposing factors for DM, such as obesity, cannot be used as an indicator of prediabetes (ie, increased future risk of DM in cats), as many individuals with diabetogenic risk factors will maintain normal glucose tolerance as long as β-cell compensation remains sufficient (see **Fig. 2**). In people, the criteria for diagnosing prediabetes vary between major health care organizations and are based on several indicators of glycemic control, including FPG, HbA$_{1c}$, and OGTT results (**Table 1**). However, the use of similar measures of glucose tolerance as accurate markers of prediabetes in cats presents challenges. Reference intervals for capillary glucose concentration both at the time of hospital admission and following an 18- to 24-hour fast have been suggested for healthy senior cats that were ≥8 years old.[78] This revealed a reference interval of 67 to 189 mg/dL (3.7–10.5 mmol/L) for admission BG, and an upper limit of 116 mg/dL (6.4 mmol/L) for fasting BG, and the authors suggested that cats with an admission BG of greater than 189 mg/dL (10.5 mmol/L) should undergo fasting glucose measurement to assess for persisting hyperglycemia. The same group also proposed a methodology and cut points for using fasting BG after an 18- to 24-hour fast, and BG 2 hours after administration of 0.5 g/kg glucose IV, to assess for prediabetes in cats.[79] This study suggested a similar upper limit for fasting glucose of 117 mg/dL (6.5 mmol/L), and an upper cut point for 2-hour glucose of 176.4 mg/dL (9.8 mmol/L). Seven of the 51 (13.7%) overweight/obese cats in this study had a 2-hour BG above the proposed upper cut point, but only one of these had increased fasting glucose. However, it is unknown whether any of these cats developed DM in the future, and the findings of this study cannot be used as diagnostic criteria for prediabetes in cats. To the authors' knowledge, no studies have prospectively examined the ability of any markers of glycemic control to predict the development of DM in cats, making it currently impossible to apply a diagnosis of prediabetes in cats as is done in people.

The appropriateness of both OGTT and IVGTT to assess glucose homeostasis in cats has been questioned by some investigators,[9,80] because carbohydrate digestion in cats bears several differences to other species as a result of cats' evolution as carnivores. In people, OGTTs are used to assess glucose tolerance as they assess the incretin effect, which accounts for a substantial component of postmeal insulin secretion. The incretin effect refers to the augmentation of insulin secretion, which is seen following an oral glucose load compared with IV glucose administration. This effect occurs because of secretion of the gastrointestinal hormones glucose-dependent insulinotropic peptide (GIP) and glucagon-like peptide-1 (GLP-1) following feeding.[81] Differences in incretin secretion between cats and people following an oral glucose load might contribute to the difficulties in interpreting OGTTs in cats. The incretin effect is estimated to account for at least 50% of total insulin secretion following glucose ingestion in healthy people,[82] but only 30% in healthy cats.[83] This difference might be caused by lack of GIP secretion following glucose ingestion in cats, whereas in people, GIP is responsible for most of the incretin response to oral glucose.[83,84] The lack of GIP response to glucose in cats might be explained by their inability to sense glucose as a result of pseudogenization of the *Tas1r2* gene, the gene encoding for

Table 1
Diagnostic tests used to identify prediabetes in people and suggested cutoffs recommended by the American Diabetes Association[3] and World Health Organization[108]

Diagnostic Test	Recommended Cutoffs for Prediabetes	
	American Diabetes Association	World Health Organization
FPG (mg/dL)	100–125 (5.6–6.9 mmol/L)	110 to 125 (6.1–6.9 mmol/L)
2-h plasma glucose during 75-g OGTT (mg/dL)	140–199 (7.8–11.0 mmol/L)	140–196.2 (7.8–10.9 mmol/L)
HbA$_{1c}$ (%)	5.7–6.4	Not recommended

Abbreviation: FPG, fasting plasma glucose (venous glucose concentration after an 8- to 12-h fast).

the sweet taste receptor.[85] One study reported substantial overlap between OGTT results in obese and lean, age-matched cats, although it was unknown how this related to these cats' insulin sensitivity. OGTT is also impractical in cats, as it requires feeding tube placement.[86]

Glycated HbA$_{1c}$ is frequently used to assess for prediabetes in people (see **Table 1**), but is not routinely used to diagnose or monitor DM in cats, mainly because of limited availability of validated assays and no clinical advantage over fructosamine measurement.[77] Serum fructosamine concentration might be of use in identifying cats with persistently elevated BG. Although fructosamine concentration was positively correlated with body weight in 1 study,[87] another study found no difference between the serum fructosamine concentrations of overweight/obese cats, who are considered to have a higher likelihood of DM, and lean counterparts.[88] It is unknown whether any cats in those studies later developed DM. Other, current hindrances to the use of fructosamine as a potential test for prediabetes in cats include a lack of standardized reference interval for feline fructosamine concentration, and that the methodology used to measure fructosamine differs between veterinary laboratories.

DIABETIC REMISSION IN CATS

If β-cell failure is the final step in the development of prediabetes/DM (see **Fig. 2**),[7] it seems reasonable that diabetic remission occurs when β-cell compensation returns to a level that can sustain glucose tolerance once again. This return of β-cell compensation might be due to improvements in β-cell function, improvement in insulin sensitivity, decreased glucose load, or a combination of these 3 factors. Two aspects, which have been considered to have an important influence on the development of feline diabetic remission, include reversal of glucotoxicity, and whether the cause of a cat's DM allows for improvements or reversal in any of the 3 factors stated above. These aspects are discussed separately below.

Reversal of Glucotoxicity

Improvement in β-cell function is increasingly recognized as an important mechanism for remission in people with type 2 DM,[89] and diabetic remission in cats is shown to be accompanied by a return of insulin secretion during IVGTT.[90] In cats, this return of β-cell function is often attributed to improvements in the reversible components of glucotoxicity, based on the findings of various studies. This includes work that has shown a greater likelihood of diabetic remission in cats that have a shorter duration of DM, that have less severe hyperglycemia at diagnosis, and that achieve good DM control more promptly.[91–93] Milder hyperglycemia, and a shorter duration of

DM, could mean that such cats are exposed to a lower degree of glucotoxicity and therefore have greater potential for β-cell recovery. In contrast, diabetic neuropathy has been associated with a decreased likelihood of remission, possibly because affected cats typically have poor long-term DM control and, therefore, a greater risk of prolonged glucotoxicity (Video 1A, B).[92]

Treatment protocols that provide effective glycemic control, as promptly as possible, are also likely to limit a cat's exposure to glucotoxicity and might encourage remission. A variety of antihyperglycemic therapies can be used to manage DM in cats, including the oral sulfonylurea glipizide, medium- or long-acting insulins and insulin analogues or, very recently, oral sodium-glucose cotransporter 2 inhibitors.[94,95] Clinical experience with the latter is still extremely limited. Recent guidelines on the treatment of feline DM typically recommend every 12-hour treatment with the long-acting insulin protamine zinc insulin (PZI), or a long-acting insulin analogue, such as insulin glargine or detemir, as the optimum choice for effective DM control in cats, including a greater potential for remission.[94] However, there is little evidence to strongly recommend the use of 1 insulin type over another. Proposals that glargine and detemir are associated with particularly high remission rates is largely based on studies that examined a select group of cats who also received intensive home BG monitoring and ultra-low-carbohydrate diet, making it challenging to extrapolate these results to other populations.[92,96] As for PZI, the evidence for achieving high remission rates can only be derived indirectly from a study looking at the effect of different dietary carbohydrate contents on remission rates. In this study, 85% of cats were treated with PZI, alongside moderate- or low-carbohydrate diet, with high remission rates achieved in both groups, although somewhat higher with the low-carbohydrate diet. However, this study was not designed to assess the effect of insulin.[97] It is assumed that the longer duration of action of glargine, detemir, and PZI when compared with lente insulin in cats[98,99] might provide better glycemic control and limit glucotoxicity. However, no adequately powered, randomized studies comparing long-acting insulin preparations and lente in cats have been published. The only study that compared glargine, PZI, and lente was not randomized, and only included 8 cats per treatment group.[93] Although this study detected higher remission rate in glargine-treated cats when compared with PZI and lente, a randomized clinical trial including 46 cats treated with either glargine or PZI showed no difference in glycemic control or remission rate between these 2 long-acting insulins over a 1-year trial period, questioning at least partially the results of the former, smaller study.[100] It is therefore currently unproven whether any single insulin type offers better control, and greater likelihood of remission, than others.[6] There is also reasonable evidence that feeding a carbohydrate-restricted diet promotes better glycemic control, and a greater chance of remission, in diabetic cats.[97] Dietary carbohydrate restriction decreases postprandial hyperglycemia and mean BG in healthy cats.[101] Similarly, beneficial effects in cats with DM could aid in reducing glucotoxicity, besides other effects, including reduced glucose load leading to decreased insulin requirements. These effects might account for why studies reporting the highest rates of feline diabetic remission have typically fed diets containing a maximum of 12% metabolizable energy as carbohydrate.[92,102]

Diabetes Mellitus Cause

Remission is likely to be encouraged by improvement, or resolution, of pathogenic factors that contribute to a cat's DM by causing IR, impaired β-cell function, or increased glucose load. Prompt recognition of such factors is therefore highly important during initial diagnosis of feline DM. Identifying and addressing these factors during treatment is likely to encourage a state whereby endogenous insulin production can maintain euglycemia without the need for antihyperglycemic medications, and remission is achieved. Examples of diabetogenic factors, which have been linked to a greater likelihood of remission if adequately treated, include obesity in cats with type 2–like DM, and several causes of "other specific types of DM," including recent glucocorticoid therapy, and the presence of HS or naturally occurring HA.

There is initial evidence to support that planned weight loss encourages remission in diabetic cats who are overweight. This could be due to improvements in obesity-related IR,[21] or resolution of other factors associated with an overweight state (see earlier section on "Obesity"). One study found a greater likelihood of remission among cats who achieved at least 2% weight loss in the first month of treatment with either every 12-hours PZI or glargine.[100] Cats with a higher percentage body fat, measured by dual-energy X-ray absorptiometry, have also been demonstrated to have a greater chance of remission, which was usually associated with an eventual reduction in their percentage body fat.[102] Controlled weight loss should therefore form part of the treatment plan for overweight or obese diabetic cats once DM-associated weight loss has stabilized.

Several etiologic causes of feline DM, which have been likened to "specific types of DM" in people, have been associated with considerable DM remission rates when these causes are adequately addressed during treatment. Cats with DM secondary to HS or naturally occurring HA typically show a poor response to standard DM management, but can achieve DM remission if their underlying HS or HA is adequately controlled. This includes DM remission rates of 60% to 90% reported in cats with HS-associated DM treated using transsphenoidal hypophysectomy (see separate article in this issue).[14,103,104] Several studies have found that diabetic cats that have previously received glucocorticoids have a greater likelihood of remission compared with cats without a history of glucocorticoid treatment,[92,105] which could be due to a return of normal glucose tolerance once the diabetogenic effects of their glucocorticoid therapy wane.

GLUCOSE TOLERANCE IN DIABETIC REMISSION

It is likely that many cats in diabetic remission have ongoing glucose intolerance despite being able to maintain euglycemia without the need for antihyperglycemic therapy. A previous study found that approximately 20% of diabetic cats in remission were hyperglycemic (defined as BG > 6.5 mmol/L [117 mg/dL]) after a 24-hour fast, and approximately 74% had abnormal glucose clearance based on IVGTTs. Diabetic cats in remission also had significantly greater serum fructosamine concentrations than healthy control cats.[106] Ongoing glucose intolerance likely contributes to the high rate of DM relapse (26%–30%) among cats in diabetic remission.[92,107] Identifying which cats in diabetic remission might have ongoing glucose intolerance is associated with the same challenges discussed under "Prediabetes in Cats." To limit the chance of DM relapse, it is advisable that potential causes of IR, increased glucose load and β-cell dysfunction, are avoided, as much as possible, in the management of cats in diabetic remission (see **Box 2**). Cats in remission should also be carefully monitored for DM relapse.

DISCLOSURE

R. Gostelow receives funding from Royal Canin, France, and both Ruth Gostelow and K. Hazuchova received funding from Boehringer Ingelheim, Germany. The authors have no other disclosures.

SUPPLEMENTARY DATA

Supplementary data related to this article can be found online at https://doi.org/10.1016/j.cvsm.2023.02.001.

REFERENCES

1. American Diabetes A. Diagnosis and classification of diabetes mellitus. Diabetes Care 2013;36(Suppl 1):S67–74.
2. ESVE. Project ALIVE. 30/09/2022, Available at: https://www.esve.org/alive/search.aspx. Accessed September 30, 2022.
3. American Diabetes Association Professional Practice C. 2. Classification and diagnosis of diabetes: standards of medical care in diabetes-2022. Diabetes Care 2022;45(Suppl 1):S17–38.
4. American Diabetes A. 2. Classification and diagnosis of diabetes: standards of medical care in diabetes-2019. Diabetes Care 2019;42(Suppl 1):S13–28.
5. Riddle MC, Cefalu WT, Evans PH, et al. Consensus report: definition and interpretation of remission in type 2 diabetes. J Clin Endocrinol Metab 2022;107(1):1–9.
6. Gostelow R, Forcada Y, Graves T, et al. Systematic review of feline diabetic remission: separating fact from opinion. Vet J 2014;202(2):208–21.
7. Schwartz SS, Epstein S, Corkey BE, et al. The time is right for a new classification system for diabetes: rationale and implications of the beta-cell-centric classification schema. Diabetes Care 2016;39(2):179–86.
8. Appleton DJ, Rand JS, Sunvold GD. Insulin sensitivity decreases with obesity, and lean cats with low insulin sensitivity are at greatest risk of glucose intolerance with weight gain. J Feline Med Surg 2001;3(4):211–28.
9. Gilor C, Niessen SJ, Furrow E, et al. What's in a name? Classification of diabetes mellitus in veterinary medicine and why it matters. J Vet Intern Med 2016;30(4):927–40.
10. Niessen SJ, Church DB, Forcada Y. Hypersomatotropism, acromegaly, and hyperadrenocorticism and feline diabetes mellitus. Vet Clin North Am Small Anim Pract 2013;43(2):319–50.
11. Nelson RW, Reusch CE. Animal models of disease: classification and etiology of diabetes in dogs and cats. J Endocrinol 2014;222(3):T1–9.
12. Osto M, Zini E, Reusch CE, et al. Diabetes from humans to cats. Gen Comp Endocrinol 2013;182:48–53.
13. Niessen SJ, Forcada Y, Mantis P, et al. Studying cat (Felis catus) diabetes: beware of the acromegalic imposter. PLoS One 2015;10(5):e0127794.
14. Valentin SY, Cortright CC, Nelson RW, et al. Clinical findings, diagnostic test results, and treatment outcome in cats with spontaneous hyperadrenocorticism: 30 cases. J Vet Intern Med 2014;28(2):481–7.
15. Slingerland LI, Fazilova VV, Plantinga EA, et al. Indoor confinement and physical inactivity rather than the proportion of dry food are risk factors in the development of feline type 2 diabetes mellitus. Vet J 2009;179(2):247–53.
16. Zini E, Lunardi F, Zanetti R, et al. Endocrine pancreas in cats with diabetes mellitus. Vet Pathol 2016;53(1):136–44.
17. Hall DG, Kelley LC, Gray ML, et al. Lymphocytic inflammation of pancreatic islets in a diabetic cat. J Vet Diagn Invest 1997;9(1):98–100.
18. Tuomi T, Santoro N, Caprio S, et al. The many faces of diabetes: a disease with increasing heterogeneity. Lancet 2014;383(9922):1084–94.

19. Ohlund M, Egenvall A, Fall T, et al. Environmental Risk Factors for Diabetes Mellitus in Cats. J Vet Intern Med 2017;31(1):29–35.

20. Narayan KM, Boyle JP, Thompson TJ, et al. Effect of BMI on lifetime risk for diabetes in the U.S. Diabetes Care 2007;30(6):1562–6.

21. Hoenig M, Thomaseth K, Waldron M, et al. Insulin sensitivity, fat distribution, and adipocytokine response to different diets in lean and obese cats before and after weight loss. Am J Physiol Regul Integr Comp Physiol 2007;292(1): R227–34.

22. Kawano Y, Nakae J, Watanabe N, et al. Colonic pro-inflammatory macrophages cause insulin resistance in an intestinal Ccl2/Ccr2-dependent manner. Cell Metabol 2016;24(2):295–310.

23. Rebello CJ, Burton J, Heiman M, et al. Gastrointestinal microbiome modulator improves glucose tolerance in overweight and obese subjects: a randomized controlled pilot trial. J Diabet Complications 2015;29(8):1272–6.

24. Williams KJ, Wu X. Imbalanced insulin action in chronic over nutrition: Clinical harm, molecular mechanisms, and a way forward. Atherosclerosis 2016;247: 225–82.

25. Gray SL, Donald C, Jetha A, et al. Hyperinsulinemia precedes insulin resistance in mice lacking pancreatic beta-cell leptin signaling. Endocrinology 2010; 151(9):4178–86.

26. James DE, Stockli J, Birnbaum MJ. The aetiology and molecular landscape of insulin resistance. Nat Rev Mol Cell Biol 2021;22(11):751–71.

27. Lebovitz HE, Banerji MA. Point: visceral adiposity is causally related to insulin resistance. Diabetes Care 2005;28(9):2322–5.

28. Hoenig M. The cat as a model for human obesity and diabetes. Review. Journal of diabetes science and technology 2012;6(3):525–33.

29. Samuel VT, Shulman GI. The pathogenesis of insulin resistance: integrating signaling pathways and substrate flux. J Clin Invest 2016;126(1):12–22.

30. Wilkins C, Long RC Jr, Waldron M, et al. Assessment of the influence of fatty acids on indices of insulin sensitivity and myocellular lipid content by use of magnetic resonance spectroscopy in cats. Am J Vet Res 2004;65(8):1090–9.

31. Czech MP. Insulin action and resistance in obesity and type 2 diabetes. Nat Med 2017;23(7):804–14.

32. Kampmann U, Christensen B, Nielsen TS, et al. GLUT4 and UBC9 protein expression is reduced in muscle from type 2 diabetic patients with severe insulin resistance. PLoS One 2011;6(11):e27854.

33. Brennan CL, Hoenig M, Ferguson DC. GLUT4 but not GLUT1 expression decreases early in the development of feline obesity. Domest Anim Endocrinol 2004;26(4):291–301.

34. Spranger J, Kroke A, Mohlig M, et al. Adiponectin and protection against type 2 diabetes mellitus. Lancet. 2003;361(9353):226–8.

35. Muranaka S, Mori N, Hatano Y, et al. Obesity induced changes to plasma adiponectin concentration and cholesterol lipoprotein composition profile in cats. Res Vet Sci 2011;91(3):358–61.

36. Bjornvad CR, Rand JS, Tan HY, et al. Obesity and sex influence insulin resistance and total and multimer adiponectin levels in adult neutered domestic shorthair client-owned cats. Domest Anim Endocrinol 2014;47:55–64.

37. Considine RV, Sinha MK, Heiman ML, et al. Serum immunoreactive-leptin concentrations in normal-weight and obese humans. N Engl J Med 1996;334(5): 292–5.

38. Freitas Lima LC, Braga VA, do Socorro de Franca Silva M, et al. Adipokines, diabetes and atherosclerosis: an inflammatory association. Front Physiol 2015; 6:304.

39. Park HK, Ahima RS. Physiology of leptin: energy homeostasis, neuroendocrine function and metabolism. Metabolism 2015;64(1):24–34.

40. Feinstein R, Kanety H, Papa MZ, et al. Tumor necrosis factor-alpha suppresses insulin-induced tyrosine phosphorylation of insulin receptor and its substrates. J Biol Chem 1993;268(35):26055–8.

41. Hoenig M, McGoldrick JB, deBeer M, et al. Activity and tissue-specific expression of lipases and tumor-necrosis factor alpha in lean and obese cats. Domest Anim Endocrinol 2006;30(4):333–44.

42. Hoenig M, Pach N, Thomaseth K, et al. Cats differ from other species in their cytokine and antioxidant enzyme response when developing obesity. Obesity 2013;21(9):E407–14.

43. Tvarijonaviciute A, Ceron JJ, Holden SL, et al. Effects of weight loss in obese cats on biochemical analytes related to inflammation and glucose homeostasis. Research Support, Non-U.S. Gov't. Domest Anim Endocrinol 2012;42(3): 129–41.

44. Bensellam M, Laybutt DR, Jonas JC. The molecular mechanisms of pancreatic beta-cell glucotoxicity: recent findings and future research directions. Mol Cell Endocrinol 2012;364(1–2):1–27.

45. Zini E, Osto M, Franchini M, et al. Hyperglycaemia but not hyperlipidaemia causes beta cell dysfunction and beta cell loss in the domestic cat. Diabetologia 2009;52(2):336–46.

46. Brunzell JD, Robertson RP, Lerner RL, et al. Relationships between fasting plasma glucose levels and insulin secretion during intravenous glucose tolerance tests. J Clin Endocrinol Metab 1976;42(2):222–9.

47. Ritzel RA, Hansen JB, Veldhuis JD, et al. Induction of beta-cell rest by a Kir6.2/ SUR1-selective K(ATP)-channel opener preserves beta-cell insulin stores and insulin secretion in human islets cultured at high (11 mM) glucose. J Clin Endocrinol Metab 2004;89(2):795–805.

48. Oslowski CM, Urano F. A switch from life to death in endoplasmic reticulum stressed beta-cells. Diabetes Obes Metab 2010;12(Suppl 2):58–65, 0 2.

49. DeFronzo RA. Dysfunctional fat cells, lipotoxicity and type 2 diabetes. Int J Clin Pract Suppl 2004;(143):9–21. https://doi.org/10.1111/j.1368-504x.2004.00389.x.

50. Poitout V, Robertson RP. Glucolipotoxicity: fuel excess and beta-cell dysfunction. Endocr Rev 2008;29(3):351–66.

51. Poitout V, Amyot J, Semache M, et al. Glucolipotoxicity of the pancreatic beta cell. Biochim Biophys Acta 2010;1801(3):289–98.

52. Nishi M, Sanke T, Nagamatsu S, et al. Islet amyloid polypeptide. A new beta cell secretory product related to islet amyloid deposits. J Biol Chem 1990;265(8): 4173–6.

53. Ahmad E, Ahmad A, Singh S, et al. A mechanistic approach for islet amyloid polypeptide aggregation to develop anti-amyloidogenic agents for type-2 diabetes. Biochimie 2011;93(5):793–805.

54. Rafacho A, Ortsater H, Nadal A, et al. Glucocorticoid treatment and endocrine pancreas function: implications for glucose homeostasis, insulin resistance and diabetes. J Endocrinol 2014;223(3):R49–62.

55. Woolcock AD, Bugbee AC, Creevy KE. Evaluation of baseline cortisol concentration to monitor efficacy of twice-daily administration of trilostane to dogs

with pituitary-dependent hyperadrenocorticism: 22 cases (2008-2012). J Am Vet Med Assoc 2016;248(7):814–21.

56. Schaefer S, Kooistra HS, Riond B, et al. Evaluation of insulin-like growth factor-1, total thyroxine, feline pancreas-specific lipase and urinary corticoid-to-creatinine ratio in cats with diabetes mellitus in Switzerland and the Netherlands. J Feline Med Surg 2017;19(8):888–96.

57. Zini E, Hafner M, Kook P, et al. Longitudinal evaluation of serum pancreatic enzymes and ultrasonographic findings in diabetic cats without clinically relevant pancreatitis at diagnosis. J Vet Intern Med 2015;29(2):589–96.

58. Almgren P, Lehtovirta M, Isomaa B, et al. Heritability and familiality of type 2 diabetes and related quantitative traits in the Botnia Study. Diabetologia 2011; 54(11):2811–9.

59. O'Neill DG, Gostelow R, Orme C, et al. Epidemiology of diabetes mellitus among 193,435 cats attending primary-care veterinary practices in England. J Vet Intern Med 2016;30(4):964–72.

60. Ohlund M, Fall T, Strom Holst B, et al. Incidence of Diabetes Mellitus in Insured Swedish Cats in Relation to Age, Breed and Sex. J Vet Intern Med 2015;29(5): 1342–7.

61. Rand JS, Bobbermien LM, Hendrikz JK, et al. Over representation of Burmese cats with diabetes mellitus. Aust Vet J 1997;75(6):402–5.

62. Prahl A, Guptill L, Glickman NW, et al. Time trends and risk factors for diabetes mellitus in cats presented to veterinary teaching hospitals. J Feline Med Surg 2007;9(5):351–8.

63. Alhaddad H, Khan R, Grahn RA, et al. Extent of linkage disequilibrium in the domestic cat, Felis silvestris catus, and its breeds. PLoS One 2013;8(1):e53537.

64. O'Leary CA, Duffy DL, Gething MA, et al. Investigation of diabetes mellitus in Burmese cats as an inherited trait: a preliminary study. N Z Vet J 2013;61(6): 354–8.

65. Kurushima JD, Lipinski MJ, Gandolfi B, et al. Variation of cats under domestication: genetic assignment of domestic cats to breeds and worldwide random-bred populations. Anim Genet 2013;44(3):311–24.

66. Forcada Y, Holder A, Church DB, et al. A polymorphism in the melanocortin 4 receptor gene (MC4R:c.92C>T) is associated with diabetes mellitus in overweight domestic shorthaired cats. J Vet Intern Med 2014;28(2):458–64.

67. Xi B, Chandak GR, Shen Y, et al. Association between common polymorphism near the MC4R gene and obesity risk: a systematic review and meta-analysis. PLoS One 2012;7(9):e45731.

68. Forcada Y, Boursnell M, Catchpole B, et al. A genome-wide association study identifies novel candidate genes for susceptibility to diabetes mellitus in non-obese cats. PLoS One 2021;16(12):e0259939.

69. Samaha G, Wade CM, Beatty J, et al. Mapping the genetic basis of diabetes mellitus in the Australian Burmese cat (Felis catus). Sci Rep 2020;10(1):19194.

70. Balmer L, O'Leary CA, Menotti-Raymond M, et al. Mapping of Diabetes Susceptibility Loci in a Domestic Cat Breed with an Unusually High Incidence of Diabetes Mellitus. Genes 2020;11(11). https://doi.org/10.3390/genes11111369.

71. Bird SR, Hawley JA. Update on the effects of physical activity on insulin sensitivity in humans. BMJ Open Sport Exerc Med 2016;2(1):e000143.

72. Panciera DL, Thomas CB, Eicker SW, et al. Epizootiologic patterns of diabetes mellitus in cats: 333 cases (1980-1986). J Am Vet Med Assoc 1990;197(11): 1504–8.

73. Chiu KC, Lee NP, Cohan P, et al. Beta cell function declines with age in glucose tolerant Caucasians. Clin Endocrinol 2000;53(5):569–75.
74. Lederer R, Rand JS, Jonsson NN, et al. Frequency of feline diabetes mellitus and breed predisposition in domestic cats in Australia. Vet J 2009;179(2):254–8.
75. Lowe AD, Graves TK, Campbell KL, et al. A pilot study comparing the diabetogenic effects of dexamethasone and prednisolone in cats. Comparative Study Research Support, Non-U.S. Gov't. J Am Anim Hosp Assoc Sep-Oct 2009; 45(5):215–24.
76. Frezoulis PS, Oikonomidis IL, Saridomichelakis MN, et al. Prevalence, association with systemic inflammatory response syndrome and outcome of stress hyperglycaemia in sick cats. J Small Anim Pract 2022;63(3):197–202.
77. Reusch C. Feline diabetes mellitus. In: Feldman EC, Nelson RW, Reusch C, et al. *Canine and feline endocrinology*, 4th edition, 2015, Elsevier Saunders, St. Louis, MO, 258–314, chap 7.
78. Reeve-Johnson MK, Rand JS, Vankan D, et al. Cutpoints for screening blood glucose concentrations in healthy senior cats. J Feline Med Surg 2017;19(12): 1181–91.
79. Reeve-Johnson MK, Rand JS, Vankan D, et al. Diagnosis of prediabetes in cats: glucose concentration cut points for impaired fasting glucose and impaired glucose tolerance. Domest Anim Endocrinol 2016;57:55–62.
80. Hoenig M. Comparative aspects of human, canine, and feline obesity and factors predicting progression to diabetes. Veterinary Sciences 2014;1(2):121–35.
81. Holst JJ, Gromada J. Role of incretin hormones in the regulation of insulin secretion in diabetic and nondiabetic humans. Am J Physiol Endocrinol Metab 2004; 287(2):E199–206.
82. Kim W, Egan JM. The role of incretins in glucose homeostasis and diabetes treatment. Pharmacol Rev 2008;60(4):470–512.
83. Gilor C, Graves TK, Gilor S, et al. The incretin effect in cats: comparison between oral glucose, lipids, and amino acids. Research Support, Non-U.S. Gov't. Domest Anim Endocrinol 2011;40(4):205–12.
84. Nauck MA, Bartels E, Orskov C, et al. Additive insulinotropic effects of exogenous synthetic human gastric inhibitory polypeptide and glucagon-like peptide-1-(7-36) amide infused at near-physiological insulinotropic hormone and glucose concentrations. J Clin Endocrinol Metab 1993;76(4):912–7.
85. Li X, Li W, Wang H, et al. Pseudogenization of a sweet-receptor gene accounts for cats' indifference toward sugar. PLoS Genet 2005;1(1):27–35.
86. Hoenig M, Jordan ET, Ferguson DC, et al. Oral glucose leads to a differential response in glucose, insulin, and GLP-1 in lean versus obese cats. Domest Anim Endocrinol 2010;38(2):95–102.
87. Gilor C, Graves TK, Lascelles BD, et al. The effects of body weight, body condition score, sex, and age on serum fructosamine concentrations in clinically healthy cats. Vet Clin Pathol 2010;39(3):322–8.
88. Hoenig M, Traas AM, Schaeffer DJ. Evaluation of routine hematology profile results and fructosamine, thyroxine, insulin, and proinsulin concentrations in lean, overweight, obese, and diabetic cats. J Am Vet Med Assoc 2013;243(9): 1302–9.
89. Suleiman M, Marselli L, Cnop M, et al. The Role of Beta Cell Recovery in Type 2 Diabetes Remission. Int J Mol Sci 2022;23(13). https://doi.org/10.3390/ijms23137435.
90. Nelson RW, Griffey SM, Feldman EC, et al. Transient clinical diabetes mellitus in cats: 10 cases (1989-1991). J Vet Intern Med 1999;13(1):28–35.

91. Tschuor F, Zini E, Schellenberg S, et al. Remission of diabetes mellitus in cats cannot be predicted by the arginine stimulation test. Research Support, Non-U.S. Gov't. J Vet Intern Med 2011;25(1):83–9.

92. Roomp K, Rand J. Intensive blood glucose control is safe and effective in diabetic cats using home monitoring and treatment with glargine. J Feline Med Surg 2009;11(8):668–82.

93. Marshall RD, Rand JS, Morton JM. Treatment of newly diagnosed diabetic cats with glargine insulin improves glycaemic control and results in higher probability of remission than protamine zinc and lente insulins. Clinical Trial Research Support, Non-U.S. Gov't. J Feline Med Surg 2009;11(8):683–91.

94. Sparkes AH, Cannon M, Church D, et al. ISFM consensus guidelines on the practical management of diabetes mellitus in cats. J Feline Med Surg 2015; 17(3):235–50.

95. Niessen S, Voth R, Kroh C, et al. Once daily oral therapy for feline diabetes mellitus: SGLT-2-inhibitor velagliflozin as stand-alone therapy compared to insulin injection therapy in diabetic cats [abstract]. J Vet Intern Med 2022;36(6): 2512–3.

96. Roomp K, Rand J. Evaluation of detemir in diabetic cats managed with a protocol for intensive blood glucose control. J Feline Med Surg 2012;14(8):566–72.

97. Bennett N, Greco DS, Peterson ME, et al. Comparison of a low carbohydrate-low fiber diet and a moderate carbohydrate-high fiber diet in the management of feline diabetes mellitus. Comparative Study Controlled Clinical Trial Randomized Controlled Trial Research Support, Non-U.S. Gov't. J Feline Med Surg 2006; 8(2):73–84.

98. Marshall RD, Rand JS, Morton JM. Glargine and protamine zinc insulin have a longer duration of action and result in lower mean daily glucose concentrations than lente insulin in healthy cats. Comparative Study Research Support, Non-U.S. Gov't. J Vet Pharmacol Therapeut 2008;31(3):205–12.

99. Gilor C, Ridge TK, Attermeier KJ, et al. Pharmacodynamics of insulin detemir and insulin glargine assessed by an isoglycemic clamp method in healthy cats. Randomized Controlled Trial Research Support, Non-U.S. Gov't. J Vet Intern Med 2010;24(4):870–4.

100. Gostelow R, Scudder C, Forcada Y, et al. One year, prospective, randomized trial comparing efficacy of glargine and protamine zinc insulins in diabetic cats [abstract]. J Vet Intern Med 2017;31:1273.

101. Farrow HA, Rand JS, Morton JM, et al. Effect of dietary carbohydrate, fat, and protein on postprandial glycemia and energy intake in cats. J Vet Intern Med 2013;27(5):1121–35.

102. Mazzaferro EM, Greco DS, Turner AS, et al. Treatment of feline diabetes mellitus using an alpha-glucosidase inhibitor and a low-carbohydrate diet. J Feline Med Surg 2003;5(3):183–9.

103. Fenn J, Kenny PJ, Scudder CJ, et al. Efficacy of hypophysectomy for the treatment of hypersomatotropism-induced diabetes mellitus in 68 cats. J Vet Intern Med 2021;35(2):823–33.

104. van Bokhorst KL, Galac S, Kooistra HS, et al. Evaluation of hypophysectomy for treatment of hypersomatotropism in 25 cats. J Vet Intern Med 2021;35(2): 834–42.

105. Gostelow R, O'Neill DG, Brodbelt DC, et al. Diabetic remission in cats examined in UK primary-care practices: Occurrence and risk factors (abstract). J Vet Intern Med 2017;31(4):1273.

106. Gottlieb S, Rand JS, Marshall R, et al. Glycemic status and predictors of relapse for diabetic cats in remission. J Vet Intern Med 2015;29(1):184–92.

107. Zini E, Hafner M, Osto M, et al. Predictors of clinical remission in cats with diabetes mellitus. J Vet Intern Med 2010;24(6):1314–21.

108. World Health Organization. Definition of diabetes mellitus and intermediate hyperglycemia: report of a WHO/IDF consultation. Geneva, Switzerland: WHO Document Production Services; 2006.

109. Nerhagen S, Moberg HL, Boge GS, et al. Prednisolone-induced diabetes mellitus in the cat: a historical cohort. J Feline Med Surg 2021;23(2):175–80.

110. Lee P, Mori A, Coradini M, et al. Potential predictive biomarkers of obesity in Burmese cats. Vet J 2013;195(2):221–7.

Diabetes Ketoacidosis and Hyperosmolar Hyperglycemic Syndrome in Companion Animals

Arnon Gal, DVM, PhD[a],*, Adesola Odunayo, DVM, MS[b]

KEYWORDS

- Diabetes • Diabetes mellitus • Diabetic ketoacidosis
- Hyperosmolar hyperglycemic state • Hyperosmolar diabetic ketoacidosis
- Eugylcemic ketoacidosis • Dog • Cat

KEY POINTS

- Diabetes ketoacidosis and hyperosmolar hyperglycemic state are life-threatening complications of diabetes that result from a variable imbalance between insulin and glucose counter-regulatory hormones.
- Diabetes ketoacidosis develops over a short period of time and often requires intensive care management with insulin and correction of deranged electrolytes, acid base, and water balance.
- Hyperosmolar hyperglycemic state develops over a longer period of time with severe dehydration being the main underlying abnormality that also requires intensive care management.
- There is a combined entity of diabetes ketoacidosis and hyperosmolar hyperglycemic state (hyperosmolar-diabetes ketoacidosis) that carries a poor prognosis.

DEFINITIONS

Diabetes ketoacidosis (DKA) is defined by the American Diabetes Association as hyperglycemia (blood glucose >200 mg/dL [11 mmol/L]), acidemia (venous pH < 7.3), low bicarbonate levels (<15 mmol/L), with ketonemia and ketonuria.[1] Euglycemic DKA (EDKA) is defined as DKA in patients with "near normal or lower than anticipated" blood glucose ≤200 to 250 mg/dL (≤11 to 14 mmol/L).[2] Hyperosmolar hyperglycemic state (HHS) is

[a] Department of Veterinary Clinical Medicine, College of Veterinary Medicine, University of Illinois at Urbana-Champaign, 1008 West Hazelwood Drive, Urbana, IL 61820, USA;
[b] Department of Small Animal Clinical Sciences, College of Veterinary Medicine, University of Florida, 2015 Southwest 16th Avenue, Gainesville, FL 32608, USA
* Corresponding author.
E-mail address: agal2@illinois.edu

Vet Clin Small Anim 53 (2023) 531–550
https://doi.org/10.1016/j.cvsm.2023.01.005
0195-5616/23/© 2023 Elsevier Inc. All rights reserved.

defined as blood glucose greater than 600 mg/dL (33.3 mmol/L), arterial pH > 7.3, bicarbonate greater than 15 mmol/L, effective osmolarity greater than 320 mOsm/kg [effective osmolarity is calculated 2 × Na (mmol/L)+glucose (mg/dL)/18], and insignificant amounts of ketone bodies.[1] Hyperosmolar DKA (H-DKA) is defined as high plasma osmolarity (>320 mOsm/kg), severe hyperglycemia (>600 mg/dL), low bicarbonate (<18 mmol/L), acidosis (pH < 7.3), ketonuria, azotemia, and severe dehydration.[3]

DEMOGRAPHICS

DKA occurs in middle-aged and older diabetic dogs and cats,[4] albeit, in one cat study, DKA occurred at a younger age than in cats with noncomplicated diabetes mellitus (DM).[5] Female dogs[4] and male cats[4,6] have a higher risk for DKA,[4] and in one study, Siamese and Abyssinian cats were overrepresented.[5] DKA is diagnosed in approximately 34% to 50% of newly diagnosed diabetic cats,[7] and 65% of newly diagnosed diabetic dogs.[8]

Cats with HHS are composed 6.4% of total ER visits of diabetic cats,[9] whereas the prevalence of canine HHS was 5% of all diabetic dogs examined at one teaching hospital.[10] Most cats with HHS were domestic shorthair cats,[9] and most dogs with HHS were of mixed breeds.[10] There were twice more diabetic male cats with HHS than females,[9] whereas 53% of diabetic dogs with HHS were neutered males, 36% neutered females, 6% intact females, and 4% intact males.[10] Diabetic cats with HHS had a mean age of 12.6 ± 3.2 years.[9] 71% of cats with HHS had already been previously diagnosed with DM with a median duration of 18 months between the onset of DM and the diagnosis of HHS, and a median (range) reported duration of illness before presentation of 3 (0 to 30) days.[9] Approximately 53% of diabetic dogs with HHS were newly diagnosed diabetics, whereas approximately 47% of diabetic dogs with HHS had been previously diagnosed with DM and had been treated with insulin for a median of 12 months. Their mean (±standard deviation [SD]) age (years) at diagnosis of HHS was 9.7 ± 3.1. Their mean (±SD) duration of clinical signs before the diagnosis of HHS was 0.3 ± 0.39 months.[10]

KETOGENESIS

Glucose is the predominant source of energy for the brain, which cannot use fatty acids for energy. When glucose is at very low levels, ketone bodies (acetoacetate [AcAc], beta-hydroxybutyrate [BHB], acetone) can be used by the brain and other tissues. Physiologic ketogenesis is considered a normal adaptive mechanism activated during nonpathologic conditions such as fasting, prolonged physical activity, pregnancy, and in neonates. Physiologic ketosis is self-limiting because basal insulin levels prevent long-lived and robust ketogenesis (**Fig. 1**). Once ketone bodies are produced, they are used by many tissues and are excreted in the urine.[11]

Ketogenesis occurs when three conditions are met: (1) constant delivery of free fatty acid (FFA) to the liver from white adipose tissue (WAT) lipolysis; (2) considerable hepatic oxidation of fatty acyl-CoA (FA-CoA); and (3) reduced availability of oxaloacetate (tricarboxylic acid cycle [TCA] intermediate). The balance between glucose counterregulatory hormones (predominantly glucagon) and insulin controls the rate of ketogenesis through regulation of the activities of (1) hormone-sensitive lipase (HSL); (2) acetyl CoA (AcCoA)-carboxylase; and (3) HMG-CoA synthase (mHS). The rate of ketogenesis is also controlled through the availability of oxaloacetate (necessary for entry of AcCoA to TCA), citrate (substrate for Malonyl-CoA synthesis), and increasing FA-CoA levels that synergistically with glucagon repress the activity of AcCoA-carboxylase.[12]

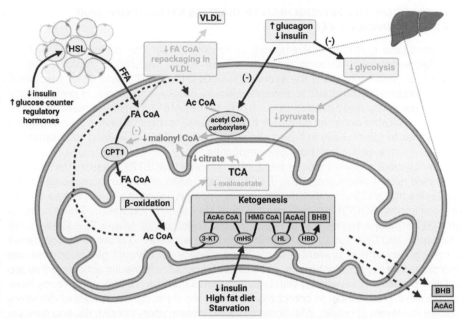

Fig. 1. Low-insulin and high-glucose counter-regulatory hormones (glucagon, cortisol, catecholamines, and GH) levels promote ketogenesis. First, WAT's HSL hydrolyses FFA from triglycerides. Released FFA reach the liver and are routed for hepatic mitochondrial oxidation instead of undergoing an ATP-dependent esterification to FA-CoA,[61] repackaged in VLDLs, and released to peripheral tissues. The mitochondrial CPT-1 shuttles FA-CoA across the inner mitochondrial membrane, where FA-CoA could be oxidized for energy via beta-oxidation. FA-CoA repackaging versus beta-oxidation is determined by Malonyl-CoA levels (intermediate of FA synthesis).[11] High Malonyl-CoA levels repress CPT-1's activity. Glucagon represses, and insulin stimulates the activity of AcCoA-carboxylase, the enzyme that converts AcCoA to Malonyl-CoA. Therefore, insulin promotes FA-CoA VLDL repackaging and prevents ketogenesis by increasing the levels of Malonyl-CoA. Glucagon has the opposite effect; it promotes FA-CoA oxidation and ketogenesis by inhibiting Malonyl-CoA synthesis.[11] Once inside the inner mitochondrial membrane, AcCoA is cleaved from FA-CoA and condenses with oxaloacetate (TCA intermediate) to enter the TCA. When insulin level is low, and glucagon level is high, the metabolism of carbohydrates is shifted from glycolysis to gluconeogenesis, which subsequently reduces the levels of oxaloacetate and diverts AcCoA away from the TCA toward the production of ketone bodies. In the process of ketogenesis, 3-KT first converts AcCoA to AcAcCoA, then mitochondrial mHS converts AcAcCoA to HMG-CoA; starvation, low levels of insulin, and high-fat diets stimulate the activity of mHS. Then HL cleaves AcAc from HMG-CoA. Lastly, HBD catalyzes the reduction of AcAc to BHB, and during this step, NADH is oxidized to NAD^+. Hepatic mitochondrial redox potential ($NADH/NAD^+$ ratio) determines the BHB/AcAc ratio. Spontaneous decarboxylation of AcAc produces small amounts of acetone.[11] 3-KT, 3-ketothiolase; AcAc, acetoacetate; AcAcCOA, acetoacetyl CoA; AcCoA, acetyl CoA; AcCoA-carboxylase, acetyl CoA carboxylase; BHB, betahydroxybutyrate; CPT1, Carnitine palmitoyl 1; FA, fatty acids; FA-CoA, fatty acyl-CoA; FFA, free fatty acids; GH, growth hormone; HBD, 3-hydroxybutyrate dehydrogenase; HL, HMG CoA lyase; HMG-CoA, 3-hydroxy-3-methylglutaryl Co A; HSL, hormone-sensitive lipase; mHS, HMG-CoA synthase; TCA, tricarboxylic acid cycle; WAT, white adipose tissue.

PREDISPOSITION AND PATHOGENESIS OF DIABETES KETOACIDOSIS AND EUGLYCEMIC DIABETES KETOACIDOSIS

Infections (and systemic inflammation) commonly trigger the development of DKA (and hyperglycemia)[1] through the induction of insulin resistance. Activated white blood cells (WBC) increases the expression of GLUT1, GLUT3, and GLUT4 isoforms on their plasma membrane[13] to enhance glucose uptake, for glucose is preferentially used by the innate and adaptive immune cells to mediate immune responses crucial to survival.[14] Another common cause for the rapid development of DKA is an inadequate level of insulin (particularly in type 1 diabetes mellitus [T1DM]) leading to unopposed glucose counter-regulatory hormone responses.[1]

Use of type-2 sodium-glucose transporter inhibitors (SGLT2i) is associated with an increased risk of developing DKA.[15] SGLT2i have been shown to increase glucagon levels directly, and indirectly through a compensatory response to increased urinary glucose losses. SGLT2i also reduces the renal clearance of ketones.[15] T1DM patients on SGLT2i have a higher risk of hypoglycemia (because of severe SGLT2i-induced glucosuria) and DKA because a lower insulin dose necessary to prevent hypoglycemia is not high enough to prevent lipolysis and ketogenesis. Chronic glucocorticoid use and drugs that may confer hepatic or peripheral resistance to insulin action predispose to DKA, particularly in patients with type 2 diabetes mellitus (T2DM) who already have severe insulin resistance. In companion animals, the unrecognized onset of diabetes, inadequate levels of insulin, infections, systemic inflammatory conditions, and concurrent endocrinopathies that confer insulin resistance have been reported to precipitate DKA.[4,5,8,16]

In DKA, decreased renal clearance and peripheral utilization of ketones (particularly in skeletal muscles) lead to severe accumulation in the blood. Ketones are weak acids and quickly exhaust the body's buffering capacity and induce a state of life-threatening metabolic acidosis (pH < 7). The metabolic acidosis results in a characteristic compensatory respiratory alkalosis (Kussmaul breathing). Lactic acid buildup from hypoperfusion and hyperchloremia from isotonic fluid administration further aggravates metabolic acidosis, whereas increased gastrointestinal and urinary losses of potassium contribute to the development of concurrent metabolic alkalosis. WAT lipolysis further exacerbates peripheral insulin resistance and decreases peripheral utilization of glucose. Enhanced gluconeogenesis and glycogenolysis simultaneously increase hepatic glucose output. Consequently, severe hyperglycemia develops. Hyperglycemic-induced diuresis and ketonemia, ketone-induced decreased fluid (and food) intake, and increased gastrointestinal fluid losses (vomiting and diarrhea) lead to severe dehydration, electrolyte losses, and intracellular, extracellular, and intravascular volume contraction. Severe electrolyte imbalances, particularly hypokalemia, and hypomagnesemia, negatively affect vascular tone, cardiac contractility, and cardiac output. Intravascular volume contraction predisposes to the development of thromboembolism and end-organ thrombosis. The combination of thromboembolism, severe dehydration and hypoperfusion, loss of vascular tone, and reduced cardiac output leads to shock, severe multiorgan failure, and death (**Fig. 2**).

In the Central Nervous System (CNS), hypertonicity leading to fluid shifts from the intracellular to the extracellular compartment results in cellular dehydration. If the correction of hyperglycemia with insulin treatment causes a rapid decrease in serum osmolarity, it can result in rapid fluid shifts back from the extracellular to the intracellular compartments. This is one presumed mechanism of cerebral edema which is commonly seen in human pediatric patients with T1DM[17] but not as frequently in

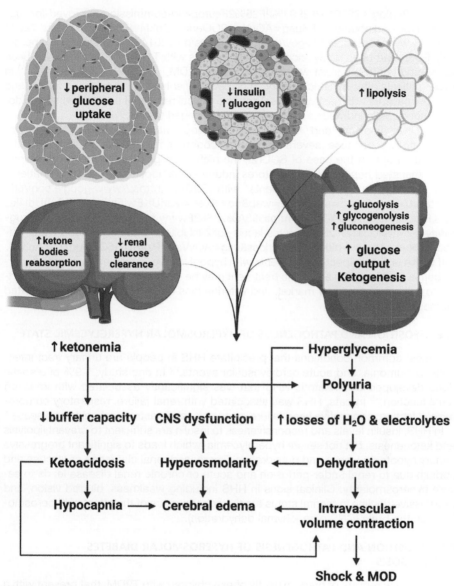

Fig. 2. Pathogenesis of DKA.

companion animals. Additional mechanisms that are thought to contribute to the pathogenesis of cerebral edema in DKA include hypoperfusion-mediated damage to the CNS (from severe dehydration and hyperventilation) followed by cerebral hyperperfusion after administration of intravenous (IV) fluids; activation of the sodium-hydrogen membrane exchanger in the CNS that mediates sodium entry and cellular edema; and administration of bicarbonate.[18]

Before the recently increased use of the SGLT2i as an adjunct therapy in T1DM (https://www.google.com/url?sa=t&rct=j&q=&esrc=s&source=web&cd=&ved=2ah UKEwjR-e_o6aP6AhWAADQIHYu8CfEQFnoECAUQAQ&url=https%3A%2F%2Fwww.

jdrf.org%2Fblog%2F2019%2F03%2F25%2Feuropean-commission-approved-forxiga-adults-type-1-diabetes%2F&usg=AOvVaw0OQerkdgCgkf4wEJnN9X27) and T2DM (https://www.accessdata.fda.gov/drugsatfda_docs/nda/2014/204629Orig1s000Approv.pdf), EDKA had been rarely encountered in patients with T1DM.[19] EDKA has also been rarely reported in pregnant women with T1DM, T2DM, and gestational diabetes,[20] in T1DM patients after bariatric surgery, in diabetic patients with insulin pump failure, and in T1DM patients with gastroparesis. There are clinical reports of euglycemic ketoacidosis in nondiabetic individuals associated with prolonged fasting.[21]

In EDKA, lipolysis and ketoacidosis develop without severe hyperglycemia (>250 mg/dL) because severe hepatic glycogen stores depletion limits hepatic glucose output. In the case of SGLT2i, the high renal glucose clearance combined with exhausted hepatic glycogen stores induce ketoacidosis, particularly in patients with T1DM[22] but also in patients with T2DM (https://www.google.com/url?sa=t&rct=j&q=&esrc=s&source=web&cd=&ved=2ahUKEwj5h6Wp9qP6AhUdl4kEHXsJBccQFnoECAsQAQ&url=https%3A%2F%2Fwww.fda.gov%2Fdrugs%2Fdrug-safety-and-availability%2Ffda-revises-labels-sglt2-inhibitors-diabetes-include-warnings-about-too-much-acid-blood-and-serious&usg=AOvVaw0PzsBD-16QObuqXMfLAu3m).

If EDKA is not suspected in patients with hypoglycemia, euglycemia, or mild hyperglycemia (<250 mg/dL) adequate treatment may be withheld. SGLT2i are slowly starting to enter the veterinary market, and veterinarians must recognize their associated increased risk for EDKA.

PREDISPOSITION AND PATHOGENESIS OF HYPEROSMOLAR HYPERGLYCEMIC STATE

The most common conditions that precipitate HHS in people are urinary tract infections, pneumonia, and acute cardiovascular events.[23] In one study, 1.9% of diabetic dogs developed a nonketotic HHS that was significantly associated with impaired renal function.[10] In cats, HHS was associated with renal failure, respiratory compromise, infection, congestive heart failure, neoplasia, and gastrointestinal tract disease.[9]

In HHS, insulin levels and responsiveness to insulin are sufficient to prevent lipolysis and ketogenesis, but not severe hyperglycemia, which leads to significant progressive urinary hypotonic losses and dehydration. Decreased renal clearance of glucose and sodium due to renal under-perfusion and acute or chronic renal disease leads to severe hyperosmolarity. Clinical signs in HHS including weakness, blurred vision, and progressive decline in mental status are the consequence of the effect of hyperosmolarity on the brain (CNS parenchymal dehydration).

PREDISPOSITION AND PATHOGENESIS OF HYPEROSMOLAR DIABETES KETOACIDOSIS

There are few reports of predominantly obese children with T2DM, that present with a hybrid between HHS and DKA. H-DKA has been associated with a high mortality rate due to multi-organ failure.[3] H-DKA develops when the conditions for DKA and HHS are present, namely (1) severe imbalance between insulin and the glucose counter-regulatory hormones leading to severe lipolysis, ketogenesis, increased hepatic glucose production, and decreased peripheral glucose utilization; and (2) severe dehydration from hypotonic urinary fluid losses and decreased renal glucose clearance.

H-DKA carries a poor prognosis in people and the prognosis is suspected to be the same in companion animals. There is only one veterinary report of dogs that may have had H-DKA. In this report, dogs with nonketotic HHS (HNK) had a similar outcome to dogs with H-DKA (HK).[10] However, the strict criteria that define HHS, DKA, and H-DKA in people were not applied to all dogs in this report.

CLINICAL HISTORY OF DIABETES KETOACIDOSIS IN DOGS AND CATS

Clinical signs of DKA in dogs and cats may be non-specific and may include polyuria, polydipsia, vomiting, anorexia, hyporexia, lethargy, weight loss, diarrhea, tachypnea, weakness, abnormal gait, or impaired jumping ability in cats.[24] Patients with HHS may also have a history of cardiac or kidney disease or newly developed neurologic signs, such as seizures, altered mentation, circling, or pacing.[25]

PHYSICAL EXAMINATION FINDINGS

Physical examination abnormalities in affected patients are non-specific and may vary depending on the patient signalment, concurrent disease (**Box 1**), hemodynamic status, severity, and chronicity of the DKA syndrome.[25] Abnormalities include evidence of dehydration, poor body condition, abdominal pain, respiratory distress, cataracts, blindness, fever, evidence of diarrhea, or an unkempt haircoat in cats.[5,26] Kussmaul respiration has been anecdotally reported in dogs and cats.[27] There are also reports of a sweet musty apple smell to the breath (indicative of exhaled acetone) although this finding is not reliably detected by all individuals.[25,26] Neurologic abnormalities may be documented in dogs and cats with DKA, H-DKA, and HHS. Those abnormalities may include change in mentation, circling, seizures, ataxia or abnormal pupillary light reflex.[9,25]

An important observation that should be made by the clinician during the physical exam is evaluation of the patient for signs of poor oxygen delivery or shock. Poor perfusion is a life-threatening condition as a result of circulatory collapse in the DKA patient secondary to maldistribution (pancreatitis, sepsis), hypovolemia (vomiting,

---

Box 1
Common comorbidities to evaluate for in patients with diabetes ketoacidosis

Acute pancreatitis

Chronic pancreatitis

Lower urinary tract infection

Pyelonephritis

Urolithiasis

Hyperadrenocorticism

Acute kidney injury

Chronic kidney disease

Neoplasia

Hepatic lipidosis

Cholangitis/hepatitis

Chronic enteropathy

Meningoencephalitis

Gingivitis

Pyoderma

Triditis in cats (pancreatitis, cholangitis and chronic enteropathy)

Obesity

diarrhea), or cardiogenic (hypertrophic cardiomyopathy, dilated cardiomyopathy) causes.[28] Physical examination indications of poor perfusion are listed in **Box 2**. Hypotension is also often present when a blood pressure is obtained. Physical exam findings of poor perfusion are very distinct from those of dehydration and the clinician should ensure those are well delineated as the treatment plan for each is very different.

CLINICAL DIAGNOSIS OF DIABETES KETOACIDOSIS

There is no clinical feature that definitively enables the diagnosis of DKA. DKA is classically diagnosed as the triad of hyperglycemia, anion gap metabolic acidosis, and ketonemia.[26,29,30] Hyperglycemia is not diagnostic of DKA without the accompanying acidosis.[29,31] Although EDKA has not been well described in veterinary patients, in one study of dogs with DKA, approximately 2% of dogs (2/120) had glucose levels within the normal reference range on presentation.[8]

The criteria for the clinical diagnosis of HHS include hyperglycemia (usually above 500 mg/dL), arterial pH > 7.3, venous pH > 7.25, serum bicarbonate greater than 15 mmol/L, small-to-absent ketonuria, absent-to-small ketonemia, effective serum osmolarity greater than 320 mOsm/kg and evidence of neurologic abnormalities (obtundation, seizures).[9,30] The categorization of the severity of DKA has not been well elucidated in veterinary patients.

The severity of DKA in human patients is categorized by the degree of acidosis:[30]

- Mild: venous pH < 7.3 or serum bicarbonate less than 15 mmol/L
- Moderate: Venous pH < 7.2 or serum bicarbonate less than 10 mmol/L
- Severe: venous pH < 7.1 or serum bicarbonate < 5 mmol/L

Serum biochemical analysis should be performed to evaluate the patient for hyperglycemia. Blood glucose concentrations may also be determined using a point-of-care glucose monitor during the triage examination. Hemoconcentration or hemodilution may not accurately reflect the patient's actual blood glucose concentration on a point-of-care monitor.[32] Other abnormalities that have been described on the serum biochemical analysis in dogs and cats with DKA/HHS include hyperbilirubinemia, hypercholesterolemia, hypertriglyceridemia, electrolyte abnormalities, azotemia, hyperphosphatemia, and increased liver enzyme activity.[25]

The presence of ketones is established by identifying ketoacids using a urine dipstick on serum or urine samples or on a point-of-care ketone meter.[9] Ketonemia

---

Box 2
Indications of poor perfusion in dogs and cats

Tachycardia

Weak or absent peripheral pulses

Pale mucous membranes

Prolonged capillary refill time

Altered mentation

Cold extremities

Hypotension

Hyperlactatemia

Bradycardia, hypothermia, and hypotension are a classic triad in cats with poor perfusion

is more specific than ketonuria to diagnose ketoacidosis and may be more helpful as an early point-of-care test for DKA.[31] Ketonuria is most commonly assessed using commercially available urine reagent strips.[33] This methodology uses a nitroprusside reaction leading to a color change as an indicator of the presence of ketones.[33] AcAa and acetone are detected using these bedside strips but BHA is not. The nitroprusside methodology has a higher affinity for AcAa compared with acetone thus the assumption is often made that urine ketone bodies detected by the nitroprusside reaction are mainly AcAa.[33] False-negative results may be seen when serum AcAa levels are not high enough to reach the renal threshold for excretion. Although it is possible to convert BHA to AcAa by adding hydrogen peroxide to the urine, the concentration of BHA needed for this reaction to happen is very high and at this high concentration, there are usually concurrently high levels of AcAa in the urine.[33,34] The same urine strips may be used to detect ketones in the plasma and serum with one study in cats showing that the sensitivity for ketone detection in plasma is higher than it is in urine.[35]

In human patients, point-of-care ketone meters have largely replaced the semi-quantitative nitroprusside method in identifying serum ketone concentrations.[34] These ketone meters are affordable, user-friendly, portable, and provide rapid results with very small concentrations of blood required for testing.[34] These meters measure BHA concentration and the type of blood (venous or capillary) in which ketones are measured do not seem to affect the ketone meters and hematocrit does not appear to affect the results.[34] Studies in dogs and cats comparing ketone meters to laboratory analyzers have shown good accuracy.[34]

Finally, blood gasses with accompanying electrolyte evaluations (sodium, potassium, chloride) are required to diagnose acidosis and the presence of a high anion gap (or the Na-Cl difference), the hallmark feature of DKA.[31] Animals with HHS may have no evidence of metabolic acidosis due to small concentrations of ketone bodies present although acidosis has been reported in cats. Profound electrolyte abnormalities (hypokalemia, hyponatremia, hypernatremia, hypomagnesemia) are common in patients with DKA. Evaluation of the blood gas should be done very soon after patient evaluation so that life-threatening electrolyte abnormalities may be promptly corrected.

OTHER DIAGNOSTIC TESTS

Complete blood counts and blood smear analysis should be evaluated routinely. Hematological changes reported in dogs and cats with DKA include neutrophilic leukocytosis with or without a left shift, stress leukogram, anemia, polycythemia, and thrombocytosis. Many of these changes are attributed to concurrent diseases associated with the DM and are often non-specific findings.[36] High-grade codocytosis may be identified more frequently in dogs with DKA.[36] A complete urinalysis should be performed to identify glucosuria, the presence of ketones as well as any evidence of bacteriuria or proteinuria. A urine culture is also strongly recommended to rule out a lower urinary tract infection or evaluate for pyelonephritis.

Other diagnostic considerations to rule out concurrent diseases (see **Box 1**) include thoracic and abdominal imaging, pancreatic lipase immunoreactivity concentrations, serum folate, and cobalamin concentrations, aspirates of lymph nodes, or other abnormalities detected on imaging tests. These tests should be performed based on the signalment, clinical history, physical examination findings, and diagnostic testing results of the patient.

Although hyperadrenocorticism is a common reason for insulin resistance in diabetic dogs, specific testing (low dose dexamethasone suppression test, Adrenocorticotropic hormone [ACTH] stimulation test) should be considered after the patient is fully recovered from the DKA crises due to the increased risk for false positive results.

CLINICAL MANAGEMENT OF DIABETES KETOACIDOSIS

Management of DKA usually involves in-patient care at a 24-h facility as the fluid, electrolyte, and insulin requirements of these patients can be very dynamic. The three main issues to be addressed in treating DKA in dogs and cats include the following:[31]

- Fluid repletion to correct poor perfusion (if present) and dehydration (often present).
- Electrolyte replacement with particular attention to life-threatening shifts in serum potassium concentrations.
- Insulin administration to resolve ketogenesis and lipolysis.

Fluid Replacement

Poor perfusion, also known as poor oxygen delivery or shock (see **Box 2**), is not uncommon in patients with DKA.[26,31] A peripheral catheter should be placed as quickly as possible for resuscitation (treatment of the intravascular space) in patients identified with poor perfusion. Intraosseous catheterization may also be considered if peripheral catheter placement is challenging.

Isotonic replacement crystalloids (Normosol R, Plasmalyte A, 0.9% sodium chloride, or Lactated Ringers Solution) are most commonly used in the resuscitation of patients with evidence of poor perfusion. Although often called "physiologic saline", 0.9% sodium chloride is a non-buffered solution and has a chloride concentration much higher than serum chloride (**Table 1**). This high chloride concentration causes an acidifying effect that may lead to a slower resolution of metabolic acidosis in patients with DKA.[37] 0.9% sodium chloride also contains no potassium and may contribute to worsening hypokalemia with rehydration and insulin therapy if potassium is not adequately supplemented. Some clinicians may choose 0.9% sodium chloride as the fluid of choice for resuscitation due to the presence of hyponatremia in the patient; however, it is important to remember that hyponatremia in DKA is often caused by concurrent hyperglycemia (causing increased serum osmolarity and subsequent fluid shifts causing dilution of serum sodium concentrations) and/or hypertriglyceridemia. Thus, whenever possible, other balanced isotonic crystalloids are preferable to 0.9% sodium chloride in treating the patient with DKA.[38]

A fraction of the shock dose of isotonic fluids (10 to 15 mL/kg in cats, 20 to 25 mL/kg in dogs) should be provided as a bolus intravenously or via an intraosseous catheter over 10 to 15 min. The patient's perfusion parameters should be reassessed after the fluid bolus (heart rate, pulse quality, blood pressure, lactate concentration, capillary

Table 1
pH and electrolyte composition of commonly used isotonic crystalloids

Fluid Type	pH	Sodium	Chloride	Potassium	Bicarbonate Precursors
0.9% sodium chloride	5.5	154	154	0	None
Plasmalyte	7.4 (6.5 to 8)	140	98	5	Acetate and gluconate
Normosol	7.4	140	98	5	Acetate and gluconate
Lactated ringers solution	3.5	130	109	4	Lactate

refill time, etc.) and an additional bolus may be provided (up to 60 mL/kg/h in cats and 80 to 90 mL/kg/h in dogs) if there is still evidence of poor perfusion. Active external heating support should be provided to cats during resuscitation and body temperature should be at least 98°F (36.7°C) before providing a 2nd isotonic crystalloid bolus.[26] Some animals with poor perfusion due to anemia may need to resuscitated with a rapid blood transfusion (10 to 15 mL/kg of packed red blood cells or whole blood over 15 min to 2 h, depending on the clinical condition of the patient). Low oncotic pressure (hypoalbuminemia) may cause relative hypovolemia in some patients with DKA due to the third spacing of fluids. In hypoalbuminemic patients with evidence of poor perfusion, rapid correction of the albumin is indicated. This may be achieved using canine albumin, human serum albumin, or less effectively, fresh/fresh frozen plasma transfusions.[39] Artificial colloids (vetstarch and hetastarch) may also be considered although their use in critically ill animals is controversial.[40] If hypotension and other parameters of poor perfusion still persist after fluid therapy, vasopressor therapy or inotropic may be indicated.

Once the patient is appropriately resuscitated and perfusion is restored, rehydration (treatment of the interstitial space) should be commenced on dehydrated patients (**Table 2**). Guidelines for treating human patients with DKA assume that all patients have at least a 5% level of dehydration on presentation to the hospital.[41] The total fluid deficit should be estimated based on the % dehydration (see **Table 2**) and this fluid deficit should be replaced over 8 to 24 h in most patients (fluid deficit (L) = % dehydration X body weight in kg). A slower rehydration rate (12 to 24 h) should be considered in patients that are potentially fluid intolerant (cats, animals with heart disease or low albumin concentration, etc.). Being intentional about the rehydration plan (calculating the fluid deficit) provides more targeted care to treating dehydration instead of an arbitrary fluid volume (eg, 60 to 180 mL/kg/d).

Fluid therapy during the rehydration period often decreases the initial glucose concentration due to increases in the glomerular filtration rate. However, fluid therapy may also cause potential alterations in electrolytes (potassium, phosphorus, and sodium) thus it is important to monitor serum electrolyte concentrations closely after initiating fluid therapy. The animal's hydration status should be re-evaluated every 6 to 12 h and the fluid rate may be adjusted depending on the physical exam findings.

The patient's maintenance fluid needs (usually approximately 45 to 60 mL/kg/d) should also be provided during the rehydration period. The hourly maintenance fluid requirement can be added to the hourly replacement fluid volume and administered

Table 2		
Clinical findings and estimation of dehydration in dogs and cats		
Percent Dehydration	**Clinical Findings**	
<5%	No physical examination abnormality observed, animal has a clinical history that suggests dehydration is likely present (vomiting, polyuria, anorexia)	
5% to 7%	Dry mucous membranes, skin tenting may be present	
7% to 9%	Dry mucous membranes, skin tenting, sunken eyes, dry corneas may be present	
9% to 12%	Dry mucous membranes, skin tenting, sunken eyes, dry corneas, signs of shock may be present	
12% to 15%	Dry mucous membranes, skin tenting, sunken eyes, dry corneas, signs of shock present	

using the same replacement fluid type and infusion pump. However, the maintenance fluid requirement may be provided using maintenance fluids (eg, 0.45% sodium chloride, Normosol M) and administered using a separate infusion pump.

Electrolyte Therapy

Normalization and supplementation of electrolytes is a major cornerstone in the therapeutic management of patients with DKA. Dogs and cats with DKA often present with a wide variety of electrolyte abnormalities, especially affecting sodium, potassium, phosphorous, calcium, and magnesium.

Dogs and cats with DKA generally tend to have a total body potassium deficit due to osmotic diuresis, excessive vomiting, volume depletion due to activation of the renin-angiotensin system, and excessive urinary potassium loss.[38,42] However, insulin deficiency and metabolic acidosis (which is present before treating patients with DKA) leads to an extracellular shift of potassium and may mask the total body potassium deficiency. However, once insulin therapy is initiated, potassium is shifted into the intracellular space leading to a drop in potassium. Significant hypokalemia may lead to muscle weakness, hypoventilation (due to respiratory muscle weakness), cardiac arrhythmias, and death.[42] Thus potassium supplementation should be initiated early (even during the rehydration phase) unless the patient is hyperkalemic or anuric.[42] Potassium supplementation should be initiated with patients with normal-to-mildly low potassium concentrations starting at 0.05 to 0.1 mEq/kg/h. K_{max} (0.4 to 0.5 mEq/kg/h) should be reserved for patients with severe hypokalemia (usually potassium concentrations less than 2.5 mEq/L) or those showing life-threatening clinical signs attributed to hypokalemia (potassium is most commonly supplemented using potassium chloride [KCl]).

The authors recommended providing potassium through a separate infusion pump so that potassium supplementation concentrations are not affected when the fluid rate is adjusted. However, if supplemental potassium is added to the patient's fluid bag, the care team should pay close attention to changes in the fluid rate to ensure there is no risk of hyperkalemia or inadequate potassium supplementation. In addition, it is important to thoroughly mix all supplemental potassium in the fluid bag to prevent excessive high concentrations of potassium from being administered.[38]

Depletion of intracellular phosphate occurs in DKA and phosphate is lost as a result of osmotic diuresis.[30] It is estimated that approximately 20% to 40% of human patients presenting with DKA are hypophosphatemic.[43] Many more patients present with hyperphosphatemia but serum levels often drop precipitously with the administration of insulin.[43] Administration of IV fluids and bicarbonate also leads to lower serum phosphate levels.[43] Lysis of red blood cells can occur when serum phosphate levels less than 1.5 mg/dL leading to hemolytic anemia. Seizures have also been reported in dogs and cats secondary to hypophosphatemia.[43]

Except in cases when the patient is hyperphosphatemic, the authors prefer to initiate phosphate supplementation either at the time of rehydration (with hypophosphatemic patients) or at the time of insulin supplementation (with normophosphatemic patients). In all cases, even when phosphorous is high on presentation, serum phosphate concentrations should be monitored every 6 to 12 h so that supplementation can be adjusted as needed. Phosphorous is usually supplemented at a dose of 0.03 to 0.12 mmol/kg/h commonly using potassium phosphate (KPO_4). Potassium phosphate can be instilled in the patient's bag with similar limitations as for KCL. Potassium phosphate is also often incompatible with many fluid types and is generally diluted or infused in 0.9% sodium chloride. An alternative is to run the KPO_4 through a separate infusion pump, usually a syringe pump. It is important to remember that KPO4 contains a small amount of potassium (4.3 mEq/mL) and this should be considered when calculating the overall potassium dose for the patient.

In human patients, there is still a lot of controversy concerning the association between the rate of fluid or sodium administration and the development of cerebral edema.[30] Recent studies and guidelines in human patients suggest that sodium restriction is not necessary for hyponatremic patients with DKA.[30,44] In many patients with DKA, severe hyperglycemia leads to an inaccurately low sodium concentration due to osmotic shifts of fluid into the intravascular space, causing dilutional hyponatremia. The patient's actual sodium concentration may be calculated using the corrected sodium equation:

Corrected sodium = measured sodium + [1.6 (glucose − 100)/100].

In hyponatremic patients, any balanced isotonic replacement crystalloid may be used to treat dehydration. The patient sodium concentration may be re-evaluated every 4 to 12 h, depending on the severity of hyponatremia present. Maintenance fluids containing higher volumes of free water (0.45% sodium chloride, 5% dextrose in water, Normosol M) may be used in patients with hypernatremia.

Insulin Therapy

Although rehydration alone frequently causes a marked decrease in blood glucose concentration, insulin therapy is essential to restore normal cellular metabolism, suppress lipolysis and ketogenesis, as well as to normalize blood glucose concentrations.[30]

In human patients, DKA is treated with an IV insulin infusion. This is considered the gold standard in human patients with DKA and has been determined to be safe and effective.[30,44] However, during the coronavirus disease-2019 (COVID-19) global pandemic, limited intensive care resources necessitated the use of subcutaneous (SC) insulin in patients with mild-to-moderate DKA, when IV insulin was not an option.[45]

Many studies have evaluated various types of insulin regimens in dogs and cats with DKA. An IV infusion was first described in 1993 by Dr. Douglass Macintire and that protocol (or its modification; **Table 3**) is still being used by many veterinarians across the world.[46] Short-acting insulin (Humulin R or regular insulin), is initiated as a constant rate infusion (CRI) at 2.2 U/kg/d in dogs and 1.1 U/kg/d in cats, although a study determined a 2.2U/kg/d in cats did not increase the frequency of adverse neurologic or biochemical events.[47] The blood glucose concentration is usually monitored every 2 h. Dextrose is supplemented in the IV fluids after the blood glucose drops to a certain level and in periods of profound hypoglycemia (glucose < 100 mg/dL), the insulin infusion is discontinued to allow the blood glucose an opportunity to come up, after which the infusion is restarted. Current modifications to this protocol discourage stopping the insulin CRI even when hypoglycemia is present. The continued infusion, even in the face of hypoglycemia, allows for ongoing resolution of metabolic acidosis. The CRI dose may be decreased with concurrently increased dextrose supplementation to allow for the uninterrupted administration of insulin.[30,44]

Rapid-acting insulin, lispro, has been investigated for IV administration in dogs and cats with DKA.[24,48] In both studies, IV administration of lispro as a CRI was equally as effective as the regular insulin CRI. There is currently no clear rationale for preferring lispro over regular insulin in dogs and cats with DKA and it is currently more expensive than regular insulin.[49] Rapid-acting insulin, asprat, has also been used intravenously in dogs with DKA with success and no adverse effects.[50]

Intramuscular (IM) and SC administration of insulin has also been described in veterinary patients with DKA. IM administration of lispro was shown to be safe and

Table 3
Insulin constant rate infusion protocol for dogs and cats using regular insulin (Humulin R)

1. Determine total daily insulin dose of patients (2.2 U/kg/d in dogs, 1.1–2.2 U/kg/d in cats)
2. Administer total daily dose of insulin into 25–250 mL of 0.9% sodium chloride (Volume of 0.9% NaCl based on the size of the animal, presence of underlying heart disease, patient's ability to tolerate large volume of fluids, etc.). Note that final recovered insulin concentrations are lower when smaller concentrations of insulin are added to large volumes of 0.9% NaCl.[62]
3. Prime the fluid administration line set with insulin CRI solution. Allow insulin CRI to saturate the fluid bag and administration line for about 30 min (insulin binds to plastic).
4. Waste about 5–50 mL of the insulin CRI- depending on the priming volume of the fluid administration line set.
5. Start insulin CRI based on volume of 0.9% NaCl insulin was diluted in that is, 1 mL/h (25 mL divided by 24 h) to 10.4 mL/h (250 mL divided by 24 h)
6. Monitor blood glucose concentrations every 2 h. Provide dextrose supplementation when glucose concentrations are lower than 250 mg/dL
7. Use chart below to adjust insulin rate.[46] Note that fluid rate in chart is based on 2.2 U/kg of insulin in 250 mL of 0.9% NaCl. Fluid rate will vary based on volume of diluent used.
8. Please note that many protocols exist for setting up a constant rate infusion (CRI) of insulin. Some protocols do not discontinue the insulin even in the face of hypoglycemia in order to promote uninterrupted resolution of ketogenesis.

Blood glucose concentration	Dextrose supplementation	Dose of insulin administered (U/kg/h)	Rate of insulin solution based on 2.2 U/kg of insulin in 250 mL of NaCl[a]
>250 mg/dL	None	0.09 U/kg/h.	10 mL/h.
200–250 mg/dL	2.5% dextrose	0.064 U/kg/h.	7 mL/h.
150–199 mg/dL	2.5% dextrose	0.045 U/kg/h.	5 mL/h.
100–149 mg/dL	5% dextrose	0.045 U/kg/h.	5 mL/h.
< 100 mg/dL	5% dextrose	Stop insulin infusion	Stop insulin infusion

9. Change out insulin CRI bag, administration line every 24 h.
10. Consider transitioning to long-acting insulin once there is voluntary oral intake of food and water and ketoacidosis has returned. Note that ketonuria may persist for several hours and should not be used as an end-point ofr determining resolution of DKA>
11. Administer first subcutaneous injection of long-acting insulin about 3–4 h before stopping the insulin infusion to allow for sufficient time for the SC insulin to be absorbed.

[a] Note that this rate is based on 2.2 U/kg of insulin in 250 mL of NaCl. Rate will be slower or faster if smaller or larger volumes of 0.9% NaCl are used as the diluent.

effective in dogs with DKA.[51] A study described a basal-bolus SC injection of long-acting insulin, glargine, in cats with DKA, combined with IM glargine injections.[52] An initial dose of 1 to 2U per cat was administered IM with 1 to 3U SC, followed by 1 to 2 U IM as needed (q 2 h or less frequently) and 1 to 2U SC q 12 h until regulated. It was considered a feasible alternative to traditional CRI of regular insulin and may be a reasonable option for clients with limited funds where intense monitoring and hospitalization may not be feasible.[26] A 2021 study compared the glargine regimen to the CRI of regular insulin in cats and found the glargine regimen to be simple, effective, and safe.[53] Another study used intermittent SC glargine and IM regular insulin and compared it to a CRI of regular insulin in cats with DKA. Although there were only eight cats in each group, cats in the SC/IM group had a significantly shorter duration of hospitalization, time of resolution of hyperglycemia, ketonemia, and normalization of pH and bicarbonate. Regular insulin (0.1 to 0.2 U/kg) has also been used intermittently IM (every 1 to 4 h) in dogs and cats with DKA.[26,54] Dextrose supplementation is always provided when hypoglycemia is present, regardless of the type of insulin chosen or the route of insulin administration.

In human patients, insulin therapy is started about an hour after fluid replacement therapy, as soon as there is enough intravascular volume expansion.[30] There is still some controversy in the veterinary community regarding the ideal time to initiate insulin therapy. Some veterinary literature recommends waiting until dehydration has been completed to initiate insulin therapy.[46] This is to mitigate the impact of rapidly decreasing the effective osmolarity and potentially causing cerebral edema.[26,46] However, in a retrospective study of dogs and cats with DKA, early initiation of insulin (<6 h) was associated with more rapid resolution of DKA without an associated increase in complication rates.[26,55] The authors generally initiate insulin therapy early (<6 h) in normovolemic patients with the main reason for delaying immediate administration being the resolution of moderate to severe hypokalemia or hypophosphatemia. In HHS patients, human guidelines recommend starting an insulin infusion when the blood glucose no longer decreases with fluids alone.[30] Early insulin administration is thought to be unnecessary in HHS patients. Similar guidelines for insulin administration are commonly used in veterinary patients with HHS.

Other Considerations

Bicarbonate administration is not recommended except for the treatment of life-threatening hyperkalemia or unusually severe acidosis (pH < 6.9) with evidence of alterations in cardiac contractility.[30] Although bicarbonate administration may be considered in patients with severe acidosis (pH 6.9), there is scant data to support or refute its use.[56] There is evidence against its use in patients with mild-to-moderately severe acidosis.[56] Adverse effects of bicarbonate administration may include delay in resolution of ketosis, refractory hypokalemia, and paradoxic acidosis in the central nervous system.[56]

Glucose concentrations should be monitored every 2 to 4 h, especially during IV administration of insulin. A central venous catheter should be considered early in dogs and cats with DKA due to the number of infusions often needed (fluids, electrolytes, and other medications like antibiotics). A central venous catheter also facilities easier sampling for blood glucose concentrations. The use of continuous glucose monitoring systems has been described in dogs and cats with DKA and is a reasonable consideration to reduce iatrogenic anemia and patient discomfort from frequent blood sampling.[57,58] The clinician should be aware of the limitations of these devices (dehydration, hypoglycemia, and cost). Serum electrolyte concentrations should also be evaluated every 4 to 12 h, depending on the severity of the abnormalities.

Nutritional supplementation should be initiated as soon as the patient is normotensive, hydrated, and electrolyte abnormalities have been stabilized (especially potassium and phosphorus). Enteral feeding is preferred to parenteral nutrition except in situations where enteral feeding is unfeasible (uncontrollable vomiting or regurgitation, altered mentation). Nasogastric and nasoesophageal tubes are most commonly used although esophagostomy tubes may also be used. Nutrition should be initiated at less than 25% of the patient's resting energy requirement, which may then be increased over time as long as the patient tolerates it.

Medications for nausea, analgesia, and poor gastrointestinal motility may be provided based on the clinical needs of the patients. Broad-spectrum antibiotics should be considered if there is suspicion of an infectious underlying cause (fever, presence of a left shift, evidence of bacteria on the urinalysis, infected wounds, etc.).

Vital signs, including heart rate, respiratory rate, temperature, blood pressure, pulse oximetry saturation, and mentation should be monitored every 1 to 8 h, depending on the patient's underlying disease and severity of signs. Physical therapy should be considered for the recumbent patient and whenever possible, dogs should be walked frequently due to increased urine production. The authors also believe frequent outdoor walks may also provide some emotional inspiration for some canine patients.

Criteria for Discharge

The patient should be transitioned into a long-acting insulin once ketoacidosis has resolved and there is consistent voluntary oral intake of food and water. Persistent ketonuria (due to measurement of AcAc and acetone) may occur several hours after serum BHA levels have returned to normal; thus, the absence of ketonuria should not be used as an end-point for determining the resolution of DKA.[30] To prevent rebound hyperglycemia, the first SC injection of a long-acting insulin should be given approximately 3 to 4 h before stopping the insulin infusion, to allow sufficient time for the SC insulin to be absorbed.[30] If the clinician decides to make a transition from an insulin infusion to intermittent regular insulin injections, the overlap period should be approximately 1 to 2 h before stopping the insulin infusion.

The patient should be monitored in the hospital for at least 12 to 24 h on a long-acting insulin protocol, largely to ensure that no periods of hypoglycemia (or marked hyperglycemia) occurs and a dose adjustment should occur only as needed. A continuous glucose monitoring device may be considered for discharge for closer glucose monitoring at home. However, clients should be educated about the goal for monitoring and strongly discouraged from making arbitrary changes to the insulin dose without veterinary advice. Most patients with DKA should be evaluated for a glucose curve approximately 10 to 14 days after discharge. A recheck plan for any other comorbidities should also be clearly laid out at the time of discharge.

OUTCOME OF DOGS AND CATS WITH DIABETES KETOACIDOSIS

The average duration of hospitalization for dogs and cats with DKA is approximately 4 to 6 days.[5,8,55] The mortality rate of DKA in dogs and cats varies depending on the study performed. Mortality rates in cats range from 26% to 41%[5,59,60], whereas mortality rates range from 16% to 30% in dogs.[8,55] Recurrence rates are reported at approximately 42%. Survival has been reported to be correlated to the degree of anemia, initial azotemia, total bilirubin concentrations, hypocalcemia, and acidosis.[5,8]

CLINICS CARE POINTS

- Diabetes ketoacidosis (DKA) is classically diagnosed as the triad of hyperglycemia, anion gap metabolic acidosis, and ketonemia (or ketonuria). Hyperosmolar hyperglycemia syndrome (HHS) is diagnosed by hyperglycemia, arterial pH > 7.3 or venous pH > 7.25, serum bicarbonate greater than 15 mmol/L, small-to-absent ketonuria, absent-to-small ketonemia, effective serum osmolarity greater than 320 mOsm/kg and evidence of neurologic abnormalities.

- A wide range of diagnostic screening tests should be considered to identify any underlying concurrent disease(s)

- Clinical management of DKA and HHS requires care in a 24-h facility. The main issues addressed during the care of affected dogs and cats include

Fluid repletion to correct poor perfusion (if present) and dehydration (often present)

Electrolyte replacement with particular attention to life-threatening shifts in serum potassium concentrations

Insulin administration to resolve ketogenesis and lipolysis

- Insulin therapy may be provided using an intravenous insulin infusion although intramuscular or subcutaneous administration techniques have been described

- Bicarbonate administration is not recommended except for treatment of life-threatening hyperkalemia or severe metabolic acidosis (pH < 6.9) with evidence of alterations in cardiac contractility

- Nutritional supplementation should be initiated as soon as the patient is normotensive, hydrated, and electrolyte abnormalities have been stabilized

- The patient should be transitioned to long-acting insulin once ketoacidosis has resolved and there is consistent voluntary oral intake of food and water

DISCLOSURE

The authors have nothing to disclose.

REFERENCES

1. American Diabetes A. 15. Diabetes Care in the Hospital: Standards of Medical Care in Diabetes-2019. Diabetes Care 2019;42(Suppl 1):S173–81.
2. Nasa P, Chaudhary S, Shrivastava PK, et al. Euglycemic diabetic ketoacidosis: A missed diagnosis. World J Diabetes 2021;12(5):514–23.
3. Brar PC, Tell S, Mehta S, et al. Hyperosmolar diabetic ketoacidosis– review of literature and the shifting paradigm in evaluation and management. Diabetes Metab Syndr 2021;15(6):102313.
4. Nelson RW. Diabetic ketoacidosis. In: Feldman EC, Nelson RW, Reusch CE, et al, editors. Canine and feline endocrinology. 4th ed. Elsevier Saunders; 2015. p. 315–47, chap 8.
5. Cooper RL, Drobatz KJ, Lennon EM, et al. Retrospective evaluation of risk factors and outcome predictors in cats with diabetic ketoacidosis (1997-2007): 93 cases. Article. J Vet Emerg Crit Care 2015;25(2):263–72.
6. Crenshaw KL, Peterson ME. Pretreatment clinical and laboratory evaluation of cats with diabetes mellitus: 104 cases (1992-1994). Article. J Am Vet Med Assoc 1996;209(5):943–9.

7. Callegari C, Mercuriali E, Hafner M, et al. Survival time and prognostic factors in cats with newly diagnosed diabetes mellitus: 114 cases (2000-2009). Article. J Am Vet Med Assoc 2013;243(1):91–5.
8. Hume DZ, Drobatz KJ, Hess RS. Outcome of dogs with diabetic ketoacidosis: 127 dogs (1993-2003). J Vet Intern Med 2006;20(3):547–55.
9. Koenig A, Drobatz KJ, Beale AB, et al. Hyperglycemic, hyperosmolar syndrome in feline diabetics: 17 Cases (1995-2001). Article. J Vet Emerg Crit Care 2004; 14(1):30–40.
10. Trotman TK, Drobatz KJ, Hess RS. Retrospective evaluation of hyperosmolar hyperglycemia in 66 dogs (1993-2008). J Vet Emerg Crit Care 2013;23(5):557–64.
11. Laffel L. Ketone bodies: a review of physiology, pathophysiology and application of monitoring to diabetes. Diabetes Metab Res Rev 1999;15(6):412–26.
12. McGarry JD, Foster DW. Ketogenesis. In: Porte D Jr, Sherwin RS, Baron A, editors. Ellenberg and Rifkin's diabetes mellitus. 6th ed. McGraw-Hill; 2003. p. 15–22, chap 2.
13. Maratou E, Dimitriadis G, Kollias A, et al. Glucose transporter expression on the plasma membrane of resting and activated white blood cells. Eur J Clin Invest 2007;37(4):282–90.
14. Chawla A, Nguyen KD, Goh YP. Macrophage-mediated inflammation in metabolic disease. Nat Rev Immunol 2011;11(11):738–49.
15. Taylor SI, Blau JE, Rother KI. SGLT2 Inhibitors May Predispose to Ketoacidosis. J Clin Endocrinol Metab 2015;100(8):2849–52.
16. O'Brien MA. Diabetic emergencies in small animals. Vet Clin North Am Small Anim Pract 2010;40(2):317–33.
17. Bohn D, Daneman D. Diabetic ketoacidosis and cerebral edema. Curr Opin Pediatr 2002;14(3):287–91.
18. Wolfsdorf JI, Allgrove J, Craig ME, et al. ISPAD Clinical Practice Consensus Guidelines 2014. Diabetic ketoacidosis and hyperglycemic hyperosmolar state. Pediatr Diabetes 2014;15(Suppl 20):154–79.
19. Munro JF, Campbell IW, McCuish AC, et al. Euglycaemic diabetic ketoacidosis. Br Med J 1973;2(5866):578–80.
20. Lucero P, Chapela S. Euglycemic Diabetic Ketoacidosis in the ICU: 3 Case Reports and Review of Literature. Case Rep Crit Care 2018;2018:1747850.
21. Mellbye FB, Pedersen MGB. [Euglycaemic ketoacidosis induced by ketogenic diet and intermittent fastingin a non-diabetic patient]. Ugeskr Laeger 2020;(30):182.
22. Musso G, Sircana A, Saba F, et al. Assessing the risk of ketoacidosis due to sodium-glucose cotransporter (SGLT)-2 inhibitors in patients with type 1 diabetes: A meta-analysis and meta-regression. PLoS Med 2020;17(12):e1003461.
23. Pasquel FJ, Umpierrez GE. Hyperosmolar hyperglycemic state: a historic review of the clinical presentation, diagnosis, and treatment. Diabetes Care 2014;37(11): 3124–31.
24. Sears KW, Drobatz KJ, Hess RS. Use of lispro insulin for treatment of diabetic ketoacidosis in dogs. J Vet Emerg Crit Care 2012;22(2):211–8.
25. Koenig A. Endocrine emergencies in dogs and cats. Veterinary clinics: Small animal practice 2013;43(4):869–97.
26. Rudloff E. Diabetic ketoacidosis in the cat: recognition and essential treatment. J Feline Med Surg 2017;19(11):1167–74.
27. Plotnick AN, Greco DS. Diagnosis of diabetes mellitus in dogs and cats: Contrasts and comparisons. Veterinary Clinics: Small Animal Practice 1995;25(3): 563–70.

28. Tiwari LK, Muralindharan J, Singhi S. Risk factors for cerebral edema in diabetic ketoacidosis in a developing country: role of fluid refractory shock. Pediatr Crit Care Med 2012;13(2):e91–6.

29. Barski L, Eshkoli T, Brandstaetter E, et al. Euglycemic diabetic ketoacidosis. Eur J Intern Med 2019;63:9–14.

30. Wolfsdorf JI, Glaser N, Agus M, et al. ISPAD Clinical Practice Consensus Guidelines 2018: Diabetic ketoacidosis and the hyperglycemic hyperosmolar state. Pediatr Diabetes 2018;19:155–77.

31. Besen BA, Ranzani OT, Singer M. Management of diabetic ketoacidosis. Intensive Care Med 2022;1–4.

32. Lane SL, Koenig A, Brainard BM. Formulation and validation of a predictive model to correct blood glucose concentrations obtained with a veterinary point-of-care glucometer in hemodiluted and hemoconcentrated canine blood samples. J Am Vet Med Assoc 2015;246(3):307–12.

33. Stojanovic V, Ihle S. Role of beta-hydroxybutyric acid in diabetic ketoacidosis: A review. Can Vet J 2011;52(4):426.

34. Chong SK, Reineke EL. Point-of-care glucose and ketone monitoring. Top Companion Anim Med 2016;31(1):18–26.

35. Zeugswetter F, Pagitz M. Ketone measurements using dipstick methodology in cats with diabetes mellitus. J Small Anim Pract 2009;50(1):4–8.

36. Slead TS, Woolcock AD, Scott-Moncrieff JC, et al. Complete Blood Counts and Blood Smear Analyses in 312 Diabetic Dogs (2007–2017). J Am Anim Hosp Assoc 2022;58(4):180–8.

37. Ramanan M, Attokaran A, Murray L, et al. Sodium chloride or Plasmalyte-148 evaluation in severe diabetic ketoacidosis (SCOPE-DKA): a cluster, crossover, randomized, controlled trial. Intensive Care Med 2021;47(11):1248–57.

38. Thomovsky E. Fluid and electrolyte therapy in diabetic ketoacidosis. Veterinary Clinics: Small Animal Practice 2017;47(2):491–503.

39. Mazzaferro EM, Rudloff E, Kirby R. The role of albumin replacement in the critically ill veterinary patient. J Vet Emerg Crit Care 2002;12(2):113–24.

40. Cazzolli D, Prittie J. The crystalloid-colloid debate: consequences of resuscitation fluid selection in veterinary critical care. J Vet Emerg Crit Care 2015;25(1):6–19.

41. Gosmanov AR, Gosmanova EO, Dillard-Cannon E. Management of adult diabetic ketoacidosis. Diabetes, Metab Syndrome Obes Targets Ther 2014;7:255.

42. Agwu JC, Ng SM. Fluid and electrolyte therapy in childhood diabetic ketoacidosis management: A rationale for new national guideline. Diabet Med 2021;38(8):e14595.

43. Schropp DM, Kovacic J. Phosphorus and phosphate metabolism in veterinary patients. J Vet Emerg Crit Care 2007;17(2):127–34.

44. Dhatariya KK, Glaser NS, Codner E, et al. Diabetic ketoacidosis. Nat Rev Dis Prim 2020;6(1):1–20.

45. Priyambada L, Wolfsdorf JI, Brink SJ, et al. ISPAD Clinical Practice Consensus Guideline: Diabetic ketoacidosis in the time of COVID-19 and resource-limited settings-role of subcutaneous insulin. Pediatr Diabetes 2020;21(8):1394–402.

46. Macintire D. Treatment of diabetic ketoacidosis in dogs by continuous low-dose intravenous infusion of insulin. J Am Vet Med Assoc 1993;202(8):1266–72.

47. Claus MA, Silverstein DC, Shofer FS, et al. Comparison of regular insulin infusion doses in critically ill diabetic cats: 29 cases (1999–2007). J Vet Emerg Crit Care 2010;20(5):509–17.

48. Malerba E, Mazzarino M, Del Baldo F, et al. Use of lispro insulin for treatment of diabetic ketoacidosis in cats. J Feline Med Surg 2019;21(2):115–23.

49. Gilor C, Graves TK. Synthetic insulin analogs and their use in dogs and cats. Veterinary Clinics: Small Animal Practice 2010;40(2):297–307.
50. Walsh ES, Drobatz KJ, Hess RS. Use of intravenous insulin aspart for treatment of naturally occurring diabetic ketoacidosis in dogs. J Vet Emerg Crit Care 2016; 26(1):101–7.
51. Malerba E, Alessandrini F, Grossi G, et al. Efficacy and Safety of Intramuscular Insulin Lispro vs. Continuous Intravenous Regular Insulin for the Treatment of Dogs With Diabetic Ketoacidosis. Front Vet Sci 2020;7:559008.
52. Marshall RD, Rand JS, Gunew MN, et al. Intramuscular glargine with or without concurrent subcutaneous administration for treatment of feline diabetic ketoacidosis. J Vet Emerg Crit Care 2013;23(3):286–90.
53. Zeugswetter FK, Luckschander-Zeller N, Karlovits S, et al. Glargine versus regular insulin protocol in feline diabetic ketoacidosis. J Vet Emerg Crit Care 2021; 31(4):459–68.
54. Chastain C, Nichols C. Low-dose intramuscular insulin therapy for diabetic ketoacidosis in dogs. J Am Vet Med Assoc 1981;178(6):561–4.
55. DiFazio J, Fletcher DJ. Retrospective comparison of early-versus late-insulin therapy regarding effect on time to resolution of diabetic ketosis and ketoacidosis in dogs and cats: 60 cases (2003–2013). J Vet Emerg Crit Care 2016;26(1):108–15.
56. Patel MP, Ahmed A, Gunapalan T, et al. Use of sodium bicarbonate and blood gas monitoring in diabetic ketoacidosis: A review. World J Diabetes 2018; 9(11):199.
57. Malerba E, Cattani C, Del Baldo F, et al. Accuracy of a flash glucose monitoring system in dogs with diabetic ketoacidosis. J Vet Intern Med 2020;34(1):83–91.
58. Silva D, Cecci G, Biz G, et al. Evaluation of a flash glucose monitoring system in dogs with diabetic ketoacidosis. Domest Anim Endocrinol 2021;74:106525.
59. Gallagher BR, Mahony OM, Rozanski EA, et al. A pilot study comparing a protocol using intermittent administration of glargine and regular insulin to a continuous rate infusion of regular insulin in cats with naturally occurring diabetic ketoacidosis. J Vet Emerg Crit Care 2015;25(2):234–9.
60. Bruskiewicz KA, Nelson RW, Feldman EC, et al. Diabetic ketosis and ketoacidosis in cats: 42 cases (1980-1995). Article. J Am Vet Med Assoc 1997;211(2):188–92.
61. Schulz H. Fatty acid oxidation. In: Lennarz WJ, Lane MD, editors. Encyclopedia of biological chemistry. 2nd ed. Academic Press; 2013. p. 281–4.
62. Clark JL, Rudloff E, Rick M. Percent recovery of insulin from two different concentrations (3 U/250 mL and 45 U/250 mL) of regular insulin solutions prepared for continuous rate infusion. J Vet Emerg Crit Care 2021;31(1):117–20.

Glucose Counterregulation

Clinical Consequences of Impaired Sympathetic Responses in Diabetic Dogs and Cats

Jocelyn Mott, DVM[a], Chen Gilor, DVM, PhD[b],*

KEYWORDS

- Hypoglycemia • Diabetes mellitus • Autonomic nervous system
- Hypoglycemic associated autonomic failure • Insulin • Glucagon • Somogyi effect

KEY POINTS

- Insulin induced hypoglycemia (IIH) is common in veterinary patients and limits ability to achieve adequate glycemic control with insulin.
- Frequency of IIH is underestimated when using blood glucose curves as a monitoring tool. Continuous glucose monitoring is superior for detecting hypoglycemic events.
- Some diabetic dogs and humans have impairment of the autonomic nervous system and are less able to respond to IIH.
- Loss of sympathetic innervation to pancreatic islets (sympathetic islet neuropathy) occurs in dogs with diabetes mellitus.
- Even when not associated with clinical signs, IIH is not benign: It lowers the threshold for sympathoadrenal defenses and increases the risk of future severe iatrogenic hypoglycemia.

INTRODUCTION

Diabetes mellitus (DM) is a disease of insulin deficiency (relative or absolute) that typically results from beta cell loss or dysfunction. However, if DM was limited to a beta cell lesion, treatment with insulin therapy would be simple because numerous neural and endocrine mechanisms exist to combat insulin-induced hypoglycemia (IIH). Instead, hypoglycemia is the limiting factor that prevents the ability to achieve adequate glycemic control during insulin therapy for DM.[1–3] This is because counterregulatory responses to IIH are often impaired in DM,[4,5] resulting in great severity of, and delayed recovery from hypoglycemia.

---

[a] College of Veterinary Medicine, University of Florida, 2015 Southwest 16th Avenue, Gainesville, FL 32610-0126, USA; [b] Small Animal Internal Medicine, College of Veterinary Medicine, University of Florida, 2015 Southwest 16th Avenue, Gainesville, FL 32610-0126, USA
* Corresponding author.
E-mail address: cgilor@ufl.edu

Vet Clin Small Anim 53 (2023) 551–564
https://doi.org/10.1016/j.cvsm.2023.01.001
0195-5616/23/© 2023 Elsevier Inc. All rights reserved.

The adverse effects of counterregulatory responses are a prime deterrent to the aggressive insulin therapy that is needed to lessen the long-term complications of the disease. Multiple mechanisms have been proposed to explain the impairment of counterregulatory responses to IIH.[6] Some of these are a consequence of the primary insult that led to the development of DM (eg, collateral damage from pancreatitis) while others are secondary to the metabolic derangements associated with DM and insulin therapy. These include hyperglycemia and hypoglycemia, both shown to cause impairment in counterregulatory responses and increase the risk of future hypoglycemia. It is therefore recognized that beyond the immediate negative consequences of hyperglycemia and hypoglycemia, and beyond the well-known long-term negative consequences of hyperglycemia, both hyperglycemia and hypoglycemia should be avoided in order to prevent future hypoglycemic crises.

IIH is also an important determinant of quality of life for both owners and their diabetic cats and dogs. In quality-of-life surveys, more than 50% of cat and dog owners say that they worry about hypoglycemia and more than a third of them suspect their pet had exhibited hypoglycemic signs.[7,8]

FREQUENCY OF INSULIN-INDUCED HYPOGLYCEMIA IN DIABETIC DOGS AND CATS

Subclinical (or "biochemical") IIH is common in diabetic cats and dogs while clinical IIH occurs less frequently. Biochemical IIH has been reported in 31%,[9] 44.3%,[10] and 64%[11] of cats treated with bovine-recombinant protamine zinc insulin, glargine or porcine zinc insulin, and human-recombinant protamine zinc insulin, respectively. The frequency of clinical IIH in 2 of the studies was 7% and 2%.[9,11] When near-euglycemia was a treatment goal (target blood glucose [BG] concentrations of 60–160 mg/dL, measured by nonveterinary glucometer), and BG was measured at home by owners 3 to 5 times a day, biochemical IIH was reported in 93% (51/55) of cats in more than 10,000 home glucose curves but the frequency of clinical hypoglycemia was still low (2%).[12]

In diabetic dogs, clinical IIH was documented or suspected in 40%,[13] 38.6%,[14] and 8.9%[15] of dogs treated with insulin detemir, porcine insulin zinc suspension, and human recombinant protamine zinc suspension, respectively. In the latter study, 5.8% of 276 dogs experienced seizures. Biochemical IIH was observed in 22%[13] and 35.8%[14] of diabetic dogs on BG curves.

What insulin formulations, diets, monitoring protocols, and other factors are associated with increased risk of IIH in cats and dogs? Currently, there are no studies that answer this question. Comparison of IIH frequency between veterinary studies is fraught with limitations such as differences in sample sizes, insulin type and dose, and study designs. Importantly, BG cutoffs used for defining IIH are arbitrary and differ among studies. The recently published Agreement Language in Veterinary Endocrinology defines hypoglycemia in DM as BG less than 3.3 mmol/L (60 mg/dL). However, varying cutoffs for hypoglycemia have been used in cats (<50,[16,17] <65,[18] and <80 mg/dL[9,11]) and dogs (<60,[14,19] <65,[20] <80,[15,21] and <89 mg/dL[13]). The American Diabetes Association (ADA) has a broader definition, stating that hypoglycemia in DM should be considered as all episodes of abnormally low plasma glucose concentrations that expose individuals to potential harm. Furthermore, the ADA recognizes that it is not possible to define hypoglycemia by a single plasma glucose concentration cutoff because glycemic responses to hypoglycemia are dynamic.[22]

Frequency and methods used to detect IIH in veterinary studies vary as well. BG curves underestimate the frequency of IIH because of their intermittent nature.[23] There are also differences between home and in-hospital BG curves due to influences of stress, exercise, and refusal to eat. Interestingly, some studies in diabetic cats[24] and dogs[25] have shown lower BG in hospital curves compared with home curves. The incidence of biochemical hypoglycemia is higher in diabetic people monitored by continuous glucose monitoring (CGM; 56.9%[26] and 59%[27]) versus self-monitored BG (SMBG; 26.4%[26] and 50%[27]), respectively. Hypoglycemia identified by CGM is undetected in 19% of patients monitored by SMBG.[27] Flash glucose monitoring systems (FGMS) are more accurate in identifying hypoglycemic events in diabetic dogs as well. Individual FGMS scans detect 60% of low interstitial glucose events compared with 9% by portable BG monitor.[28] All of these factors "muddy the waters" in determining the frequency of IIH and its risk factors in diabetic dogs and cats.

CLINICAL SIGNS OF INSULIN-INDUCED HYPOGLYCEMIA IN DIABETIC DOGS AND CATS

Diabetic dogs and cats with IIH can present with a wide array of clinical signs and severity ranging from subclinical to coma and death. If the brain does not receive an adequate supply of glucose, neuroglycopenic signs occur. Deprivation of glucose in the brain causes activation of the autonomic nervous system and neurogenic signs (**Fig. 1**) such as vocalizing, restlessness, shaking, pacing, nervousness, tachypnea, panting, tachycardia, vomiting, diarrhea, and/or ptyalism.[29] In people, these clinical signs "raise the alarm"[30] and invoke the behavioral response of feeding. Some diabetic dogs and cats with IIH do not develop neurogenic warning signs or the signs are not recognized by owners before the onset of neuroglycopenia.[31] In fact, less than 50% of cat owners reported neurogenic signs in their diabetic cats with IIH.[18] In people, approximately 25% of insulin-treated diabetics do not exhibit neurogenic

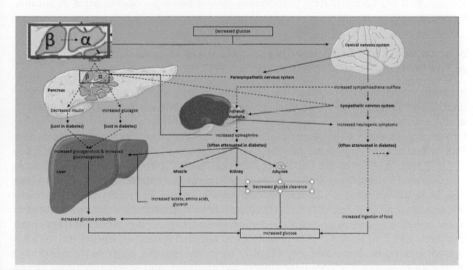

Fig. 1. Counterregulatory responses to hypoglycemia. As glucose levels decrease, sequential glucose counterregulatory responses are activated in healthy individuals to maintain euglycemia. The red arrow represents inhibition of pancreatic α cells by pancreatic β cells. Dashed arrows represent responses that are often attenuated or lost in patients with diabetes. (*Adapted from* Cryer PE. Hypoglycemia. In: *Williams Textbook of Endocrinology.* Elsevier; 2016:1585. https://doi.org/10.1016/B978-0-323-29738-7.00034-4 with permission. The figure was partly generated using Servier Medical Art, provided by Servier, licensed under a Creative Commons Attribution 3.0 unported license.)

signs because of attenuation of sympathoadrenal responses known as "hypoglycemia unawareness."[30] This can lead to lack of correction, allowing the hypoglycemia to become more severe. Prolonged and severe hypoglycemia can result in seizures, coma, brain damage, and death. Bradycardia and circulatory collapse have also been reported.[32] Diabetic dogs and cats that develop chronic or recurrent hypoglycemia may also develop "hypoglycemia unawareness."[31] As such, the incidence and prevalence of IIH in diabetic dogs and cats is likely underestimated because clinical signs are sometimes not recognized or exhibited.

In cats presented for IIH, neurologic signs are common. In one study of 30 hypoglycemic cats, 14 (47%) presented with weakness/ataxia and mental dullness with 6 of the 14 presenting blind and 5 presenting with excessive vocalization. Fifteen cats presented in a state of stupor, coma, or seizures and were all blind.[18] Other common clinical signs included inability to walk, lethargy, twitching, panting, drooling, diarrhea, inappropriate urination, failure to respond to stimulus and hyporexia.[18] Four of the 30 cats had a history of vomiting but it could not be established whether the hypoglycemia led to vomiting or vomiting led to decreased carbohydrate absorption, which then led to hypoglycemia. In an experimental set up, however, when IIH is induced in healthy cats, vomiting occurs when BG is decreased to less than 55 mg/dL (unpublished data).

Diabetic dogs with IIH may be asymptomatic or present with anorexia, diarrhea, weakness, lethargy, ataxia, pacing, restlessness, tremors, disorientation, head tilt, blindness, seizures, collapse, coma, and death.[31] It is hypothesized that the degree and duration of hypoglycemia, rate of BG drop, and counterregulatory responses determine the severity of clinical signs in IHH diabetic dogs and cats.[29] However, an individual diabetic dog or cat experiencing chronic or repeated IIH may be asymptomatic at a BG concentration that causes severe neuroglycopenic signs in another individual.

GLUCAGON RESPONSES TO HYPOGLYCEMIA ARE LARGELY MEDIATED BY ACTIVATION OF THE AUTONOMIC NERVOUS SYSTEM

In health, physiologic and behavioral defenses are sequentially activated as BG concentrations decline (see **Fig. 1**). First, when BG reduces to low normal (80–85 mg/dL), endogenous insulin secretion decreases, releasing pancreatic α cells from the inhibitory paracrine effect of insulin and allowing the secretion of glucagon to occur (see **Fig. 1**, **Table 1**).[3,33] Glucagon secretion is the first line of defense during hypoglycemia[34]: It results in increased hepatic glucose production through hepatic glycogenolysis followed by hepatic gluconeogenesis and decreased hepatic glucose uptake (see **Fig. 1**). By the time glucose concentrations have fallen to ~70 mg/dL, insulin secretion is totally shut off (see **Table 1**).[35,36] Therefore, other mechanisms must be recruited in order to further increase glucagon secretion when glucose level reduces to less than this threshold. The activation of the autonomic nervous system by the central nervous system makes an important contribution to increased glucagon secretion during moderate-to-severe IIH: parasympathetic, sympathetic, and adrenomedullary inputs to the islet are activated by IIH and all 3 of these are capable of stimulating glucagon secretion (see **Fig. 1**).[37]

In nondiabetic animals, each of the 3 autonomic inputs to the islet is capable, by itself, of mediating most of the increase of glucagon in response to IIH. By blocking all 3 of these inputs to the islet, it was demonstrated that the activation of the autonomic nervous system mediates most of the glucagon response to IIH in healthy animals,[38–41] including, nondiabetic dogs.[42] Parasympathetic nerves innervating the islets become

Table 1
Physiologic responses to progressive hypoglycemia in health

Glycemic Thresholds (mg/dL)	System Activated (A)/ Inhibited (I)	Response
80–85	β cells (partially I)/α cells (A)	Decrease endogenous insulin secretion Stimulate glucagon secretion
70	β cells (I)	Insulin secretion shut off
<70	Parasympathetic (A)	Stimulate glucagon secretion
<60	Adrenal medulla (A)	Epinephrine release Stimulate glucagon secretion
50–55	Sympathetic neural (A)	Neurogenic clinical signs Ingestion of food
<40	Sympathetic (A)	Stimulate glucagon secretion Decreased cognition, seizures, coma
10–20		Neuronal cell death

Adapted from Cryer PE. Hypoglycemia. In: *Williams Textbook of Endocrinology.* Elsevier; 2016:1584. https://doi.org/10.1016/B978-0-323-29738-7.00034-4 with permission; and Martín-Timón I. Mechanisms of hypoglycemia unawareness and implications in diabetic patients. *World Journal of Diabetes.* 2015;6(7):914. https://doi.org/10.4239/wjd.v6.i7.912.

activated when BG level decreases to less than ~70 mg/dL (see **Table 1**). The threshold for epinephrine (EPI) release from the adrenal medulla is a BG level less than ~60 mg/dL (see **Table 1**). Finally, sympathetic nerves innervating the islets are activated when BG level decreases to less than ~40 mg/dL (see **Table 1**).[6] The behavioral response (sympathetic neural) to hypoglycemia (50–55 mg/dL) is ingestion of food (see **Table 1**, see **Fig. 1**).[3,43] These physiologic and glucose counterregulatory responses in healthy animals combat IIH and result in euglycemia.

IMPAIRED COUNTERREGULATORY RESPONSES TO HYPOGLYCEMIA IN DIABETES MELLITUS

Unfortunately, counterregulatory responses to IIH are often impaired in diabetics. With exogenous insulin therapy, a decrease in insulin levels depends on the rate of absorption and clearance of insulin and not on the level of hypoglycemia.[43] Therefore, the inhibitory effect of insulin on α cells does not subside in IIH. In addition, dysfunction of sympathoadrenal system contributes to a defective glucagon response to IIH. The sympathoadrenal response is attenuated through mechanisms such as antecedent hypoglycemia, diabetic autonomic neuropathy (DAN), sympathetic islet neuropathy (humans and dogs), exercise, and sleep[3,43] (see **Fig. 1**). The activation thresholds of different branches of the autonomic system are not fixed; they shift either to higher BG levels in poorly controlled hyperglycemic patients or to lower BG levels following episodes of hypoglycemia.[44,45]

Mechanisms of Impaired Counterregulatory Responses

In hyperglycemia
Both short-term and long-term exposures to hyperglycemia impair autonomic responses. DAN results from prolonged exposure to hyperglycemia, increased oxidative stress, and suppression of peripheral autonomic activity.[46] Short-term (7 days) exposure to hyperglycemia leads to the suppression of sympathetic ganglionic neurotransmission and impairments of plasma norepinephrine and glucagon responses to

preganglionic nerve stimulation.[47] The site of ganglionic suppression has been localized within a specific subunit of the nicotinic receptor.

In hypoglycemia

Hypoglycemia-associated autonomic failure (HAAF; **Fig. 2**) is a reversible phenomenon that is caused by earlier episodes of hypoglycemia[48] that are related to either sporadic or chronic overuse of insulin.[6] Although the exact mechanism(s) have yet to be elucidated,[49] under experimental conditions, exposure to as few as 2 episodes of earlier hypoglycemia is sufficient to reduce indices of autonomic neural activation (ie, PP, NE, and EPI responses) of all 3 autonomic branches during a subsequent episode in humans.[48] Cortisol responses to IIH are also impaired in HAAF (at least partially).[50–52] The attenuated sympathetic neural response and associated neurogenic signs can result in hypoglycemia unawareness.[22] Without perception of hypoglycemia, prompt behavioral defense of carbohydrate ingestion to help restore euglycemia does not occur. Antecedent hypoglycemia lowers glycemic thresholds for both sympathoadrenal defenses and recognition of neurogenic and neuroglycopenic signs.[30,45] This results in an increased risk for subsequent severe hypoglycemia in humans by 6-fold in type 1 DM (T1DM)[53] and 17-fold in type 2 DM (T2DM).[54] Strict avoidance of hypoglycemia for 2 to 3 weeks can reverse HAAF and hypoglycemia unawareness. As such, ADA stresses that episodes of hypoglycemia, including asymptomatic ones, are not benign and can compromise glucose counterregulatory responses and pose an increased risk of imminent severe iatrogenic hypoglycemia.[22]

Hypoglycemia counterregulation is impaired in dogs with diabetes mellitus

Using the hyperinsulinemic-hypoglycemic clamp method, it was recently demonstrated that as in diabetic people, diabetic dogs also suffer from diminished hypoglycemia counterregulation. As in people, this is caused by impairment of multiple branches of the autonomic system. Of 13 dogs with naturally occurring DM, glucagon responses to hypoglycemia (BG ~40 mg/dL) were absent or severely diminished compared with healthy controls. In only 5 of the 13 diabetic dogs, glucagon responses

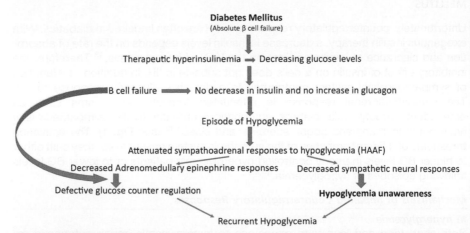

Fig. 2. Schematic of HAAF in humans with DM. Individuals with type 1 diabetes mellitus or advanced type 2 diabetes mellitus (β cell failure) are at increased risk of developing hypoglycemia unawareness and recurrent episodes of hypoglycemia. (*Adapted from* Cryer PE. Hypoglycemia. In: *Williams Textbook of Endocrinology.* Elsevier; 2016:1582-1607. https://doi.org/10.1016/B978-0-323-29738-7.00034-4 with permission.)

were in the range of healthy controls.[55] The 8 diabetic "nonresponders" exhibited impaired norepinephrine, EPI, and cholinergic responses to IIH compared with controls. These impairments were not observed in the diabetics that mounted a normal response to IIH. Interestingly, dogs in this study did not exhibit impaired plasma cortisol responses to IIH as reported in the syndrome of HAAF in people.

Early sympathetic islet neuropathy

Early sympathetic islet neuropathy (eSIN) is a selective loss of sympathetic nerves innervating the pancreatic islets that is not affecting the exocrine pancreas. eSIN occurs early in T1DM and it seems to be sustained long after the primary insult to the islets is gone.[56] eSIN is triggered by the lymphocytic infiltration of the islet, involves subsequent activation of the p75 neurotrophin receptor residing on sympathetic nerves, and ultimately results in the destruction of a vast majority of proximal sympathetic nerve terminals within the islet.[57] eSIN immediately precedes the development of diabetic hyperglycemia and seems to coincide with the autoimmune attack on islet beta cells.[58] eSIN has been documented in humans and in several rodent models of T1DM[58–60] but not in T2DM and in models of toxin induced DM.[61] Yet, it has not been determined whether eSIN might occur secondary to other inflammatory diseases in which lymphocytes do not necessarily predominate (such as pancreatitis).

Sympathetic islet neuropathy in dogs

Loss of sympathetic innervation to pancreatic islets in dogs has been recently demonstrated.[62] This lesion was found in all dogs with naturally occurring DM, including those that also suffered from pancreatitis, and in dogs with toxin-induced DM. Using the pan-leukocyte cell surface marker CD-45 as a sensitive marker of inflammation, no evidence was observed for leukocytes involvement in the selective loss of beta cells in diabetic dogs, differentiating this neuropathy from eSIN that is observed in models of T1DM.[62] Interestingly, a marked reduction in islet sympathetic innervation was also observed in dogs suffering from pancreatitis that had no history of DM.[62]

THE "Somogyi EFFECT": TIME TO LET IT GO

In 1959, Dr Michael Somogyi, a chemist, published an article titled "Exacerbation of diabetes by excess insulin action", in which he concluded that even mild and subclinical hypoglycemia leads to hyperglycemia and worsening of signs of DM. Dr Somogyi hypothesized that this occurs because of activation of stress hormones.[63] Later, this became the "Somogyi effect" and the definition was reduced to "Early morning hyperglycemia due to treatment with excessive amount of exogenous insulin."[64] Although some early studies supported Somogyi's hypothesis, in recent years, overwhelming evidence accumulated contradicting it. Studies in diabetic people repeatedly demonstrate the existence of diminished or absent counterregulatory responses to hypoglycemia. For example, in a study of diabetic children, the counterregulatory response to hypoglycemia was shown to be defective, resulting in prolonged nocturnal hypoglycemia.[65] Although EPI increased because of hypoglycemia, the threshold for its response was remarkably low (34 mg/dL [1.9 mmol/L]). In the same study, nocturnal hypoglycemia did not result in an increase in norepinephrine, glucagon, and cortisol. Growth hormone did increase after nocturnal hypoglycemia but this could have been a normal nocturnal response (Dawn effect).[65] More recent studies using CGM in hundreds of patients demonstrate that nocturnal hypoglycemia is not associated with morning hyperglycemia but rather with morning hypoglycemia.[66–68]

Using CGM systems, recent studies have demonstrated that hypoglycemic events are more common than previously realized; in one study, patients were unaware of

75% of the hypoglycemic events recorded by CGM.[69] Importantly, higher glucose variability indices including higher mean absolute glucose values have recently been shown to predict episodes of nocturnal hypoglycemia in insulin-treated people.[70] Individuals with increased glycemic variability therefore may present with poor diabetic control due to the occurrence of frequent hyperglycemia, whereas most of the hypoglycemic events are associated with no clinical signs and would be missed by standard intermittent BG monitoring. Nevertheless, the frequent hypoglycemia can induce physiologic unawareness of hypoglycemia and impaired glucose counterregulation, which in turn predisposes to an increased risk of neuroglycopenia.[71]

No Evidence for the "Somogyi Effect" in Dogs and Cats

Insulin-induced hyperglycemia, or "rebound hyperglycemia" (RH) was erroneously reported in 8 diabetic dogs and 6 diabetic cats from the 1980s.[72,73] In these reports, a high dose of insulin was administered and hypoglycemia was recorded, followed by hyperglycemia.[72,73] A cause and effect between hypoglycemia and hyperglycemia was not demonstrated in these studies, and in fact, hypoglycemia was often prolonged (especially in dogs, sometimes lasting hours) without evidence of an acute counterregulatory response. No hormones were measured in these studies: The possibility that hyperglycemia was caused simply by insulin wearing off or by absorption of carbohydrates from the GI tract was not ruled out and the plausibility that hyperglycemia was caused by increased counterregulatory hormones was not demonstrated. In the canine study, dogs were fed only one-fourth of their daily caloric intake when their standard insulin dose was administered at 8:00 AM. Hyperglycemia was consistently documented although not shortly after hypoglycemia was recorded but rather after 5:00 PM when the dogs were fed three-fourths of their daily caloric intake (without being treated with insulin again). In the feline study, it is unclear whether the quicker resolution of hypoglycemia (and development of hyperglycemia) was the result of feeding because feedings were not standardized as in the dog study. It is therefore likely that after observing hypoglycemia (reported as low as 38 mg/dL), clinicians immediately fed their patients.

The assertion that these cases represented insulin-induced hyperglycemia was supported by improvement in clinical signs (and in some cases by lesser fluctuations in BG level based on glucose curves) after insulin dose was decreased. Indeed, the main importance of these studies is in describing clinical cases that presented for signs that were consistent with insulin deficiency but benefited from a reduction in insulin dose. It is possible that these cases represent the subset of diabetic patients in which glucagon responses are still intact. In these patients, an insulin overdose should result in perceived "shortening" of insulin duration of effect because of counterregulatory hormones raising BG level before insulin wears off. Indeed, most of these cases were diagnosed with insulin-induced hyperglycemia when their dose of insulin was quite high.

After the publication of these small case series, it was asserted that "secretion of diabetogenic hormones during the Somogyi response may induce insulin resistance which can last 24 to 72 hours after the hypoglycemic episode."[2] Induction of insulin resistance would be an important reason to consider the diagnosis of the "Somogyi effect" because if real, it would be the only differential diagnosis for insulin resistance that requires the clinician to reduce the dose of insulin in the face of hyperglycemia. Contrary to historic veterinary dogma,[2,72,74] however, there is no evidence in any published study that exaggerated and prolonged stress responses in dogs or cats can lead to prolonged insulin resistance. In a more recent study, 10,767 home glucose curves from 55 cats were collected from a web-based cat DM forum.[16] RH was defined in this study as a hypoglycemic event (BG < 50 mg/dL) that is followed by a

BG level greater than 300 mg/dL within 4 to 10 hours. If the BG level remained greater than 250 mg/dL for at least 24 hours, the event was labeled as RH with insulin resistance. In this context, RH was observed in 0.42% of the glucose curves, and there was no difference in the frequency or magnitude of hyperglycemia between posthypoglycemia events and posteuglycemia events, suggesting that hyperglycemia was not caused by hypoglycemia. Only 4 of the 10,767 curves were suggestive of "RH with insulin resistance"; however, day-to-day variations related to insulin absorption, inconsistent feedings, and other factors were not accounted for.[16]

The term posthypoglycemic-hyperglycemia (PHH) has been used instead of RH to indicate temporal correlation versus causation in another recent study. In that study, PHH was reported in 25% of diabetic cats with IIH but there was no comparison of hyperglycemic events that followed hypoglycemia versus euglycemia. Therefore, causation could not be established.[10]

SUMMARY

Hypoglycemia begets hypoglycemia, not hyperglycemia. There is no evidence in dogs, cats, or in other species that in DM, counterregulatory hormones are released excessively in response to hypoglycemia. The opposite is true: hypoglycemia counterregulatory responses are impaired in DM. Better glycemic control and avoidance of hypoglycemia might minimize this impairment. To some degree, however, this impairment is associated with the underlying pathologic condition leading to DM and is irreversible once DM has been established. Clinically, it is important to recognize that episodes of IIH in veterinary patients are not without consequences and have long-term effects. Antecedent IIH attenuates the sympathoadrenal responses and sets the patient up for an increased risk of severe future iatrogenic hypoglycemia.

CLINICS CARE POINTS

- IIH is common in veterinary patients and dogs and cats may or may not exhibit clinical signs.
- The frequency of IIH is underestimated when using BG curves as a monitoring tool.
- Some diabetic dogs have impairment of the autonomic nervous system and are less able to respond to IIH. The same is true in humans. No data on this are available for diabetic cats.
- Episodes of subclinical IIH are not benign: they lower the glycemic threshold for sympathoadrenal responses and increase the risk of future severe hypoglycemic crises.
- Hypoglycemia begets hypoglycemia, not hyperglycemia. There is no evidence for "Somogyi effect" or "rebound hyperglycemia" in dogs or cats.

DISCLOSURE

The authors have nothing to disclose.

REFERENCES

1. Fleeman LM, Rand JS. Management of canine diabetes. Vet Clin North Am Small Anim Pract 2001;31(5):855–80, vi.
2. Nelson RW. Canine diabetes mellitus. In: Feldman E, Nelson RW, editors. Canine and feline endocrinology. 4th edition. Philadelphia, PA: Saunders; 2015. p. 213–57.

3. Cryer PE. The barrier of hypoglycemia in diabetes. Diabetes 2008;57(12): 3169–76.

4. Bolli G, de Feo P, Compagnucci P, et al. Abnormal glucose counterregulation in insulin-dependent diabetes mellitus. Interaction of anti-insulin antibodies and impaired glucagon and epinephrine secretion. Diabetes 1983;32(2): 134–41.

5. Gerich JE, Langlois M, Noacco C, et al. Lack of glucagon response to hypoglycemia in diabetes: evidence for an intrinsic pancreatic alpha cell defect. Science 1973;182(4108):171–3.

6. Taborsky GJ, Mundinger TO. Minireview: The Role of the Autonomic Nervous System in Mediating the Glucagon Response to Hypoglycemia. Endocrinology 2012; 153(3):1055–62.

7. Niessen SJM, Powney S, Guitian J, et al. Evaluation of a quality-of-life tool for cats with diabetes mellitus. J Vet Intern Med 2010;24(5):1098–105.

8. Niessen SJM, Powney S, Guitian J, et al. Evaluation of a Quality-of-Life Tool for Dogs with Diabetes Mellitus. J Vet Intern Med 2012;26(4):953–61.

9. Nelson RW, Lynn RC, Wagner-Mann CC, et al. Efficacy of protamine zinc insulin for treatment of diabetes mellitus in cats. J Am Vet Med Assoc 2001;218(1): 38–42.

10. Zini E, Salesov E, Dupont P, et al. Glucose concentrations after insulin-induced hypoglycemia and glycemic variability in healthy and diabetic cats. J Vet Intern Med 2018;32(3):978–85.

11. Nelson RW, Henley K, Cole C. Field safety and efficacy of protamine zinc recombinant human insulin for treatment of diabetes mellitus in cats. J Vet Intern Med 2009;23(4):787–93.

12. Roomp K, Rand J. Intensive blood glucose control is safe and effective in diabetic cats using home monitoring and treatment with glargine. J Feline Med Surg 2009;11(8):668–82.

13. Fracassi F, Corradini S, Hafner M, et al. Detemir insulin for the treatment of diabetes mellitus in dogs. J Am Vet Med Assoc 2015;247(1):73–8.

14. Monroe WE, Laxton D, Fallin EA, et al. Efficacy and safety of a purified porcine insulin zinc suspension for managing diabetes mellitus in dogs. J Vet Intern Med 2005;19(5):675–82.

15. Ward CR, Christiansen K, Li J, et al. Field efficacy and safety of protamine zinc recombinant human insulin in 276 dogs with diabetes mellitus. Domest Anim Endocrinol 2021;75:106575.

16. Roomp K, Rand J. Rebound hyperglycaemia in diabetic cats. J Feline Med Surg 2016;18(8):587–96.

17. Marshall RD, Rand JS, Morton JM. Treatment of newly diagnosed diabetic cats with glargine insulin improves glycaemic control and results in higher probability of remission than protamine zinc and lente insulins. J Feline Med Surg 2009; 11(8):683–91.

18. Viebrock KA, Dennis J. Hypoglycemic episodes in cats with diabetes mellitus: 30 cases (2013-2015). J Feline Med Surg 2018;20(6):563–70.

19. Mori A, Kurishima M, Oda H, et al. Comparison of glucose fluctuations between day- and night-time measured using a continuous glucose monitoring system in diabetic dogs. J Vet Med Sci 2013;75(1):113–7.

20. Shea EK, Hess RS. Assessment of postprandial hyperglycemia and circadian fluctuation of glucose concentrations in diabetic dogs using a flash glucose monitoring system. J Vet Intern Med 2021;35(2):843–52.

21. della Maggiore A, Nelson RW, Dennis J, et al. Efficacy of protamine zinc recombinant human insulin for controlling hyperglycemia in dogs with diabetes mellitus. J Vet Intern Med 2012;26(1):109–15.

22. Workgroup on Hypoglycemia, American Diabetes Association. Defining and reporting hypoglycemia in diabetes: a report from the American Diabetes Association Workgroup on Hypoglycemia. Diabetes Care 2005;28(5):1245–9.

23. DeClue AE, Cohn LA, Kerl ME, et al. Use of continuous blood glucose monitoring for animals with diabetes mellitus. J Am Anim Hosp Assoc 2004;40(3): 171–3.

24. Casella M, Hässig M, Reusch CE. Home-monitoring of blood glucose in cats with diabetes mellitus: evaluation over a 4-month period. J Feline Med Surg 2005;7(3): 163–71.

25. Casella M, Wess G, Hässig M, et al. Home monitoring of blood glucose concentration by owners of diabetic dogs. J Small Anim Pract 2003;44(7): 298–305.

26. Zick R, Petersen B, Richter M, et al. Comparison of Continuous Blood Glucose Measurement with Conventional Documentation of Hypoglycemia in Patients with Type 2 Diabetes on Multiple Daily Insulin Injection Therapy. Diabetes Technol Ther 2007;9(6):483–92.

27. Pazos-Couselo M, García-López JM, González-Rodríguez M, et al. High Incidence of Hypoglycemia in Stable Insulin-Treated Type 2 Diabetes Mellitus: Continuous Glucose Monitoring vs. Self-Monitored Blood Glucose. Observational Prospective Study. Can J Diabetes 2015;39(5):428–33.

28. del Baldo F, Canton C, Testa S, et al. Comparison between a flash glucose monitoring system and a portable blood glucose meter for monitoring dogs with diabetes mellitus. J Vet Intern Med 2020;34(6):2296–305.

29. Idowu O, Heading K. Hypoglycemia in dogs: Causes, management, and diagnosis. Can Vet J 2018;59(6):642–9.

30. Sankar A, Khodai T, McNeilly AD, et al. Experimental Models of Impaired Hypoglycaemia-Associated Counter-Regulation. Trends Endocrinol Metab 2020;31(9):691–703.

31. Whitley NT, Drobatz KJ, Panciera DL. Insulin overdose in dogs and cats: 28 cases (1986-1993). J Am Vet Med Assoc 1997;211(3):326–30.

32. Little CJL. Hypoglycaemic bradycardia and circulatory collapse in a dog and a cat. J Small Anim Pract 2005;46(9):445–8.

33. Zhou H, Tran POT, Yang S, et al. Regulation of alpha-cell function by the beta-cell during hypoglycemia in Wistar rats: the "switch-off" hypothesis. Diabetes 2004; 53(6):1482–7.

34. Rizza RA, Cryer PE, Gerich JE. Role of Glucagon, Catecholamines, and Growth Hormone in Human Glucose Counterregulation. J Clin Invest 1979;64(1):62–71.

35. Banarer S, McGregor VP, Cryer PE. Intraislet Hyperinsulinemia Prevents the Glucagon Response to Hypoglycemia Despite an Intact Autonomic Response. Diabetes 2002;51(4):958–65.

36. Sherck SM, Shiota M, Saccomando J, et al. Pancreatic response to mild non-insulin-induced hypoglycemia does not involve extrinsic neural input. Diabetes 2001;50(11):2487–96.

37. Havel PJ, Taborsky GJ. The contribution of the autonomic nervous system to changes of glucagon and insulin secretion during hypoglycemic stress. Endocr Rev 1989;10(3):332–50.

38. Havel PJ, Akpan JO, Curry DL, et al. Autonomic control of pancreatic polypeptide and glucagon secretion during neuroglucopenia and hypoglycemia in mice. Am J Physiol 1993;265(1 Pt 2):R246–54.

39. Havel PJ, Parry SJ, Stern JS, et al. Redundant parasympathetic and sympathoadrenal mediation of increased glucagon secretion during insulin-induced hypoglycemia in conscious rats. Metabolism 1994;43(7):860–6.

40. Havel PJ, Valverde C. Autonomic mediation of glucagon secretion during insulin-induced hypoglycemia in rhesus monkeys. Diabetes 1996;45(7):960–6.

41. Havel PJ, Ahren B. Activation of autonomic nerves and the adrenal medulla contributes to increased glucagon secretion during moderate insulin-induced hypoglycemia in women. Diabetes 1997;46(5):801–7.

42. Havel PJ, Veith RC, Dunning BE, et al. Role for autonomic nervous system to increase pancreatic glucagon secretion during marked insulin-induced hypoglycemia in dogs. Diabetes 1991;40(9):1107–14.

43. Cryer PE. Mechanisms of Hypoglycemia-Associated Autonomic Failure in Diabetes. N Engl J Med 2013;369(4):362–72.

44. Boyle PJ, Schwartz NS, Shah SD, et al. Plasma glucose concentrations at the onset of hypoglycemic symptoms in patients with poorly controlled diabetes and in nondiabetics. N Engl J Med 1988;318(23):1487–92.

45. Amiel SA, Sherwin RS, Simonson DC, et al. Effect of intensive insulin therapy on glycemic thresholds for counterregulatory hormone release. Diabetes 1988;37(7): 901–7.

46. Brownlee M. Biochemistry and molecular cell biology of diabetic complications. Nature 2001;414(6865):813–20.

47. Mundinger TO, Cooper E, Coleman MP, et al. Short-term diabetic hyperglycemia suppresses celiac ganglia neurotransmission, thereby impairing sympathetically mediated glucagon responses. Am J Physiol Endocrinol Metab 2015;309(3): E246–55.

48. Heller SR, Cryer PE. Reduced neuroendocrine and symptomatic responses to subsequent hypoglycemia after 1 episode of hypoglycemia in nondiabetic humans. Diabetes 1991;40(2):223–6.

49. Lontchi-Yimagou E, You JY, Carey M, et al. Potential approaches to prevent hypoglycemia-associated autonomic failure. J Investig Med 2018;66(3):641–7.

50. Davis SN, Tate D, Hedrington MS. Mechanisms of hypoglycemia and exercise-associated autonomic dysfunction. Trans Am Clin Climatol Assoc 2014;125: 281–91, discussion 291-2.

51. Seaquist ER, Moheet A, Kumar A, et al. Hypothalamic Glucose Transport in Humans During Experimentally Induced Hypoglycemia-Associated Autonomic Failure. J Clin Endocrinol Metab 2017;102(9):3571–80.

52. Moheet A, Kumar A, Eberly LE, et al. Hypoglycemia-associated autonomic failure in healthy humans: comparison of two vs three periods of hypoglycemia on hypoglycemia-induced counterregulatory and symptom response 5 days later. J Clin Endocrinol Metab 2014;99(2):664–70.

53. Geddes J, Schopman JE, Zammitt NN, et al. Prevalence of impaired awareness of hypoglycaemia in adults with Type 1 diabetes. Diabet Med 2008;25(4):501–4.

54. Schopman JE, Geddes J, Frier BM. Prevalence of impaired awareness of hypoglycaemia and frequency of hypoglycaemia in insulin-treated type 2 diabetes. Diabetes Res Clin Pract 2010;87(1):64–8.

55. Gilor C, Duesberg C, Elliott DA, et al. Co-impairment of autonomic and glucagon responses to insulin-induced hypoglycemia in dogs with naturally occurring

insulin-dependent diabetes mellitus. Am J Physiol Endocrinol Metab 2020;319(6): E1074–83.

56. Mundinger TO, Taborsky GJ. Early sympathetic islet neuropathy in autoimmune diabetes: lessons learned and opportunities for investigation. Diabetologia 2016;59(10):2058–67.

57. Taborsky GJ, Mei Q, Bornfeldt KE, et al. The p75 neurotrophin receptor is required for the major loss of sympathetic nerves from islets under autoimmune attack. Diabetes 2014;63(7):2369–79.

58. Taborsky GJ, Mei Q, Hackney DJ, et al. Loss of islet sympathetic nerves and impairment of glucagon secretion in the NOD mouse: relationship to invasive insulitis. Diabetologia 2009;52(12):2602–11.

59. Mei Q, Mundinger TO, Lernmark A, et al. Early, selective, and marked loss of sympathetic nerves from the islets of BioBreeder diabetic rats. Diabetes 2002; 51(10):2997–3002.

60. Mundinger TO, Mei Q, Figlewicz DP, et al. Impaired glucagon response to sympathetic nerve stimulation in the BB diabetic rat: effect of early sympathetic islet neuropathy. Am J Physiol Endocrinol Metab 2003;285(5):E1047–54.

61. Mundinger TO, Mei Q, Foulis AK, et al. Human Type 1 Diabetes Is Characterized by an Early, Marked, Sustained, and Islet-Selective Loss of Sympathetic Nerves. Diabetes 2016;65(8):2322–30.

62. Gilor C, Pires J, Greathouse R, et al. Loss of sympathetic innervation to islets of Langerhans in canine diabetes and pancreatitis is not associated with insulitis. Sci Rep 2020;10(1):19187.

63. SOMOGYI M. Exacerbation of diabetes by excess insulin action. Am J Med 1959; 26(2):169–91.

64. Rybicka M, Krysiak R, Okopień B. The dawn phenomenon and the Somogyi effect - two phenomena of morning hyperglycaemia. Endokrynol Pol 2011;62(3): 276–84.

65. Matyka KA, Crowne EC, Havel PJ, et al. Counterregulation during spontaneous nocturnal hypoglycemia in prepubertal children with type 1 diabetes. Diabetes Care 1999;22(7):1144–50.

66. Guillod L, Comte-Perret S, Monbaron D, et al. Nocturnal hypoglycaemias in type 1 diabetic patients: what can we learn with continuous glucose monitoring? Diabetes Metab 2007;33(5):360–5.

67. Choudhary P, Davies C, Emery CJ, et al. Do high fasting glucose levels suggest nocturnal hypoglycaemia? The Somogyi effect-more fiction than fact? Diabet Med 2013;30(8):914–7.

68. Høi-Hansen T, Pedersen-Bjergaard U, Thorsteinsson B. The Somogyi phenomenon revisited using continuous glucose monitoring in daily life. Diabetologia 2005; 48(11):2437–8.

69. Gehlaut RR, Dogbey GY, Schwartz FL, et al. Hypoglycemia in Type 2 Diabetes–More Common Than You Think: A Continuous Glucose Monitoring Study. J Diabetes Sci Technol 2015;9(5):999–1005.

70. Klimontov V v, Myakina NE. Glucose variability indices predict the episodes of nocturnal hypoglycemia in elderly type 2 diabetic patients treated with insulin. Diabetes Metab Syndr 2017;11(2):119–24.

71. Fanelli CG, Porcellati F, Pampanelli S, et al. Insulin therapy and hypoglycaemia: the size of the problem. Diabetes Metab Res Rev 2004;20(Suppl 2):S32–42.

72. Feldman EC, Nelson RW. Insulin-induced hyperglycemia in diabetic dogs. J Am Vet Med Assoc 1982;180(12):1432–7.

73. McMillan FD, Feldman EC. Rebound hyperglycemia following overdosing of insulin in cats with diabetes mellitus. J Am Vet Med Assoc 1986;188(12): 1426–31.

74. Reusch Claudia. Feline diabetes mellitus. In: Feldman E, Nelson RW, editors. *Canine and feline endocrinology*. 4th edition. St. Louis, MO: Saunders; 2015. p. 258–308.

Diabetes Mellitus and the Kidneys

Arnon Gal, DVM, PhD[a],*, Richard K. Burchell, BSc, BVSc, MMedVet, DECVIM-CA[b]

KEYWORDS

- Diabetes mellitus • Diabetic nephropathy • Diabetic kidney disease
- Companion animals

KEY POINTS

- Evidence of chronic kidney disease (CKD) in cats with diabetes mellitus (DM) is variable.
- There is currently no clinical evidence of an association of DM and CKD in dogs.
- Criteria for diagnosing diabetic kidney disease have not been established in dogs and cats.
- Monitoring for CKD in cats with DM might be warranted.

INTRODUCTION

Diabetic kidney disease (DKD) is a chronic progressive kidney disease that is the most common cause of end-stage renal failure in people in the western world.[1] DKD results from multifactorial pathophysiological mechanisms and clinically manifests with proteinuria, subsequent progressive decline in glomerular filtration rate (GFR), and ultimately progression to end-stage renal disease.[2] There is minimal published information about DKD in companion animals in the veterinary literature. The first part of this review will focus on the pathophysiology of DKD, derived mainly from the human medical literature and rodent models of DKD. Wherever there was corresponding information relevant to companion animals, we mentioned it. The second part of this review focuses on the limited veterinary literature that loosely supports the existence of DKD as a clinical entity in companion animals.

Proposed Molecular Pathomechanisms of Diabetic Kidney Disease

Hyperglycemia

DKD does not develop in people in the absence of persistent hyperglycemia (ie, HbA1c <5.7%),[3] illustrating the importance of persistent hyperglycemia in the pathogenesis

[a] Department of Veterinary Clinical Medicine, College of Veterinary Medicine, University of Illinois at Urbana-Champaign, 1008 West Hazelwood Drive, Urbana, IL 61802, USA; [b] North Coast Veterinary Specialist and Referral Centre, 5/30 Chancellor Village, Sippy Downs, Sunshine Coast 4556, Australia
* Corresponding author.
E-mail address: agal2@illinois.edu

Vet Clin Small Anim 53 (2023) 565–580
https://doi.org/10.1016/j.cvsm.2023.01.006
0195-5616/23/© 2023 Elsevier Inc. All rights reserved.

vetsmall.theclinics.com

of DKD. Microalbuminuria (proxy of early DKD) is already present in 15% to 20% of people with prediabetes (HbA1c 5.7%–6.4%).[3] In a human clinical trial of type-1 diabetes mellitus (T1DM) strict glycemic control (HbA1c <6.5%[4]) decreased the incidence of microalbuminuria by 50%.[5] In contrast, the incidence of microalbuminuria increased steeply when HbA1c was greater than 7%. In a human clinical trial of type-2 diabetes mellitus (T2DM), reduction of HbA1c by 1% decreased the risk for microalbuminuria by 33%.[6]

Hyperglycemia influences the normal intrarenal adaptive physiologic mechanisms that regulate glomerular hemodynamics and renal blood flow. Glucose uptake by renal cells is insulin-independent and increases in proportion to blood glucose levels.[7] Glucose uptake in the renal proximal tubules (PCTs) is coupled to sodium absorption via sodium-glucose co-transporters (SGLTs).[7] There are 2 SGLTs: type 1 (SGLT1), which is a high-affinity, low-capacity glucose/galactose transporter, and type 2 (SGLT2), which is a high-capacity, low-affinity glucose transporter; the latter being the predominant PCT SGLT and accounting for approximately 90% of glucose reabsorption in the PCTs.[7]

Sodium absorption by the PCTs affects the levels of sodium delivered to the distal tubule. Specialized distal tubular cells (macula densa cells of the juxtaglomerular apparatus) sense sodium levels and regulate the tone of the afferent and efferent glomerular arterioles via tubuloglomerular feedback (TGF).[8] TGF is an important evolutionary survival mechanism of terrestrial species intended to conserve body salt and maintain intravascular volume.[8] Low or high levels of sodium chloride in the distal segment signal intravascular volume contraction or expansion, respectively. In the case of volume contraction, the TGF decreases the local conversion of ATP to adenosine and increases the production of intrarenal renin/angiotensin, which results in afferent arteriole vasodilation and efferent arteriole vasoconstriction effectively increasing renal perfusion and intraglomerular pressure. The opposite occurs in the case of volume expansion.[8–10] This physiologic adaptive mechanism positively affects the host in the short term. However, it could have deleterious outcomes when it develops into a sustained maladaptive response, as in DKD.

In an experiment in which single nephron proximal tubules were infused with glucose,[9] high intratubular glucose levels led to increased PCT glucose-coupled sodium absorption and decreased downstream sodium chloride delivery. The subsequent activation of TGF resulted in an increased intraglomerular pressure (glomerular hypertension), and resulted in renal hyperfiltration. In a rodent model of streptozotocin (STZ)-induced DM, tubular glucose overload led to a compensatory proximal tubular hypertrophy within days,[11] and similarly, people with DM have an increase in renal tubular mass early in the development of DM.[2,11,12] Renal tubular hypertrophy is considered a predictor of poor renal outcomes in people with DKD,[13,14] because it further accentuates intraglomerular hypertension and renal hyperfiltration, thus contributing to the progressive development of glomerulosclerosis and proteinuria. Nevertheless, strict glycemic control in people with T1DM DKD can reverse and normalize renal mass and GFR within 3 months.[15] Multiple growth factors including insulin growth factor 1, vascular endothelial growth factor (VEGF), platelet-derived growth factor, epidermal growth factor, transforming growth factor β1 (TGFβ1), and connective tissue growth factor are involved in the process of tubular hypertrophy in DKD. Unlike tubular hypertrophy, a reversible process, glomerular hypertrophy is an irreversible process, which is in part mediated by intrarenal activation of renin-angiotensin-aldosterone system (RAAS), resulting in the local production of the potent growth factor angiotensin II (AGII). Hence, hyperglycemia leads to a domino effect in which increased PCT glucose absorption leads to decreased sodium chloride absorption in the distal tubule and TGF activation that alters glomerular hemodynamics, and leads to irreversible glomerular hypertrophy. The ensuing tubular hypertrophy further aggravates the glomerular hypertrophy and culminates in glomerulosclerosis.

In people, the differences between T1DM and T2DM in the age of onset of diabetes (young vs old) and treatment (insulin vs metformin and GLP-1 analogs) are thought to explain the fundamental structural differences in DKD: predominance of glomerulo-sclerosis in T1DM DKD versus predominance of tubulointerstitial lesions in T2DM DKD.[16,17] The reason for these differences is inherent to the ability of the maladaptive TGF to alter the glomerular hemodynamics. Glomerular hyperfiltration is more common in patients with T1DM because of their younger age, higher age-related baseline GFR and renal plasma flow (RPF), lower renal vascular resistance (RVR), and because they are treated with insulin, which is a potent vasodilator.[18] In contrast, patients with T2DM have a "protective" decreased capacity to alter glomerular hemodynamics because of older age, lower GFR, RPF, and higher RVR. Dogs and cats, which are exclusively treated with insulin and have disease onset at an older age, have structural changes that combine those of T1DM and T2DM DKD seen in people.[19–21]

Hyperglycemic-induced tubular hypertrophy also increases proximal tubular oxygen consumption by ~40% (based on rodent models[22]) because the sodium-glucose coupled absorption increases the activity of the basolateral Na-K ATPase pumps (an ATP-dependent process). Consequently, there are substantial mismatches between increasing tubular oxygen demands and decreased oxygen delivery to the kidneys. The intimate linkage between renal hypoxia and enhanced tubular sodium-glucose uptake was confirmed in an STZ-induced diabetic rat model in which renal oxygen demands were normalized following treatment with phlorizin (a nonspecific sodium-glucose cotransporter inhibitor).[23] Renal hypoxia in DKD increases hypoxia-inducible factor 1α (HIF1α) gene expression but fails to stimulate HIF1α downstream signaling (including production of erythropoietin), thus effectively contributing to decreased renal oxygen delivery.[24,25] Renal hypoxia is a potent signal for the recruitment of inflammatory cells and extracellular matrix remodeling. Hence, the global effect of renal hypoxia contributes to progressive glomerular mesangial remodeling and tubulointerstitial inflammation and fibrosis.

Unregulated renal glucose uptake during periods of sustained hyperglycemia overwhelms the glomerular and tubular cells with glucose, oversaturates their glycolytic pathway, and leads to diversion of glucose metabolism into nonglycolytic pathways, including the hexosamine, aldose reductase (polyol), pentose phosphate, advanced glycation endproducts (AGEs), and protein kinase C (PKC) pathways.

Activation of the polyol pathway is a commonly suggested mechanism of renal injury in DKD,[26] in which, glucose is metabolized to sorbitol by aldose reductase, which is then metabolized to fructose by sorbitol dehydrogenase. Fructose is then metabolized by fructokinase (ketohexokinase [KHK]). Metabolism of the fructose by KHK in the proximal tubule leads to transient depletion of intracellular phosphate and ATP, oxidative stress, and mitochondrial injury.[27,28] Moreover, activation of the polyol pathway leads to substantial consumption of nicotinamide adenine dinucleotide phosphate (NADPH) (derived from the pentose phosphate pathway and critical for the replenishment of reduced glutathione) and excessive production of nicotinamide adenine dinucleotide (NADH), which is taken up by the mitochondrial respiratory chain and increases the production of superoxide.[29] Thus, chronic activation of the polyol pathway culminates in renal injury, inflammation, and fibrosis.

The PKC signaling pathway is a potent activator of NADPH oxidase, a cytosolic enzyme complex in mesangial cells, proximal tubular epithelium, vascular smooth myocytes, endothelium, and fibroblasts.[30] Hyperglycemia, AGII, and TGF-β are potent inducers of PKC. Activation of the PKC pathway results in large amounts of NADPH oxidase-derived reactive oxygen species (ROS)[31] and is considered an important underlying mechanism of endothelial dysfunction in DKD.

AGEs are molecules generated from nonenzymatic covalent bonding of glucose residues to free amino groups of proteins, lipids, and nucleic acids (ie, the Maillard reaction). AGEs are filtered in the glomerulus and bind to their receptor RAGE on the tubular epithelium. RAGE activates NADPH oxidase, which generates ROS, and activates the nuclear factor kappa B (NFκB) signaling pathway, which produces inflammatory cytokines and mitochondrial-derived ROS through electrons leakage.[32]

The hexosamine pathway generates uridine-5-diphosphate-N-acetylglucosamine (UDP-GlucNAc) from fructose-6-phosphate and glutamine. UDP-GlucNAc is the amino sugar precursor used to synthesize glycoproteins, glycolipids, and proteoglycans. The hexosamine pathway is activated in DKD and results in hyperglycemia-induced renal production of TGF-β and activation of the PKC pathway, resulting in renal ROS-mediated damage, inflammation, and fibrosis.[33]

Thus, glucose shunting from the glycolytic pathway to the alternative pathways leads to altered gene expression, mitochondrial dysfunction and oxidative stress, glycosylation of proteins and activation of RAGE, and endothelial injury, which synergistically promote renal glomerular and tubular cellular injury, inflammation, and fibrosis.

Preliminary results from a recent untargeted metabolomic study in cats with diabetes demonstrated that the diversion of glucose to alternative glucose metabolizing pathways also occurs in cats with diabetes as serum metabolites of the above pathways were abundant in the serum of cats with diabetes compared with that of control cats.[34]

Glucose uptake by the endothelium is an insulin-independent process. Sustained high intraendothelial glucose fluxes lead to increased intracellular glucose levels and subsequent activation of NADPH oxidase and uncoupling of endothelial nitric oxide (NO) synthases, which results in the generation of ROS.[35] Similarly, enhanced mitochondrial substrate oxidation results in increased mitochondrial membrane potential and subsequent overproduction of superoxide. ROS-mediated NF-κB signaling then leads to inflammation. ROS also cause DNA strand breaks that stimulate the DNA repair enzyme poly(ADP ribose) polymerase 1, which in turn inhibits the glycolytic enzyme glyceraldehyde-3-phosphate dehydrogenase (GAPDH) by polyADP-ribosylation. The inhibition of GAPDH diverts glucose metabolism to the hexosamine, aldose reductase (polyol), pentose phosphate, AGE, and PKC pathways.[36] ROS-mediated injury and diversion of glucose to alternative metabolic pathways lead to endothelial dysfunction and renal ischemic microangiopathy.

Chronic hyperglycemia affects the nutrient sensors mammalian target of rapamycin, 5' AMP-activated protein kinase, and the sirtuins with subsequent downregulation of autophagy (necessary for normal mitochondrial health), and reduced mitochondrial regeneration and biogenesis.[37,38] Patients with DKD have been shown to have decreased expression of peroxisome-proliferator-activated receptor-γ coactivator-1 alpha (PGC-1α; a master regulator of mitochondrial biogenesis) and reduced mitochondrial proteins and DNA. Moreover, increased mitochondrial fission results in increased numbers of nonfunctional mitochondria. Mitochondrial dysfunction of PCT and podocytes contributes to the development and progression of DKD through ROS-mediated oxidative stress, energy depletion, impaired energy-dependent repair mechanisms, and cell death.

Systemic and Intraglomerular Hypertension

After hyperglycemia, hypertension is the next most important factor in the development and progression of DKD because normotensive diabetic people with DKD progress at a lower rate than hypertensive patients with DKD.[39,40] Systemic hypertension contributes to the development and progression of DKD through progressive glomerular injury and proteinuria. The optimal target blood pressure has yet to be determined for managing diabetic people with DKD but the general consensus is to maintain it at less than 130/80 mm Hg to less than 140/90 mm Hg.

Activation of the RAAS in patients with diabetes is one of the underlying reasons for developing systemic hypertension. However, RAAS activation also directly contributes to intraglomerular hypertension (and injury) through additional mechanisms (see later discussion) independent of systemic hypertension. Therefore, angiotensin-converting enzyme (ACE) inhibitors (ACEi), AGII receptor blockers, and aldosterone antagonists are thought to improve outcomes in human patients with DKD by reducing intraglomerular hypertension, fibrosis, and inflammation.[41,42]

We provide a short review of RAAS below to highlight the intricacies of the intrarenal RAAS and their effects on the development of DKD. ACE converts angiotensin I (AGI) to AGII, which acts on the AGII type 1 receptor (AT1R). Chronic maladaptive activation of AT1R leads to vasoconstriction, inflammation, fibrosis, oxidative stress, and cellular proliferation.[43] Unlike the AT1R, the AGII type 2 receptor (AT2R) has vasodilatory, anti-inflammatory, antifibrotic, antioxidative, and antiproliferative effects.[44,45] AGII has lower affinity to AT2R than to AT1R and is converted by angiotensin-converting enzyme-related carboxypeptidase 2 (ACE2) to angiotensin (1–7),[46,47] which has a high-affinity to and acts on the Mas receptor (MASR) that has the same renoprotective effects as the AT2R.[48] ACE2 can also convert AGI to angiotensin (1–9), which is then converted by ACE or neprilysin (NEP) to angiotensin (1–7); NEP can also directly convert AGI to angiotensin (1–7).[49] Therefore, the ratio of activated AT1R versus AT2R/MASR has a critical effect on the development of DKD, with the former promoting DKD and the latter protecting against it.

ACE also has non-RAAS renal effects; ACE's N-domain cleaves its natural substrate N-acetyl-seryl-aspartyl-lysyl-proline (Ac-SDKP) into inactive fragments.[50,51] Nephrons release Ac-SDKP to prevent renal fibrosis[52,53] through the antifibrotic microRNAs (miR-29s and miR-let-7s)-mediated downregulation of dipeptidyl peptidase-4 and suppression of the TGF-β signaling pathway.[54] Thus, therapeutically, ACEi may have an antifibrotic effect outside of the RAAS by increasing the levels of renal Ac-SDKP.

Unlike ACE, ACE2 only has the C-catalytic domain that degrades angiotensins. Rodent models of DKD indicated that increased levels of ACE2 combined with decreased levels of ACE have renoprotective effects.[55] Immunogold electron microscopy localization study in rodents showed that ACE2 is localized to the podocytes and ACE to the glomerular endothelium.[56] It is speculated that ACE2 protects the podocytes and the glomerular filtration barrier from the deleterious effects that ensue with diabetes.

Histopathologic Changes in Diabetic Kidney Disease

The glomeruli in people with DKD have a set of characteristic morphologic changes,[16] including increased glomerular size (hypertrophy), mostly due to nodular (Kimmelstiel-Wilson) or diffuse deposition of mesangial hyaline matrix; thickening of endothelial basement membrane (BM) with occasional narrowing of capillary lumina; podocyte foot fusion or effacement and decreased podocyte density (podocyte death); and afferent and efferent arteriolar hyalinosis (progressive replacement of arteriolar wall myocytes by hyaline matrix composed of immunoglobulins, complement, and plasma proteins). The mesangium expansion could lead to abnormalities of the glomerular-tubular junction with focal adhesions, obstruction of the proximal tubular take-off from the glomerulus, and detachment of the tubule from the glomerulus (atubular glomeruli).[16] Tubular lesions involve focal to diffuse proximal tubular atrophy and interstitial fibrosis and are more characteristic of patients with T2DM.

To our knowledge, there are 3 reports with detailed pathologic condition of the kidneys of dogs and cats with spontaneous onset of DM[19–21] and 8 reports describing renal pathologic condition of dogs with experimentally induced DM.[57–64] Overall, the observed changes are reminiscent of those described above in people.[16] The changes in cats involve mild diffuse mesangial thickening with a Periodic acid–Schiff (PAS)-positive material, tubular atrophy, and tubulointerstitial inflammation. In dogs, the changes were predominantly restricted to the glomerulus and afferent arterioles, were uncommon, and included nodular or diffuse PAS-positive thickening of the mesangium and the afferent arteriolar wall.

Alloxan-induced or progestogen-induced DM resulted in similar changes in the kidneys. In 2 dogs with progestogen-induced diabetes, the changes in the glomeruli after 2 years of DM involved deposition of PAS-positive material in the mesangium (both nodular and diffuse forms) and thickening of the capillary BM. There were also multifocal subendothelial foci of fibrin deposition. These changes (excluding fibrin deposition) are similar to those also seen in dogs treated with porcine growth hormone and in dogs with experimentally induced DM following bovine pituitary growth hormone administration. Dogs with alloxan-induced DKD also exhibited periglomerular tubular atrophy and arteriolar hyalinosis.

Lipotoxicity and Inflammation

The glomerulosclerotic changes seen in DKD are not pathognomonic and share some overlapping features with obesity-associated nephropathy.[65,66] The overlap between obesity and T2DM (ie, lipotoxicity) is thought to contribute directly to the development of DKD and also through interference with insulin actions. Glomerular lipotoxic damage to the podocytes is thought to occur through formation of ROS from dysfunctional mitochondria, endoplasmic reticulum stress, and interference with the podocyte insulin signaling (which is considered an antiapoptotic signal[67]), all of which could lead to podocyte apoptosis, podocyte foot fusion, or foot retraction. Five hyperlipidemic cats with lipoprotein-lipase deficiency[68] had renal changes similar to those seen in DKD, suggesting that lipotoxicity mediates glomerular injury in DKD and in cats.

Monocytes and macrophages propagate the inflammation in DKD through releasing lysosomal enzymes, NO, ROS, TGFβ, VEGF, tumor necrosis factor, interleukin-1, and interferon gamma and targeting podocytes. During the development and progression of renal disease, macrophages are recruited to the kidney by the C-C chemokine receptor type 2. Interference of macrophage recruitment improved renal outcomes in mouse models of DKD and in human patients with T2DM DKD.[69,70] The NF-κB signaling pathway is activated in DKD. It mediates the inflammatory cascade and the Janus kinase (JAK)-STAT signaling pathway that is overactive in podocytes, mesangial cells, and renal tubular cells in DKD.[71,72] Furthermore, suppressors of cytokine signaling (SOCS1 and SOCS3) are underexpressed in DKD, and their negative feedback on the JAK-STAT signaling pathway is removed, thus accentuating the inflammatory process.[73,74]

Proteinuria and Renal Fibrosis

Alterations in the glomerular filtration barrier in the form of podocyte death, podocyte foot fusion or effacement, and loss of the glycocalyx component heparan sulfate (providing charge selectivity) result in albuminuria and are associated with urinary albumin excretion in T1DM and T2DM DKD.[75,76] In the glomerulus, albuminuria induces the production of the hyaline matrix by the mesangial cells. In the tubules, uptake of albumin leads to overwhelming of the lysosomal degradation process and to cell death. Hence, proteinuria promotes the development of inflammation and subsequent fibrosis.

Renal fibrosis is considered the final stage of DKD and is mediated by activated myofibroblasts. They are recruited to the renal interstitium from the transformation of mesenchymal stem cells and resident fibroblasts, recruitment of fibroblasts from the bone marrow, and tubuloepithelial to mesenchymal transdifferentiation.[77]

Clinical Perspective of Diabetic Kidney Disease in Dogs and Cats

Given the kidneys' massive reserve capacity and nephron redundancy, attrition of enough nephrons has to exhaust the renal reserve before chronic kidney disease (CKD) ensues. This presents a clinical challenge to assessing the longitudinal relationship of DM and CKD because the hyperfiltration associated with diabetic glucosuria might reduce renal filtration markers and thus a creatinine level might not be an accurate measure of nephron mass under these circumstances. Furthermore, there is overlap in the clinical signs between DM and CKD, and thus, early onset CKD clinical signs might be overlooked as poorly managed DM.

Potential Role of Inflammation

Both CKD[78,79] and obesity[80] have been shown to be associated with chronic inflammation. Understanding the cause-and-effect relationship between chronic disease and chronic inflammation is challenging because it is difficult to ascertain if the inflammatory state caused or was caused by the chronic disease process. In human medicine, both type 1 and type 2 DM have been shown to be associated with proinflammatory chemokine and cytokine signatures.[81] Obesity, which is strongly implicated in type 2 DM in people, is also considered a chronic inflammatory state.[80] Of interest in humans, the incidence of diabetic nephropathy in T2DM was twice that of type 1 diabetes in an age-matched cohort of patients aged younger than 30 years. In humans, there has been a steady increase in the number of cases of T2DM, and it is estimated that greater than 50% of human patients requiring renal replacement therapy have T2DM.[82]

Fluid Imbalances in Diabetes Mellitus and Chronic Kidney Disease

A further contributing factor in the development of CKD in dogs and cats could be explained by dehydration and fluid imbalances associated with DM. Dogs and cats diagnosed with DM tend to be older and therefore at a higher risk of CKD, and therefore, dehydration and fluid imbalance might exacerbate kidney disease. This is especially true in the case of DKA where severe fluid imbalances lead to hypovolemia necessitating volume resuscitation. DKA represents a potential double hit to the kidney because it is associated with both severe fluid imbalances and inflammation both of which could be injurious to the kidney. In 2 previous studies, 65% of dogs[83] and 61% of cats[84] with DKA were in newly diagnosed diabetics.

Urinary Tract Infections in Diabetes Mellitus and Chronic Kidney Disease

Concerns over the role of urinary tract infection (UTI) in the exacerbation of CKD in DM also deserve mention. In our experience, some veterinarians occasionally screen patients for UTIs in CKD due to a concern that a UTI could result in an ascending infection, exacerbating CKD. Because glucose is an excellent growth medium for bacteria many veterinarians have been taught that diabetics have a higher risk of UTI. However,

2 earlier studies in cats with CKD[85,86] showed no association with the presence of a UTI as defined by a positive urine culture and severity of azotemia and survival. In both studies, the authors acknowledged that antimicrobial treatment of UTI might have influenced the lack of association seen but the authors speculated that subclinical bacteriuria in CKD is unlikely to be a significant driver in the exacerbation of CKD. This is further supported by the fact that human patients with T2DM with asymptomatic bacteriuria (ASB) do not seem to be associated with adverse outcomes.[87] Furthermore, although it is intuitively logical that glucosuric patients are at an increased risk of a UTI, there is conflicting evidence on the role of glucosuria in DM and the etiopathogenesis of UTI in human patients with DM is complex.[87] In an in vitro study on uropathogenic bacterial growth in urine samples, glucose concentrations ranging between 100 and 1000 mg/dL enhanced bacterial growth but a decrease in bacterial growth was seen in when urinary glucose concentrations were very high (10,000 mg/dL).[88] Another clinical study in humans also showed an association between glucosuria and ASB in people[89] but this association was not seen in another large study in women with DM with ASB and was also not seen in another cohort of human patients with symptomatic UTIs.[90]

There is a paucity of veterinary studies pertaining to the incidence and risk factors of UTIs in DM. Furthermore, although there are parallels between humans and pets, the term ASB does not apply to pets and the term subclinical bacteriuria is used. It is more difficult to establish the presence of a clinical UTI in a nonverbal patient, and clinicians are often reliant on information from the client, which can be influenced by the owner's bias. In a retrospective study in cats,[91] the authors documented positive urine cultures in 12% of cats with diabetes with one cat displaying signs consistent with a UTI. These data were collected as part of the standard of care of that institution for cats with diabetes, and thus, cats were not specifically sampled if they had poor diabetic control or signs of lower UTIs. Therefore, it is plausible that most of the cats in this study might be more consistent with subclinical bacteriuria and might not represent a true UTI. These results were similar to another study with positive urinary cultures in 13% of 141 cats with diabetes.[92] In this study, the criteria for culture differed slightly from that of Mayer and colleagues[91] in that urine was collected for culture in cats that had signs of UTIs, poorly controlled diabetics or newly diagnosed diabetics. Unsurprisingly, the incidence of clinical UTIs (with signs consistent with lower urinary tract disease [LUTD]) was higher in this study where 44% had clinical signs attributable to LUTD. Bailiff and colleagues[92] documented an incidence of urine culture positivity in 11% of newly diagnosed cats with diabetes and suggested that because so many cases were subclinical that a UTI should not be excluded because of the absence of clinical signs. Interestingly, in this same study, 100% of cats with LUTD signs (8 out of 18 positive cases) had positive urine cultures. These studies highlight the need for further studies and standardized definitions in veterinary medicine. Both studies were conducted by reputable organizations and skilled clinicians, but the varied data are in part attributable to the variations in the criteria for testing, where in one institution it was part of a routine assessment for diabetics and in another the criteria for testing were more narrowly defined. We frequently encounter cases from referring veterinarians where they are unsure how to treat a recurring UTI in a veterinary patient with a recurrent positive culture and on further questioning, we determine that culture was performed with very little evidence of a LUTD as part of a geriatric assessment, for example, The ISCAID consensus statement on the management of UTIs is a useful resource for practitioners who are seeking guidance in managing UTIs in dogs and cats.[93]

As mentioned previously, ASB was not associated with adverse outcomes in T2DM human patients,[87] and treatment of ASB in DM has been shown to increase the risk for adverse events.[94] Therefore, subclinical bacteriuria is unlikely to be a significant contributor to the progression of renal disease. Urine culture should be performed when there are signs of LUTD. Other clinical scenarios where testing is sensible would be DKA, poorly controlled diabetics and cases with worsening renal parameters, or ultrasonographic evidence of upper or lower UTD.

Making a Diagnosis

In human medicine, the diagnostic criteria for diabetic nephropathy are a persistent estimated GFR (eGFR) of less than 60 mL/min/1.73 m² or an urinary albumin excretion of more than 30 mg/g or both.[82] Urinary protein loss is a major hallmark of diabetic nephropathy; however, recently there has been an observed increase in the proportion of patients with T2DM with nonalbuminuric CKD. The exact causes of this are unknown but are thought to be related in part to successful management of blood pressure and dyslipidemias in patients with T2DM and also an aging population where around 25% of individuals aged older than 65 years without T2DM have an eGFR of less than 60 mL/min/1.73 m².[82]

In small animal patients, the IRIS staging system to diagnose and manage CKD http://www.iris-kidney.com/guidelines/staging.html. Detecting and managing proteinuria is considered important due to the association with progression of CKD. The role of proteinuria and progression in CKD is particularly pertinent in the case of DM and CKD in pets because it highlights several gaps in our understanding. Although the association of proteinuria and CKD progression has been well established in the veterinary literature,[95,96] the causal relationship between the 2 remains unknown. It is possible that proteinuria could be associated with CKD progression due to nephron injury but it is also equally plausible that proteinuria is a marker of more severe renal injury that is more likely to progress. This has implications for the management of CKD because if proteinuria is merely an injury marker, ameliorating proteinuria might improve renal outcomes. Indeed, some previous studies suggest that this might be the case, where a reduction of proteinuria in patients was not associated with an improved outcome.[97] Furthermore, proteinuria does not seem to be consistently associated with renal disease progression in other disease states associated with CKD such as hyperthyroidism in cats.[98] As more effective pharmacologic and dietary strategies for the amelioration of proteinuria emerge, it will hopefully become evident if therapeutic reduction of proteinuria has a clinical benefit.

The confounding effect of glucosuria on urine specific gravity (USG) also could complicate the diagnosis of early CKD in DM. However, a recent study showed that the addition of glucose to urine did not significantly increase in USG, which suggests that USG is still a useful marker in the evaluation of a patient with CKD. Dogs and cats with DM tend to have USGs greater than 1.020[99] and therefore persistently isosthenuric urine in a patient with pu/pd should raise the concern for CKD in these cases. Clinicians should suspect CKD in well-controlled diabetic cases with persistent Pu/Pd.

Diabetic Kidney Disease and Diabetes Mellitus in Dogs and Cats

Only a few studies of DM and CKD in dogs and cats are available. In one study that investigated risk factors associated with CKD progression and survival,[100] DM was not identified as a comorbidity; however, this study was not designed to identify DKD. In another longitudinal study that was conducted during 2 years in 11 dogs with diabetes, 44% of dogs had proteinuria[101] but none of the dogs developed azotemia or signs of CKD during the study period. Of interest, as previously mentioned people with T1DM are half as likely to develop DKD compared with type 2.[82] In addition, it is plausible that dogs with diabetic that tend to be older, do not live long enough to develop azotemic DKD. The presence of proteinuria in the previously mentioned study was persistent in 36% of dogs, which would be classified as DKD in people. In another dog study, ultrasonographic evidence of renovascular resistance was shown using the resistive index.[102] This study also showed a positive correlation between increasing the renovascular resistance and glycated hemoglobin but the increased renovascular resistance was not correlated with systemic blood pressure or proteinuria.

Therefore, the presence of proteinuria and increased renovascular resistance seen in dogs with diabetes might increase the risk for DKD but the progression to CKD has not been shown to our knowledge.

Cats would be expected to be at a greater risk of DKD because their diabetes more closely resembles T2DM in people. Two retrospective studies in cats failed to show and association between DM and CKD in cats.[103,104] The retrospective nature of these studies does limit the inferences that can be derived from them but it should be noted that Green and colleagues (2014) involved a large number of cats (1230 cats) for a veterinary study. The data from this study was obtained from 755 primary care practices and thus represents the typical clinical presentation of cats with CKD. Interestingly, in this study, an earlier diagnosis of DM was associated with lower odds of CKD but the authors concluded that DM was unlikely to have a protective effect on the kidneys. The findings of these 2 retrospective studies differ from a more recent retrospective study in 561 cats presented to 2 referral hospitals.[105] In this study, 67 cats were diagnosed with CKD and 16 with DM. Furthermore, 44% of the DM cats were diagnosed with CKD and a multivariate analysis showed a significant association between DM and CKD. Another reason for the observed difference could in part be due to the fact that in one study, the data were obtained from primary care practices,[104] and in the other the study, data were derived from a university teaching hospital and an endocrinology clinic,[105] which might have resulted in some differences in the sample populations of cats.

SUMMARY

In conclusion, some clinical evidence in dogs and cats suggests that DKD might occur in some individuals. Based on these data, occasionally screening for CKD in pets with diabetes might be warranted. In many cases, biochemistry and urinalysis are performed 2 to 3 times a year in patients with diabetes depending on the level of control.

CLINICS CARE POINTS

- Although the pathomechanisms implicated in development of diabetic kidney disease in people are also present in companion animals with DM, there is no evidence that companion animals with diabetes will develop CKD leading to renal failure in their lifetime.
- Monitoring for CKD in cats and dogs with diabetes might be warranted based on the human literature and a paucity of studies in companion animals.

DECLARATION OF INTERESTS

The authors declare no competing interests.

REFERENCES

1. Gilbertson DT, Liu J, Xue JL, et al. Projecting the number of patients with end-stage renal disease in the United States to the year 2015. J Am Soc Nephrol 2005;16(12):3736–41.
2. Umanath K, Lewis JB. Update on Diabetic Nephropathy: Core Curriculum 2018. Am J Kidney Dis 2018;71(6):884–95.
3. Markus MRP, Ittermann T, Baumeister SE, et al. Prediabetes is associated with microalbuminuria, reduced kidney function and chronic kidney disease in the general population: The KORA (Cooperative Health Research in the Augsburg Region) F4-Study. Nutr Metab Cardiovasc Dis 2018;28(3):234–42.
4. American Diabetes A. 6. Glycemic Targets: Standards of Medical Care in Diabetes-2018. Diabetes Care 2018;41(Suppl 1):S55–64.
5. Diabetes C, Complications Trial Research G, Nathan DM, et al. The effect of intensive treatment of diabetes on the development and progression of long-term complications in insulin-dependent diabetes mellitus. N Engl J Med 1993;329(14):977–86.
6. Stratton IM, Adler AI, Neil HA, et al. Association of glycaemia with macrovascular and microvascular complications of type 2 diabetes (UKPDS 35): prospective observational study. BMJ 2000;321(7258):405–12.
7. Alsahli M, Gerich JE. Renal glucose metabolism in normal physiological conditions and in diabetes. Diabetes Res Clin Pract 2017;133:1–9.
8. Thomson SC, Blantz RC. Glomerulotubular balance, tubuloglomerular feedback, and salt homeostasis. J Am Soc Nephrol 2008;19(12):2272–5.
9. Sallstrom J, Carlsson PO, Fredholm BB, et al. Diabetes-induced hyperfiltration in adenosine A(1)-receptor deficient mice lacking the tubuloglomerular feedback mechanism. Acta Physiol (Oxf) 2007;190(3):253–9.
10. Vallon V, Schroth J, Satriano J, et al. Adenosine A(1) receptors determine glomerular hyperfiltration and the salt paradox in early streptozotocin diabetes mellitus. Nephron Physiol 2009;111(3):p30–8.
11. Vallon V, Blantz RC, Thomson S. Glomerular hyperfiltration and the salt paradox in early [corrected] type 1 diabetes mellitus: a tubulo-centric view. J Am Soc Nephrol 2003;14(2):530–7.
12. Tonneijck L, Muskiet MH, Smits MM, et al. Glomerular Hyperfiltration in Diabetes: Mechanisms, Clinical Significance, and Treatment. J Am Soc Nephrol 2017; 28(4):1023–39.
13. Altay S, Onat A, Ozpamuk-Karadeniz F, et al. Renal "hyperfiltrators" are at elevated risk of death and chronic diseases. BMC Nephrol 2014;15:160.
14. Rigalleau V, Garcia M, Lasseur C, et al. Large kidneys predict poor renal outcome in subjects with diabetes and chronic kidney disease. BMC Nephrol 2010;11:3.
15. Tuttle KR, Bruton JL, Perusek MC, et al. Effect of strict glycemic control on renal hemodynamic response to amino acids and renal enlargement in insulin-dependent diabetes mellitus. N Engl J Med 1991;324(23):1626–32.
16. Fioretto P, Mauer M. Histopathology of diabetic nephropathy. Semin Nephrol 2007;27(2):195–207.
17. Fioretto P, Mauer M, Brocco E, et al. Patterns of renal injury in NIDDM patients with microalbuminuria. Diabetologia 1996;39(12):1569–76.
18. Steinberg HO, Brechtel G, Johnson A, et al. Insulin-mediated skeletal muscle vasodilation is nitric oxide dependent. A novel action of insulin to increase nitric oxide release. J Clin Invest 1994;94(3):1172–9.

19. Gepts W, Toussaint D. Spontaneous diabetes in dogs and cats. A pathological study. Diabetologia 1967;3(2):249–65.
20. Nakayama H, Uchida K, Ono K, et al. Pathological observation of six cases of feline diabetes mellitus. Nihon Juigaku Zasshi 1990;52(4):819–22.
21. Zini E, Benali S, Coppola L, et al. Renal morphology in cats with diabetes mellitus. Vet Pathol 2014;51(6):1143–50.
22. Layton AT, Laghmani K, Vallon V, et al. Solute transport and oxygen consumption along the nephrons: effects of Na+ transport inhibitors. Am J Physiol Renal Physiol 2016;311(6):F1217–29.
23. Vallon V, Richter K, Blantz RC, et al. Glomerular hyperfiltration in experimental diabetes mellitus: potential role of tubular reabsorption. J Am Soc Nephrol 1999;10(12):2569–76.
24. Garcia-Pastor C, Benito-Martinez S, Moreno-Manzano V, et al. Mechanism and Consequences of The Impaired Hif-1alpha Response to Hypoxia in Human Proximal Tubular HK-2 Cells Exposed to High Glucose. Sci Rep 2019;9(1): 15868.
25. Persson P, Palm F. Hypoxia-inducible factor activation in diabetic kidney disease. Curr Opin Nephrol Hypertens 2017;26(5):345–50.
26. Lanaspa MA, Ishimoto T, Cicerchi C, et al. Endogenous fructose production and fructokinase activation mediate renal injury in diabetic nephropathy. J Am Soc Nephrol 2014;25(11):2526–38.
27. Cirillo P, Gersch MS, Mu W, et al. Ketohexokinase-dependent metabolism of fructose induces proinflammatory mediators in proximal tubular cells. J Am Soc Nephrol 2009;20(3):545–53.
28. Ishimoto T, Lanaspa MA, Le MT, et al. Opposing effects of fructokinase C and A isoforms on fructose-induced metabolic syndrome in mice. Proc Natl Acad Sci U S A 2012;109(11):4320–5.
29. Brownlee M. Biochemistry and molecular cell biology of diabetic complications. Nature 2001;414(6865):813–20.
30. Griendling KK, Minieri CA, Ollerenshaw JD, et al. Angiotensin II stimulates NADH and NADPH oxidase activity in cultured vascular smooth muscle cells. Circ Res 1994;74(6):1141–8.
31. Cave AC, Brewer AC, Narayanapanicker A, et al. NADPH oxidases in cardiovascular health and disease. Antioxid Redox Signal 2006;8(5–6):691–728.
32. Singh DK, Winocour P, Farrington K. Oxidative stress in early diabetic nephropathy: fueling the fire. Nat Rev Endocrinol 2011;7(3):176–84.
33. Schleicher ED, Weigert C. Role of the hexosamine biosynthetic pathway in diabetic nephropathy. Kidney Int Suppl 2000;77:S13–8.
34. Gal A. Gut Microbial Whole-Genome Gene Networks and Metabolic Pathways Analysis in Diabetic Cats. 2022:52. doi:10.1111/jvim.16541.
35. Inoguchi T, Li P, Umeda F, et al. High glucose level and free fatty acid stimulate reactive oxygen species production through protein kinase C--dependent activation of NAD(P)H oxidase in cultured vascular cells. Diabetes 2000;49(11): 1939–45.
36. Schaffer SW, Jong CJ, Mozaffari M. Role of oxidative stress in diabetes-mediated vascular dysfunction: unifying hypothesis of diabetes revisited. Vascul Pharmacol 2012;57(5–6):139–49.
37. Ding Y, Choi ME. Autophagy in diabetic nephropathy. J Endocrinol 2015;224(1): R15–30.

38. Xin W, Li Z, Xu Y, et al. Autophagy protects human podocytes from high glucose-induced injury by preventing insulin resistance. Metabolism 2016; 65(9):1307–15.
39. Group AS, Cushman WC, Evans GW, et al. Effects of intensive blood-pressure control in type 2 diabetes mellitus. N Engl J Med 2010;362(17):1575–85.
40. Xie X, Atkins E, Lv J, et al. Effects of intensive blood pressure lowering on cardiovascular and renal outcomes: updated systematic review and meta-analysis. Lancet 2016;387(10017):435–43.
41. Bolignano D, Palmer SC, Navaneethan SD, et al. Aldosterone antagonists for preventing the progression of chronic kidney disease. Cochrane Database Syst Rev 2014;29(4):CD007004.
42. Ruggenenti P, Cravedi P, Remuzzi G. The RAAS in the pathogenesis and treatment of diabetic nephropathy. Nat Rev Nephrol 2010;6(6):319–30.
43. Forrester SJ, Booz GW, Sigmund CD, et al. Angiotensin II Signal Transduction: An Update on Mechanisms of Physiology and Pathophysiology. Physiol Rev 2018;98(3):1627–738.
44. Horiuchi M, Akishita M, Dzau VJ. Recent progress in angiotensin II type 2 receptor research in the cardiovascular system. Hypertension 1999;33(2):613–21.
45. Kaschina E, Namsolleck P, Unger T. AT2 receptors in cardiovascular and renal diseases. Pharmacol Res 2017;125(Pt A):39–47.
46. Donoghue M, Hsieh F, Baronas E, et al. A novel angiotensin-converting enzyme-related carboxypeptidase (ACE2) converts angiotensin I to angiotensin 1-9. Circ Res 2000;87(5):E1–9.
47. Hamming I, Cooper ME, Haagmans BL, et al. The emerging role of ACE2 in physiology and disease. J Pathol 2007;212(1):1–11.
48. Rodrigues Prestes TR, Rocha NP, Miranda AS, et al. The Anti-Inflammatory Potential of ACE2/Angiotensin-(1-7)/Mas Receptor Axis: Evidence from Basic and Clinical Research. Curr Drug Targets 2017;18(11):1301–13.
49. Rice GI, Thomas DA, Grant PJ, et al. Evaluation of angiotensin-converting enzyme (ACE), its homologue ACE2 and neprilysin in angiotensin peptide metabolism. Biochem J 2004;383(Pt 1):45–51.
50. Fuchs S, Xiao HD, Cole JM, et al. Role of the N-terminal catalytic domain of angiotensin-converting enzyme investigated by targeted inactivation in mice. J Biol Chem 2004;279(16):15946–53.
51. Fuchs S, Xiao HD, Hubert C, et al. Angiotensin-converting enzyme C-terminal catalytic domain is the main site of angiotensin I cleavage in vivo. Hypertension 2008;51(2):267–74.
52. Romero CA, Kumar N, Nakagawa P, et al. Renal release of N-acetyl-seryl-aspartyl-lysyl-proline is part of an antifibrotic peptidergic system in the kidney. Am J Physiol Renal Physiol 2019;316(1):F195–203.
53. Zuo Y, Chun B, Potthoff SA, et al. Thymosin beta4 and its degradation product, Ac-SDKP, are novel reparative factors in renal fibrosis. Kidney Int 2013;84(6): 1166–75.
54. Srivastava SP, Goodwin JE, Kanasaki K, et al. Inhibition of Angiotensin-Converting Enzyme Ameliorates Renal Fibrosis by Mitigating DPP-4 Level and Restoring Antifibrotic MicroRNAs. Genes 2020;11(2). https://doi.org/10.3390/genes11020211.
55. Ye M, Wysocki J, Naaz P, et al. Increased ACE 2 and decreased ACE protein in renal tubules from diabetic mice: a renoprotective combination? Hypertension 2004;43(5):1120–5.

56. Ye M, Wysocki J, William J, et al. Glomerular localization and expression of Angiotensin-converting enzyme 2 and Angiotensin-converting enzyme: implications for albuminuria in diabetes. J Am Soc Nephrol 2006;17(11):3067–75.

57. Bloodworth JM Jr, Engerman RL, Powers KL. Experimental diabetic microangiopathy. I. Basement membrane statistics in the dog. Diabetes 1969;18(7): 455–8.

58. Engerman RL, Kern TS. Hyperglycemia and development of glomerular pathology: diabetes compared with galactosemia. Kidney Int 1989;36(1):41–5.

59. Engerman RL, Kern TS, Garment MB. Capillary basement membrane in retina, kidney, and muscle of diabetic dogs and galactosemic dogs and its response to 5 years aldose reductase inhibition. J Diabetes Complications 1993;7(4):241–5.

60. Gaber L, Walton C, Brown S, et al. Effects of different antihypertensive treatments on morphologic progression of diabetic nephropathy in uninephrectomized dogs. Kidney Int 1994;46(1):161–9.

61. Kern TS, Engerman RL. Kidney morphology in experimental hyperglycemia. Diabetes 1987;36(2):244–9.

62. Molon-Noblot S, Laroque P, Prahalada S, et al. Morphological changes in the kidney of dogs chronically exposed to exogenous growth hormone. Toxicol Pathol 2000;28(4):510–7.

63. Sloan JM, Oliver IM. Progestogen-induced diabetes in the dog. Diabetes 1975; 24(4):337–44.

64. Steffes MW, Buchwald H, Wigness BD, et al. Diabetic nephropathy in the uninephrectomized dog: microscopic lesions after one year. Kidney Int 1982;21(5): 721–4.

65. Chen HM, Liu ZH, Zeng CH, et al. Podocyte lesions in patients with obesity-related glomerulopathy. Am J Kidney Dis 2006;48(5):772–9.

66. de Vries AP, Ruggenenti P, Ruan XZ, et al. Fatty kidney: emerging role of ectopic lipid in obesity-related renal disease. Lancet Diabetes Endocrinol May 2014; 2(5):417–26.

67. Jiang T, Wang Z, Proctor G, et al. Diet-induced obesity in C57BL/6J mice causes increased renal lipid accumulation and glomerulosclerosis via a sterol regulatory element-binding protein-1c-dependent pathway. J Biol Chem 2005;280(37): 32317–25.

68. Thompson JC, Johnstone AC, Jones BR, et al. The ultrastructural pathology of five lipoprotein lipase-deficient cats. J Comp Pathol 1989;101(3):251–62.

69. Awad AS, Kinsey GR, Khutsishvili K, et al. Monocyte/macrophage chemokine receptor CCR2 mediates diabetic renal injury. Am J Physiol Renal Physiol 2011;301(6):F1358–66.

70. You H, Gao T, Cooper TK, et al. Macrophages directly mediate diabetic renal injury. Am J Physiol Renal Physiol 2013;305(12):F1719–27.

71. Berthier CC, Zhang H, Schin M, et al. Enhanced expression of Janus kinase-signal transducer and activator of transcription pathway members in human diabetic nephropathy. Diabetes 2009;58(2):469–77.

72. Woroniecka KI, Park AS, Mohtat D, et al. Transcriptome analysis of human diabetic kidney disease. Diabetes 2011;60(9):2354–69.

73. Ortiz-Munoz G, Lopez-Parra V, Lopez-Franco O, et al. Suppressors of cytokine signaling abrogate diabetic nephropathy. J Am Soc Nephrol 2010;21(5):763–72.

74. Zhang H, Nair V, Saha J, et al. Podocyte-specific JAK2 overexpression worsens diabetic kidney disease in mice. Kidney Int 2017;92(4):909–21.

75. Pagtalunan ME, Miller PL, Jumping-Eagle S, et al. Podocyte loss and progressive glomerular injury in type II diabetes. J Clin Invest 1997;99(2):342–8.

76. Steffes MW, Schmidt D, McCrery R, et al. International Diabetic Nephropathy Study G. Glomerular cell number in normal subjects and in type 1 diabetic patients. Kidney Int 2001;59(6):2104–13.

77. Thomas MC, Brownlee M, Susztak K, et al. Diabetic kidney disease. Nat Rev Dis Primers 2015;1:15018.

78. Habenicht LM, Webb TL, Clauss LA, et al. Urinary cytokine levels in apparently healthy cats and cats with chronic kidney disease. J Feline Med Surg 2013; 15(2):99–104.

79. Ebert T, Pawelzik S-C, Witasp A, et al. Inflammation and Premature Ageing in Chronic Kidney Disease. Toxins 2020;12(4):227.

80. Rohm TV, Meier DT, Olefsky JM, et al. Inflammation in obesity, diabetes, and related disorders. Immunity 2022;55(1):31–55.

81. Herder C, Hermanns N. Subclinical inflammation and depressive symptoms in patients with type 1 and type 2 diabetes. Semin Immunopathol 2019;41(4): 477–89.

82. Thomas MC, Cooper ME, Zimmet P. Changing epidemiology of type 2 diabetes mellitus and associated chronic kidney disease. Nat Rev Nephrol 2016;12(2): 73–81.

83. Hume DZ, Drobatz KJ, Hess RS. Outcome of dogs with diabetic ketoacidosis: 127 dogs (1993-2003). J Vet Intern Med 2006;20(3):547–55.

84. Bruskiewicz KA, Nelson RW, Feldman EC, et al. Diabetic ketosis and ketoacidosis in cats: 42 cases (1980-1995). J Am Vet Med Assoc 1997;211(2):188–92.

85. Hindar C, Chang Y-M, Syme HM, et al. The association of bacteriuria with survival and disease progression in cats with azotemic chronic kidney disease. J Vet Intern Med 2020;34(6):2516–24.

86. White JD, Stevenson M, Malik R, et al. Urinary tract infections in cats with chronic kidney disease. J Feline Med Surg 2013;15(6):459–65.

87. Geerlings S, Fonseca V, Castro-Diaz D, et al. Genital and urinary tract infections in diabetes: Impact of pharmacologically-induced glucosuria. Diabetes Res Clin Pract 2014;103(3):373–81.

88. Geerlings SE, Brouwer EC, Gaastra W, et al. Effect of glucose and pH on uropathogenic and non-uropathogenic Escherichia coli: studies with urine from diabetic and non-diabetic individuals. J Med Microbiol 1999;48(6):535–9.

89. Turan H, Serefhanoglu K, Torun AN, et al. Frequency, risk factors, and responsible pathogenic microorganisms of asymptomatic bacteriuria in patients with type 2 diabetes mellitus. Jpn J Infect Dis 2008;61(3):236–8.

90. Geerlings SE, Stolk RP, Camps MJ, et al. Risk factors for symptomatic urinary tract infection in women with diabetes. Diabetes Care 2000;23(12):1737–41.

91. Mayer-Roenne B, Goldstein RE, Erb HN. Urinary tract infections in cats with hyperthyroidism, diabetes mellitus and chronic kidney disease. J Feline Med Surg 2007;9(2):124–32.

92. Bailiff NL, Nelson RW, Feldman EC, et al. Frequency and Risk Factors for Urinary Tract Infection in Cats with Diabetes Mellitus. J Vet Intern Med 2006;20(4):850.

93. Weese JS, Blondeau J, Boothe D, et al. International Society for Companion Animal Infectious Diseases (ISCAID) guidelines for the diagnosis and management of bacterial urinary tract infections in dogs and cats. Vet J 2019;247:8–25.

94. Luu T, Albarillo FS. Asymptomatic Bacteriuria: Prevalence, Diagnosis, Management, and Current Antimicrobial Stewardship Implementations. Am J Med 2022; 135(8):e236–44.

95. Chakrabarti S, Syme HM, Elliott J. Clinicopathological Variables Predicting Progression of Azotemia in Cats with Chronic Kidney Disease. J Vet Intern Med 2012;26(2):275–81.

96. Miyakawa H, Ogawa M, Sakatani A, et al. Evaluation of the progression of non-azotemic proteinuric chronic kidney disease in dogs. Res Vet Sci 2021; 138:11–8.

97. King JN, Font A, Rousselot JF, et al. Effects of Benazepril on Survival of Dogs with Chronic Kidney Disease: A Multicenter, Randomized, Blinded, Placebo-Controlled Clinical Trial. J Vet Intern Med 2017;31(4):1113–22.

98. Williams TL, Peak KJ, Brodbelt D, et al. Survival and the Development of Azotemia after Treatment of Hyperthyroid Cats. J Vet Intern Med 2010;24(4): 863–9.

99. Feldman EC. Textbook of Veterinary Internal Medicine. Polyuria and polydipsia, 1. Elsevier; 2009.

100. O'Neill DG, Elliott J, Church DB, et al. Chronic Kidney Disease in Dogs in UK Veterinary Practices: Prevalence, Risk Factors, and Survival. J Vet Intern Med 2013;27(4):814–21.

101. Herring IP, Panciera DL, Werre SR. Longitudinal Prevalence of Hypertension, Proteinuria, and Retinopathy in Dogs with Spontaneous Diabetes Mellitus. J Vet Intern Med 2014;28(2):488–95.

102. Priyanka M, Jeyaraja K, Thirunavakkarasu PS. Abnormal renovascular resistance in dogs with diabetes mellitus: correlation with glycemic status and proteinuria. Iran J Vet Res. Fall 2018;19(4):304–9.

103. Bartlett PC, Van Buren JW, Bartlett AD, et al. Case-control study of risk factors associated with feline and canine chronic kidney disease. Vet Med Int 2010; 20:2010.

104. Greene JP, Lefebvre SL, Wang M, et al. Risk factors associated with the development of chronic kidney disease in cats evaluated at primary care veterinary hospitals. J Am Vet Med Assoc 2014;244(3):320–7.

105. Pérez-López L, Boronat M, Melián C, et al. Assessment of the association between diabetes mellitus and chronic kidney disease in adult cats. J Vet Intern Med 2019;33(5):1921–5.

Anesthetic Considerations in Dogs and Cats with Diabetes Mellitus

Renata S. Costa, DVM, MPhil, GradDipEd, MANZCVS, DACVAA[a],*,
Teela Jones, DVM, MVetSc, DACVAA[b]

KEYWORDS

- Anesthesia • Diabetes mellitus • Dog • Cat • Insulin • Glucose

KEY POINTS

- Whenever possible, procedures for diabetic patients should be performed early in the day to ensure a rapid return to the patient's normal feeding, and insulin regimen and allow for close postoperative monitoring.
- Stabilization of hydration and acid–base status, electrolytes, and blood glucose in diabetic patients before anesthesia is paramount.
- Although there is no consensus regarding preoperative insulin protocol, administration of one-fourth to one-half of the patient's regular dose may result in superior glycemic control compared with withholding insulin or administration of the patients' full dose.
- Blood glucose monitoring every 30 to 60 min will direct additional insulin and dextrose therapy.
- There are no contraindications to any specific anesthetic, analgesic, or sedative agents. Care should be taken with the administration of alpha-2 agonists because they might result in a transient increase in blood glucose. Anesthetic protocols should be tailored to the patient's overall health status, level of anticipated pain, and duration of the procedure.

INTRODUCTION

Dogs and cats with diabetes mellitus (DM) may require anesthesia or sedation for medical and surgical procedures. These procedures may be needed to treat conditions that contribute to insulin resistance such as dental disease, to treat comorbidities secondary to DM, such as cataracts, or they may not be directly related to the disease process. An understanding of the impact of DM on hydration, electrolyte,

[a] Specialty Medicine, Midwestern University, 5715 West Utopia Road, Office 323-K, Glendale, AZ 85308, USA; [b] Anesthesiologist, Summit Veterinary Referral Center, 2505 South 80th Street, Tacoma, WA 98409, USA
* Corresponding author.
E-mail address: Renata.costa.vaa@gmail.com

Vet Clin Small Anim 53 (2023) 581–589
https://doi.org/10.1016/j.cvsm.2023.01.002
0195-5616/23/© 2023 Elsevier Inc. All rights reserved.

and acid–base status is necessary to properly manage these animals during the perioperative period.

DM commonly affects middle-aged-to-geriatric dogs and cats. In dogs, the disease occurs following pancreatic beta cell loss, resulting in inadequate insulin secretion and hyperglycemia. The canine form of DM bears some phenotypic resemblance to type 1 DM in people (but the underlying cause of beta cell loss is yet undetermined). In most cats, DM resembles type 2 DM in people in that it is the result of impaired insulin secretion and the inability to increase insulin production to adequately compensate for insulin resistance.[1-5] In approximately one-fourth of cats, DM is secondary to hypersomatotropism. Although the causes of canine and feline DM are different, the initial management may include the administration of exogenous insulin to maintain blood glucose (BG) homeostasis and close monitoring is needed to assess treatment adequacy.[6] Stabilization of BG concentrations and resolution of clinical signs indicate successful management. It is important to note that even in treated and stable diabetic dogs, tight glycemic control (euglycemia with BG levels of 60 to 130 mg/dL) may not be achieved. Glycemic levels of well-controlled DM dogs vary throughout the day and BG excursions of 400 to 600 mg/dL could occur. Serial BG monitoring during the perioperative period with the understanding of this expected BG fluctuations throughout the day should guide therapy. Careful administration of exogenous insulin will decrease the risk of the development of hypoglycemic episodes.

Hyperglycemia (BG > 200 mg/dL in dogs and > 270 mg/dL in cats with classic clinical signs of hyperglycemia) is the hallmark of diagnosis of DM and results from impaired uptake of glucose into tissues and increased hepatic gluconeogenesis.[7] Other common serum biochemistry abnormalities include increased liver enzyme activity, cholesterol, and triglycerides. Glucosuria occurs when plasma glucose concentrations exceed the renal threshold. These changes often result in osmotic diuresis, polyuria, and polydipsia (PU/PD). Hyperglycemia increases serum osmolality. Cellular dehydration due to fluid shift from the intracellular into the intravascular space, systemic dehydration, and hypovolemia might ensue. Common electrolyte imbalances in patients with DM include hypokalemia, hypernatremia, hyponatremia, hypophosphatemia, and hypochloremia.[8-13] In dogs, higher morbidity, depression of leukocyte function, increased wound infections, and decreased tissue perfusion have been associated with high BG concentrations.[9,10] Chronic hyperglycemia (>5 years) might lead to retinopathy in dogs with poorly controlled diabetes.[9] As a catabolic condition, DM leads to a reduction in energy stores, protein mass, and ultimately weight loss. These possible alterations in homeostasis increase the overall anesthetic risk in animals with DM.

Diabetic ketoacidosis (DKA) is a decompensated form of DM. This condition occurs when free fatty acids are used as an energy source. Under the influence of low insulin and high glucagon concentrations (relative to one another), free fatty acids are broken down into ketoacids. Excessive accumulation of ketoacids and glucose in the blood results in life-threatening metabolic disturbances such as metabolic acidosis and hypovolemia. Another less common but possible form of decompensation of animals with DM is a hyperglycemic hyperosmolar syndrome (HHS). This syndrome occurs due to persistent hyperglycemia with BG levels reaching more than 600 mg/dL and decreased access to water followed by decreased glomerular filtration rate. Animals with DKA, HHS, or both, are rarely anesthetized until after emergent treatment of fluid and electrolyte imbalances is performed and insulin is administered to control profound hyperglycemia. Whenever possible, stabilization of animals with severe or uncontrolled disease processes should be performed.

ANESTHETIC CONSIDERATIONS AND MANAGEMENT

Planned procedures for animals with DM should be performed early in the day to allow for rapid return to normal feeding and insulin regimens post-procedure and aimed to minimize the influence of circadian changes in BG concentrations.[14–18] Complete physical examination including baseline blood pressure (BP) and blood work (complete blood count and biochemistry with electrolytes) should be obtained in all dogs and cats with DM before anesthesia. Diabetic patients might be dehydrated, hypovolemic, or both, especially if fasted or anorexic for long periods of time and if PU/PD is still present. Therefore, before anesthesia or sedation, fluid therapy to correct dehydration and electrolyte imbalances should be instituted. Hydration status, acid–base status, and electrolyte imbalances assessment and correction are also imperative in severely hyperglycemic animals and those with DKA or HHS. Dogs with insulin resistance might have concurrent hyperadrenocorticism.[11] This would also require management before anesthesia when possible.

BG concentrations should be closely monitored and will help ensure the appropriate insulin therapy required for each individual patient. Note that a single morning preoperative BG concentration higher than 300 mg/dL does not necessarily mean inadequate glycemic control. Stress hyperglycemia during hospitalization and before procedures may result in increased BG levels. BG should be re-measured in a calmer place within 30 min and further increases in BG may indicate the need for insulin administration before anesthesia.[12–14]

Preoperative Fasting and Insulin Regimen

Although various fasting times and insulin administration protocols have been recommended before anesthesia, there is no consensus statement in veterinary medicine.[12–16,19] In addition, data on pre-anesthetic fasting duration and the incidence of perioperative complications such as regurgitation and gastroesophageal reflux (GER) are controversial. A study in healthy dogs suggested that shorter fasting times (2 to 4 h vs 12 to 18 h) decrease the risk of GER.[20] However, another study reported that consumption of a light meal 3 h (vs 18 h) before anesthesia was associated with greater odds of GER and regurgitation in dogs.[21] In a study of diabetic dogs, no differences in perioperative complications and perioperative BG concentrations were found in animals that were fasted for 12 h and received one-half of their usual insulin dose, and those that were fasted for 6 h and received their full insulin dose.[19] The authors' clinical approach is to aim for fasting times no longer than 12 h to avoid prolonged food withholding and, also, to minimize the risk of subclinical dehydration. For morning procedures, food may be withheld the evening before surgery after 10 pm but a small amount of food could be given in the morning before insulin administration. The optimal fasting time should be determined independently of a patient's daily insulin regimen. Regardless of the daily insulin regimen, adjustments to dose, frequency, or insulin formulation can be made to fast the patient safely for as long as is recommended by the anesthesiologist. More details on managing insulin in a fasted patient can be found elsewhere (Insulin therapy part 1: General Principles, Insulin therapy part 2: Dogs, and Insulin therapy part 3: Cats).

A target BG of 150 to 250 mg/dL has been recommended[12] for patients under anesthesia. There are currently no data, however, on the association between levels of glycemic control and post-procedural or long-term outcomes. Based on the available literature, administration of one-fourth to one-half of the usual insulin dose before anesthesia might provide superior perioperative glycemic control in comparison to withholding insulin completely.[15,16] This recommendation though, is only relevant to patients that are treated with intermediate-acting insulin formulations. In patients treated with basal insulin, there is typically no need for dose reduction in preparation for fasting. Stress-induced-hyperglycemia and increased catecholamine release can promote glycogenolysis, gluconeogenesis, and ketogenesis, which can increase insulin requirements. Preoperative hyperglycemia can result in hyperosmolar diuresis, dehydration, and hypovolemia increasing the risk and severity of intraoperative hypotension.[14,22–24]

Some authors recommend dosing insulin based on baseline BG measurements obtained on the morning of the procedure.[12–14] The same authors, however, recognize the limitations of using single BG measurements to predict insulin requirements. This is even more critical considering the unpredictable pharmacodynamics of most insulin formulations used in veterinary medicine. Careful glucose monitoring is required peri-operatively. We recommend the administration of one-half of the usual insulin dose before anesthesia and another one-fourth dose of insulin if baseline morning BG level is above 250 mg/dL. A safer but more elaborate approach would be to maintain BG concentration either with a CRI of insulin or by administering an ultra-rapid-acting insulin formulation and adjusting the insulin dose based on continuous monitoring. Regardless of the chosen protocol, overzealous insulin administration is best avoided to decrease the risk of hypoglycemia intra- and postoperatively.

Perioperative Blood Glucose Monitoring

BG should be monitored before and after induction of anesthesia, and every 30 to 60 min intraoperatively. Frequency of monitoring may vary depending on BG measured and patient's stability. Continuous glucose monitoring (CGM) device provides close monitoring capabilities and, therefore, if already present, could be used to monitor BG levels throughout anesthesia. If the BG concentration 30 min after induction of anesthesia is similar to the baseline value and within 150 to 250 mg/dL, glucose can be rechecked after 60 min instead of 30 min. However, if BG concentrations show large fluctuations, closer monitoring and possible interventions may be needed. Persistent hyperglycemia above 300 mg/dL may be treated with regular insulin intravenous (IV) or intramuscular (IM) at 20% of the patient's usual dosage of long-acting insulin.[12] Alternatively, the authors also suggest managing persistent hyperglycemia with the administration of 0.1 U/kg IM regular insulin. Development of hypoglycemia necessitates treatment with dextrose infusions (usually 2.5% to 5% at a rate of 5 to 10 mL/kg/h for dogs and 3 to 5 mL/kg/h for cats). Patients with DKA or HHS require more intensive monitoring, regular insulin, and/or dextrose administration, particularly in emergency situations when stabilization of acid–base status and electrolyte abnormalities were not performed preoperatively.

Intraoperative Anesthetic Management

Hypotension and bradycardia are the most commonly reported intraoperative complications in diabetic dogs undergoing phacoemulsification surgery and are reported more frequently in diabetic compared with nondiabetic dogs.[23] This higher risk of hypotension might be due to preexisting hypovolemia secondary to hyperglycemia and osmotic diuresis.[23] Cardiac index of parasympathetic activity was found to be lower in diabetic dogs compared with nondiabetic dogs, although the influence of this lower vagal tone on the development of hypotension was not investigated.[23] Goal-directed IV fluid therapy should be instituted in animals with DM undergoing any procedure. Crystalloid fluids (ie, LRS or Normosol-R) at 5 to 10 mL/kg/h for dogs and 3 to 5 mL/kg/h for cats is adequate for surgical fluid rates in most cases. However, other comorbidities such as heart disease and hydration status need to be considered when selecting the most appropriate fluid rate. It is vital that ECG and BP be closely monitored throughout anesthesia.

Dogs with DM may have other comorbidities present such as hypertension.[25] Systemic hypertension, possibly due to increases in peripheral vascular resistance, has been reported in 46% (23/50) of dogs with diabetes.[26,27] Some animals require treatment with antihypertensive medications that could result in severe or refractory hypotension intraoperatively.[28,29] In these cases, positive inotropic agents and/or vasopressors in addition to appropriate volume repletion may be required to manage BP. Invasive BP monitoring, which is the gold standard of BP monitoring is recommended in hypertensive patients, and in any case considered severe or challenging. Noninvasive oscillometric or Doppler BP monitoring and capnography would suffice in absence of invasive pressures.

Perioperative hypothermia is a common complication of anesthesia and sedation, and it can be exacerbated by the low body condition scores of some animals with DM.[23] Hypothermia results in several adverse effects including impaired wound healing and infections. Animals with DM might already be predisposed to delayed wound healing and infections, which is partly due to decreased tissue perfusion. Therefore, active warming should be instituted throughout the anesthetic period. In addition, normal body temperature will support the maintenance of normal physiological variables such as HR and BP and will increase the likelihood of smooth and rapid anesthetic recoveries.

Some dogs and cats with DM are obese, which could affect ventilation during anesthesia. Hypoventilation, especially when a patient is positioned in dorsal recumbency, could be managed with intermittent positive pressure ventilation. Preoxygenation is also recommended to increase the time to desaturation during induction of anesthesia and before endotracheal intubation.[30] Pulse oximetry and capnography are important to assess oxygenation and ventilation during anesthesia. Oxygen supplementation during the recovery period may also be advised, particularly in animals that are hypothermic and shivering, and if desaturation is observed on pulse oximetry.

Anesthetic Protocol

There are no absolute drug contraindications for diabetic patients and a balanced anesthetic protocol with reversible, short-acting drugs that do not, or minimally, affect the glycemic index is preferred. Drug protocols should be selected for each patient based on health status, required procedure, the expected level of pain, and concurrent comorbidities present.

Premedication

Premedication with reversible agents such as pure-mu opioid receptor agonists and benzodiazepines often allows for fast recoveries.[14] For animals requiring more restraint, or animals that are difficult to handle, extra-label IM alfaxalone could be considered as part of a premedication protocol to facilitate IV catheter placement or to allow for short procedures to be performed.[31,32] For example, for an older diabetic cat requiring sedation for a short, minimally invasive procedure, 1 to 2 mg/kg of alfaxalone combined with 0.3 to 0.4 mg/kg of butorphanol IM might suffice. Alpha-2 receptor agonists, common premedication agents, result in transient increases in plasma glucose concentrations.[33,34] In healthy cats, dexmedetomidine administration resulted in a decrease in plasma glucagon and no change in plasma insulin concentrations.[33] Whether or not the effect of dexmedetomidine on hyperglycemia is mediated exclusively by insulin and glucagon or also by a direct effect on gluconeogenesis in the liver and kidneys is currently unknown. Especially in dogs with DM in which beta cells are largely absent by the time clinical disease is apparent, the clinical effects of the transient increase in BG following administration of drugs such as dexmedetomidine and medetomidine is unlikely to be relevant. However, care should be taken with overzealous insulin administration especially in the presence of alpha-2 agonists as hypoglycemia may ensue once the effects of the alpha-2 agonists wane. The addition of the peripheral alpha-2 antagonist, vatinoxan or MK-467, to alpha-2 agonists appears to inhibit this increase in plasma glucose while maintaining the central sedative effects of the alpha-2 agonist.[34] A new FDA-approved drug for IM canine procedural sedation, Zenalpha, consists of medetomidine combined with vatinoxan, and its use might not result in the transient increase in BG seen when medetomidine is administered alone. However, its effect on glycemic control has not been evaluated in diabetic patients and the drug is not recommended as a premedication before general anesthesia.

Induction of anesthesia
Induction of anesthesia of animals with DM can be performed with any agent used for induction of anesthesia in nondiabetic animals (eg, propofol, alfaxalone, ketamine/midazolam, and ketamine/propofol). The choice of induction agent depends on the animal's health status in general and possible comorbidities with no particular preference with respect to DM.

Anesthesia maintenance
Anesthesia maintenance of animals with DM can be performed with any inhalant anesthetics (isoflurane, sevoflurane, desflurane). Constant rate infusions (CRIs) and/or locoregional anesthesia may allow for the reduction in minimum alveolar concentration (MAC), better cardiovascular stability, and provide multi-modal analgesia. MAC-reducing techniques alleviate the negative cardiovascular effects of inhalant anesthetics which are particularly important in patients with comorbidities, dehydration, acid–base, and electrolyte abnormalities that are common in diabetic patients. For example, a maropitant could be administered as part of an anesthetic protocol. It has antiemetic, anti-nausea, and MAC-sparing effects.[35] Decreases in inhalant anesthetic agent requirements may help preserve normal body temperature and maintain more stable and normal BPs during anesthesia. Agents such as ketamine and lidocaine not only provide MAC-sparing effects but also have analgesic properties. The authors often add ketamine to anesthetic protocols (loading dose 0.5 to 1 mg/kg followed by 0.6 to 1.2 mg/kg/h) of dogs and cats undergoing invasive or painful procedures. In addition, in dogs, lidocaine (loading dose 1 to 2 mg/kg followed by 50 mcg/kg/min) has also been used to provide balanced anesthesia.[36] Locoregional anesthesia should be performed whenever possible as it provides reliable MAC-sparing effect and analgesia and has minimal systemic side effects. However, in animals with diabetic neuropathy, regional anesthesia should be avoided in the affected limb(s). The incidence of peripheral neuropathy in dogs is rare and in diabetic cats is approximately 10%.[37]

Adequate analgesia perioperatively will result in smoother procedures and may improve recoveries reducing time to return to normal function, eating, and insulin regimen. Regional anesthesia is completed using bupivacaine, ropivacaine, or lidocaine and is effective at reducing MAC and providing effective analgesia. Ophthalmic nerve blocks (retrobulbar, peribulbar, etc.) before painful procedures such as enucleation are beneficial and should be performed by experienced personnel.[38] Possible risks of such blocks include stimulation of the oculocardiac reflex, globe perforation, intravascular injection, hemorrhage, and nerve damage. Infiltration of liposomal encapsulated bupivacaine (Nocita) can provide up to 72 h of postoperative analgesia.[39]

Neuromuscular blocking agents may be required, particularly in ophthalmic proced-ures to immobilize the globe. A high proportion of diabetic dogs, approximately 75%, develop cataracts within 1 year of diagnosis and thus require surgery such as phaco-emulsification.[40,41] Atracurium has a similar duration of action in diabetic and non-diabetic dogs,[42] whereas vecuronium has been reported to have a shorter duration of action in patients with DM.[43] Diabetic dogs undergoing phacoemulsification may require higher infusion rates of rocuronium than nondiabetic dogs.[44]

Recovery

To ensure continued control of BG, once recovered from anesthesia, it is recommen-ded to feed the patient a small amount of food and return to their usual insulin regimen as soon as possible.[14] Because uncontrolled diabetic patients are prone to immune dysfunction and reduced wound healing, a rapid return to normal glycemic control is recommended. Adequate analgesia has been associated with improved recovery. Therefore, pain evaluations with multidimensional pain scales and an appropriate analgesic plan during the postoperative period should be instituted. To avoid hypo-, hyperglycemia, or development of DKA, BG monitoring, dextrose, and insulin admin-istration should be continued for patients that are not eating. Follow-up communica-tion should be instituted with clients after patients have returned home. Recheck evaluations should be performed for any patient that has not returned to normal eating and insulin regimen the following day.

DISCLOSURE

The authors have no commercial or financial conflicts of interest.

REFERENCES

1. Hoenig M. Comparative aspects of diabetes mellitus in dogs and cats. Mol Cell Endocrinol 2002;197:221–9.
2. Nelson RW. Canine diabetes mellitus. In: Ettinger SJ, Feldman EC, editors. Text-book of veterinary internal medicine. 7th edn. St Louis, MO: Saunders Elsevier; 2010. p. 1782–96.
3. Sparkes AH, Cannon M, Church D, et al. ISFM Consensus guidelines on the prac-tical management of diabetes mellitus in cats. J Feline Med Surg 2015;17: 235–50.
4. Reusch C. Feline diabetes mellitus. In: Ettinger SJ, Feldman EC, editors. Text-book of veterinary internal medicine. 7th edn. St Louis, MO: Saunders Elsevier; 2010. p. 1796–816.
5. O'Brien TD. Pathogenesis of feline diabetes mellitus. Mol Cell Endocrinol 2002; 197:213–9.
6. Rucinsky R, Cook A, Haley S, et al. American animal hospital association AAHA diabetes management guidelines. J Am Anim Hosp Assoc 2010;46(3):215–24.
7. Niessen SJM, Bjornvad C, Church DB, et al. Agreeing Language in Veterinary Endocrinology (ALIVE): diabetes mellitus a modified Delphi-method-based sys-tem to create consensus disease definitions. Vet J 2022;289:105910.
8. Greco DS. Diagnosis of diabetes mellitus in cats and dogs. Vet Clin North Am Small Anim Pract 2001;31:845–53.
9. Nishikawa T, Ederlstein D, Brownlee M. The missing link: a single unifying mech-anism for diabetic complications. Kidney Int Suppl 2000;77:S-26–S30.
10. Torre DM, deLaforcade AM, Chan DL. Incidence and clinical relevance of hyper-glycemia in critically ill dogs. J Vet Intern Med 2007;21:971–5.

11. Miceli DD, Pignataro OP, Castillo VA. Concurrent hyperadrenocorticism and diabetes mellitus in dogs. Res Vet Sci 2017;115:425–31.
12. Nelson RW. Canine diabetes mellitus. In: Feldman EC, Nelson RW, editors. Canine and feline endocrinology and reproduction. 4th edn. St Louis, MO: Saunders Elsevier; 2015. p. 213–57.
13. Behrend E, Holford A, Lathan P, et al. 2018 AAHA diabetes managements guidelines for dogs and cats. J Am Anim Hosp Assoc 2018;54:1–21.
14. Veres-Nyéki KO. Endocrine disease. In: Duke-Novakovski T, de Vries M, Seymour C, editors. BSAVA manual of canine and feline anaesthesia and analgesia. 3rd edn. Quedgeley: British Small Animal Veterinary Association; 2016. p. 375–90.
15. Adami C, Haynes RS, Sanchez RF, et al. Effect of insulin and fasting regimen on blood glucose concentrations of diabetic dogs during phacoemulsification. J Am Anim Hosp Assoc 2020;56:1–6.
16. Kronen PWM, Moon-Massat RF, Ludders JW, et al. Comparison of two insulin protocols for diabetic dogs undergoing cataract surgery. Vet Anaesth Analg 2001; 28:146–55.
17. Halter JB, P£ug AE. Relationship of impaired insulin secretion during surgical stress to anesthesia and catecholamine release. J Endocrin Metab 1980;51: 1093–8.
18. Campbell PJ, Bolli GE, Cryer PE, et al. Pathogenesis of the dawn phenomenon in patients with insulin dependent diabetes mellitus. N Engl J Med 1985;312: 1473–9.
19. Norgate DJ, Nicholls D, Geddes RF, et al. Comparison of two protocols for insulin administration and fasting time in diabetic dogs anesthetized for phacoemulsification: a prospective clinical trial. Vet Rec 2021;188(11):e81.
20. Savas I, Raptopoulos D. Incidence of gastro-oesophageal reflux during anaesthesia, following two different fasting times in dogs. Vet Anaesth Analg 2000; 27:54–62.
21. Viskjer S, Sjöström L. Effect of the duration of food withholding before anesthesia on gastroesophageal reflux and regurgitation in healthy dogs undergoing elective orthopedic surgery. Am J Vet Res 2017;78:144–50.
22. Pascoe PJ. Perioperative management of fluid therapy. In: DiBartola SP, editor. Fluid, electrolyte, and acid–base disorders in small animal practice. 4th edn. St Louis, MO: Saunders Elsevier; 2012. p. 405–35.
23. Oliver JA, Clark L, Corletto F, et al. A comparison of anesthetic complications between diabetic and nondiabetic dogs undergoing phacoemulsification cataract surgery: a retrospective study. Vet Ophthalmol 2010;13:244–50.
24. Kenefick S, Parker N, Slater L, et al. Evidence of cardiac autonomic neuropathy in dogs with diabetes mellitus. Vet Rec 2007;161:83–8.
25. Herring IP, Panciera DL, Were SR. Longitudinal prevalence of hypertension, proteinuria, and retinopathy in dogs with spontaneous diabetes mellitus. J Vet Intern Med 2014;28(2):488–95.
26. Struble AL, Feldman EC, Nelson RW, et al. Systemic hypertension and proteinuria in dogs with diabetes mellitus. J Am Vet Med Assoc 1998;213:822–5.
27. Littman MP. Hypertension. In: Ettinger SJ, Feldman EC, editors. Textbook of veterinary internal medicine. diseases of the dog and cat. 5th edn. Philadelphia, PA: Saunders Elsevier; 2000. p. 179–82.
28. Zuo L, Dillman D. Endocrine disease. In: Hines RL, Jones SB, editors. Stoelting's anesthesia and co-existing disease. 8th edn. Philadelphia: Saunders Elsevier; 2022. p. 439–64.

29. Hopper K, Brown S. Hypertensive crisis. In: Silverstein D, Hopper K, editors. Small animal critical care medicine. 2nd edn. St Louis, MO: Saunders Elsevier; 2015. p. 51–4.

30. Ambros B, Carrozzo MV, Jones T. Desaturation times between dogs preoxygenated via face mask or flow-by technique before induction of anesthesia. Vet Anaesth Analg 2018;45:452–8.

31. Tamura J, Ishizuka T, Fukui S, et al. Sedative effects of intramuscular alfaxalone administered to cats. J Vet Med Sci 2015;77(8):897–904.

32. Murdock MA, Riccó Pereira CH, Aarnes TK, et al. Sedative and cardiorespiratory effects of intramuscular administration of alfaxalone and butorphanol combined with acepromazine, midazolam, or dexmedetomidine in dogs. Am J Vet Res 2020;81(1):65–76.

33. Bouillon J, Duke T, Focken AP, et al. Effects of dexmedetomidine on glucose homeostasis in healthy cats. J Feline Med Surg 2020;22:344–9.

34. Restitutti F, Raekallio M, Vainionpää M, et al. Plasma glucose, insulin, free fatty acids, lactate and cortisol concentrations in dexmedetomidine-sedated dogs with or without MK-467: a peripheral α-2 adrenoceptor antagonist. Vet J 2012; 193(2):481–5.

35. Boscan P, Monnet E, Mama K, et al. Effect of maropitant, a neurokinin 1 receptor antagonist, on anesthetic requirements during noxious visceral stimulation of the ovary in dogs. Am J Vet Res 2011;72(12):1576–9.

36. Ortega M, Cruz I. Evaluation of a constant rate infusion of lidocaine for balanced anesthesia in dogs undergoing surgery. Can Vet J 2011;52:856–60.

37. Estrella JS, Nelson RN, Sturges BK, et al. Endoneurial microvascular pathology in feline diabetic neuropathy. Microvasc Res 2008;75(3):403–10.

38. Shilo-Benjamini Y. A review of ophthalmic local and regional anesthesia in dogs and cats. Vet Anaesth Analg 2019;46:14–27.

39. Lascelles BDX, Rausch-Derra LC, Wofford JA, et al. Pilot, randomized, placebo-controlled clinical field study to evaluate the effectiveness of bupivacaine liposome injectable suspension for the provision of post-surgical analgesia in dogs undergoing stifle surgery. BMC Vet Res 2016;12.

40. Beam S, Correa MT, Davidson MG. A retrospective-cohort study on the development of cataracts in dogs with diabetes mellitus: 200 cases. Vet Ophthalmol 1999;2(3):169–72.

41. Plummer CE, Specht A, Gelatt KN. Ocular manifestations of endocrine disease. Compendium Continuing Educ Vet 2007;29(12):733–43.

42. Leece EA, Clark L. Diabetes mellitus does not affect the neuromuscular blocking action of atracurium in dogs. Vet Anaesth Analg 2017;44:697–702.

43. Clark L, Leece EA, Brearly JC. Diabetes mellitus affects the duration of action vecuronium in dog. Vet Anaesth Analg 2012;39:472–9.

44. Haga HA, Bettembourg V, Lervik A. Rocuronium infusion: a higher rate is needed in diabetic than nondiabetic dogs. Vet Anaesth Analg 2019;46:28–35.

Continuous Glucose Monitoring in Dogs and Cats
Application of New Technology to an Old Problem

Francesca Del Baldo, DVM, MRCVS, PhD*, Federico Fracassi, DVM, PhD

KEYWORDS

- Continuous glucose monitoring system • FreeStyle Libre • Diabetes mellitus
- Monitoring • Glycemic variability

KEY POINTS

- Regular monitoring of the insulin therapy is vital to successfully control diabetic patients.
- Continuous glucose monitoring systems are nowadays used to monitor insulin therapy in small animals and can eliminate the need to rely on single blood glucose curves without the need for serial venipuncture.
- These systems have adequate clinical accuracy both in dogs and cats.
- They provide detailed glucose profiles, allowing accurate identification of glycemic excursions occurring throughout the day, as well as of glucose variations during consecutive days, thus enabling the clinician to make a more informed insulin treatment decision.

 Video content accompanies this article at http://www.vetsmall.theclinics.com.

INTRODUCTION

Insulin is the mainstay of treatment in canine and feline diabetic patients with diabetes mellitus (DM), often combined with dietary modification.[1] Successful management of DM is indicated by minimal or no clinical signs, restoration of a normal body condition score, avoidance of complications such as diabetic ketoacidosis and hypoglycemia, and owner perception of a good quality of life for the animal.[2] Regular monitoring to ensure an appropriate insulin dose is vital to successfully achieving these aims. Blood glucose curves (BGCs) are an important tool for monitoring insulin response. The evaluation of BGCs allows clinicians to determine glucose nadir, time to nadir, and mean blood glucose (BG) concentration as well as to assess the degree of variation in BG

Department of Veterinary Medical Science, University of Bologna, via Tolara di Sopra, 40066, Ozzano dell'Emilia, Bologna, Italy
* Corresponding author.
E-mail address: francesca.delbaldo2@unibo.it

Vet Clin Small Anim 53 (2023) 591–613
https://doi.org/10.1016/j.cvsm.2023.01.008
0195-5616/23/© 2023 Elsevier Inc. All rights reserved.

vetsmall.theclinics.com

concentration, thus allowing rational adjustments in insulin therapy.[3,4] Up to few years ago, BGCs could only be performed by measuring BG intermittently with some obvious limitations: the time and labor commitment required, combined with the stress of hospitalization, restraint, and the multiple needle punctures needed to obtain capillary blood. In addition, stress-induced hyperglycemia may result in inaccurate results in cats.[5] To overcome some of these problems, home BG monitoring became popular several years ago.[6] This method might circumvent the stress-induced inaccuracies of in-clinic glucose values; however, it requires pet owners to master certain technical skills. A comparison of a hypothetical BGC and CGMS-derived data is shown in **Fig. 1**. It is evident that BGCs, due to low sampling frequency, fail to give a complete BG concentration profile and, therefore, cannot reveal all critical episodes occurring throughout the day. Moreover, BGCs are unable to detect glucose variability observed over several days.[1,6–9]

In recent years, glucose monitoring has been revolutionized by the development of CGMSs, wearable non/minimally-invasive devices that measure glucose concentration almost continuously (1 to 5 min sampling interval) for several consecutive d/wk, mitigating the need for repeated venipuncture and greatly increasing information regarding glucose fluctuations and trends. **Fig. 1** shows that a CGMS reveals hypo-and hyperglycemic events not detected by BGCs. These systems are nowadays used with increasing frequency to monitor both canine and feline diabetic patients and seem to offer a solution to the problem of interpreting a classical 12-h-BGC and avoiding serial venipuncture. The devices are generally well tolerated and easy to place, and recent research has shown that they can play an important role in veterinary diabetic management.

CONTINUOUS GLUCOSE MONITORING SYSTEMS
A Brief History of the Technology

CGMS emerged in 1999 as an innovative technology with the potential of revolutionizing diabetes management.[10] Since their introduction, significant technological advancements have been made, resulting in the commercialization of CGMSs with

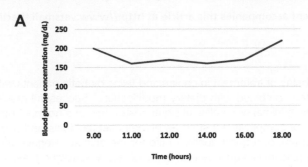

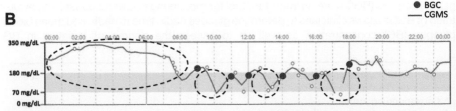

Fig. 1. Representative glucose monitoring data obtainable with intermittent measurements of blood glucose using a PBGM (*A* and *red circles* in *B*) and using a CGMS (*blue line* in [*B*]). Dotted circles in Figure B denote hyperglycemic and hypoglycemic episodes that, using only intermittent PBGM measurements, are not detectable. BGC, blood glucose curve.

improved versatility, new indications, and greater accuracy.[11,12] Major developments in the use of CGMSs in clinical practice have included (1) by 2006, a shift in CGMS assessment from a retrospective to a real-time methodology for obtaining real-time glucose readings; (2) in 2014, the development of the first flash glucose monitoring system (FGMS) which operate without the need to calibrate the interstitial glucose (IG) value to the capillary BG and provision of ambulatory glucose profile (AGP) (**Box 1, Fig. 2**) as a scientifically accurate and clinically reasonable method of reporting the dynamic properties of glucose metabolism[10,13,14]; (3) the possibility of connecting the CGMS with a mobile device (smartphone) and elimination of the need for carrying a separate receiver in 2015 and (4) in 2016, the introduction of the first implantable glucose sensor (Eversense; Senseonics) with a 90-day lifespan that was prolonged to 180 days 1 year later,[15] thus becoming the longest-lasting glucose sensor available on the market.

Technology

Continuous glucose monitoring systems measure IG concentration using transcutaneous or subcutaneous sensors. These devices have a sterile single-use sensor, a glucose monitor which records data, and a communication device for data download. Wireless devices utilize a transmitter to distribute information from the sensor to the monitor. The first-generation systems allowed only a retrospective analysis of the IG concentration after disconnecting the sensor and uploading the data (retrospective CGMS). Newer devices (real-time CGMSs) measure and display data immediately, allowing direct intervention. The most commonly used CGMSs detect glucose using technologies similar to portable blood glucose meters (PBGMs).[16] The sensor is composed of a platinum electrode and a glucose diffusion limiting membrane containing glucose oxidase. In the presence of oxygen, when the membrane is

---

Box 1
Ambulatory glucose profile report: what exactly does it show

Glucose Statistics and Targets: this section displays metrics including:
- Average glucose
- Glucose variability (GV): expressed as CV% (=SD/MG x 100)
- Glucose Management Indicator (GMI) (used in humans to predict HbA1c)
- Dates and number of days in the report
- Percentage of time that the CGM was used to collect data

Time in Ranges: this is a color-coded bar chart that helps to visualize the percentage of time spent above and below the target range:
- Time above range (TAR): percentage of time glucose is more than 180 mg/dL[a]
- Time in range (TIR): percentage of time glucose is within 70 to 180 mg/dL[a]
- Time below range (TBR): percentage of time glucose is less than 70 mg/dL[a]

Ambulatory Glucose Profile: this graph combines all the glucose readings over time to display the trends across a 24-h period:
- Blue line: the median of all the readings. Half of the glucose values are above the middle black line and half are below
- Green lines: target glucose range
- Dark blue area: 50% of glucose values lie in this area
- Light blue area: 90% of glucose values lie in this area
- Dotted blue lines: 5% of the highest and lowest glucose values are above and below this line, respectively

[a] These are established values for diabetic people. If necessary, these cut-offs can be modified and adapted to the needs of the veterinarian.

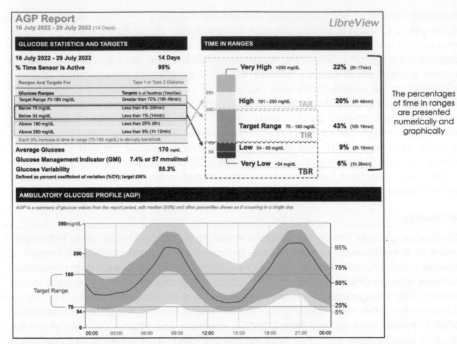

Fig. 2. AGP report. See **Box 1** for the detailed description.

exposed to glucose in the interstitium, glucose is oxidized producing gluconic acid and hydrogen peroxide. The generated hydrogen peroxide reacts with the electrode, generating a current proportional to the IG concentration.[16] This current is sampled by the monitor every few seconds, and a mean value is recorded every few minutes. Other systems use a microdialysis technique in which the microdialysis fiber unit is implanted in the subcutaneous space, and is separated from the biosensor so that reactive substances, such as hydrogen peroxide (a waste product of the enzymatic reaction), cannot diffuse into the tissues. The main advantage of this construction is that, unlike needle-type glucose electrodes, it avoids foreign body reactions and sensor fouling, which can significantly interfere with the performance of the glucose sensor.[17,18] Glucose-oxidase-based electrochemical sensors suffer from several limitations such as their non-linear response within the biologically relevant range, possible interference by active agents (eg, acetaminophen, ascorbate) and, most importantly, dependence of both sensitivity and specificity on the enzyme availability on the electrode surface. Moreover, IG concentration readings provided by glucose-oxidase-based CGM sensors are affected by delay artifacts including the time lag that results from glucose diffusion time into the sensor as well as the equilibrium lag between glucose concentrations in the interstitial fluid (ISF) and blood.[11] The ISF-plasma-glucose relationship can be explained by a 2-compartment model in which the capillary wall separating the plasma from the ISF acts as a barrier to glucose diffusion.[19,20] In this model, changes in IG are determined by the rate of glucose diffusion across the capillary wall and the rate of glucose clearance from the ISF. ISF glucose clearance is determined by the insulin-mediated glucose uptake of the surrounding cells. Clearance rates are proportional to the IG concentration and the rate of uptake by the cells. If the rate of glucose uptake by the surrounding cells is negligible, and the diffusion rates between plasma and ISF are constant, a steady-state relationship develops.[19,20] However, the diffusion of glucose from plasma into ISF is not immediate, and a corresponding lag phase exists between rapid changes in BG and the delayed change in IG. The delay has been described to be 5 to 12 min in dogs[19,21] and 5 to 11 min in cats.[22,23] The lag phase can also be affected by the diffusion of glucose from the ISF into the sensor; however, the CGMSs available have digital filters designed to compensate for this delay.

Next-generation CGMS development involves the exploration of new glucose-sensing technologies beyond glucose-oxidase. In this regard, glucose sensors based on optical sensing have recently been proposed.[11] These sensors have the benefit of being free from electromagnetic interference, simple to design and handle, and characterized by low manufacturing cost. On the basis of these principles, the first implantable CGMS based on fluorescence sensing has recently been developed (Eversense; Senseonics).[24,25]

Overview Current Continuous Glucose Monitoring Systems Used in Dogs and Cats

Several made-for-human CGMSs are commercially available and have been studied for use in dogs and cats: iPro (Medtronic), Guardian Real Time (Medtronic), MiniMed Gold (Medtronic), GlucoDay (Menarini diagnostic), FreeStyle Libre (Abbott) and Eversense (Senseonics).[22,23,26–33] The main characteristics in terms of features, accuracy, and limitations of the first devices evaluated in dogs and cats are reported in **Tables 1** and **2**. These older models have limitations regarding clinical use. They require calibration two to three times/d by measuring the BG concentration with a PBGM. Thus, using CGMSs still requires periodically obtaining a drop of blood; the recording range is 40 to 400 mg/ dL. To see results outside this range, they must be downloaded. If the BG concentration is outside this range, the system cannot be calibrated until the BG is in the working range. Finally, the sensors are quite expensive and can be used for only a few days.

FLASH GLUCOSE MONITORING SYSTEMS

The main difference between FGMSs and CGMSs is that, with a CGMS, the IG concentration is displayed on a monitoring device automatically or transmitted by Bluetooth to a cell phone or other device. With an FGMS, the IG readings are displayed only when the sensor is scanned by the reader or the mobile phone with the compatible app. The Abbott FreeStyle Libre is currently the only FGMS studied in dogs and cats. Freestyle Libre 1 is composed of a small, lightweight disc-shaped sensor (35 mm × 5 mm), which measures the IG concentration by means of a small, subcutaneous catheter (0.4 mm × 5 mm). The system has several features that differentiate it from existing technologies. It provides comprehensive glucose data without the need for calibration, and it can be worn for up to 14 days. Glucose detection is based on Wired Enzyme Technology that consists of both enzymatic (glucose oxidase) and amperometric (electrodes) systems.[37] The detection limits of the sensor are between 20 and 500 mg/dL; measurements outside this range are recorded as "LO" or "HI," respectively. The sensor begins recording data 1 h after its application and automatically measures the IG concentration every minute. The IG concentration is transferred from the sensor to a reader when the user brings the hand-held reader into close proximity to the sensor. The hand-held reader then displays the current sensor IG concentration and an IG trend arrow as well as the IG concentration (averaging each 15 min readings into a single reading) over the preceding 8 h. The FreeStyle LibreLink mobile app, available for both Android and iOS operating systems, can be used as an alternative to the reader. Scanning can be performed as often as is needed to measure the current IG concentration; otherwise, the measurements are automatically recorded

Table 1
Summary of the main characteristics in terms of features, technology, and limitations of the first-generation continuous glucose monitoring systems evaluated in dogs and cats

Device	Features	Technology	Main Limitations
MiniMed Gold (Medtronic)	Retrospective CGMS Recording range: 40 to 400 mg/dL Sensor lifetime: 3 d Sensor initialization period 1h Calibration two to three times per 24 h Monitor weight 113 g Monitor size 9.1 × 2.3 × 7.1 cm Data collected every 10 s, mean value reported every 5 min	Amperometric electrochemical sensor; glucose oxidase	High cost Need for calibration Only retrospective analysis Large dimensions of the monitor
Guardian Real Time (Medtronic)	Real-time CGMS Recording range: 40 to 400 mg/dL Sensor lifetime: 3 d Sensor initialization period 2 h Calibration 2 h after insertion, within the next 6 h, then every 12 h Sensor/transmitter weight 79 g Sensor/transmitter size 4.2 × 3.6 × 0.9 cm Monitor weight 114 g Monitor size 8.1 × 2.0 × 5.1 cm Data collected every 10 s, mean value reported every 5 min Data transmitted wirelessly up to 23 m	Amperometric electrochemical sensor; glucose oxidase	High cost Need for calibration

i-Pro (Medtronic)	Retrospective CGMS	Amperometric electrochemical sensor;	High cost
	Recording range: 40 to 400 mg/dL	glucose oxidase	Need for calibration
	Two sensors available: Sofsensor, Enlitesensor		Only retrospective analysis
	Sensor lifetime: 7 d		
	Sensor initialization period 1h		
	Calibration 1 and 3 h after insertion, then a		
	minimum of once every 12 h		
	Sensor/transmitter weight 79 g		
	Sensor/transmitter size 4.2 × 3.6 × 0.9 cm		
	Absence of a monitor		
	Data collected every 10 s, mean value reported		
	every 5 min		
GlucoDay (Menarini diagnostic)	Real-time CGMS	Amperometric electrochemical sensor;	Need for calibration
	Recording range 20 to 600 mg/dL	glucose oxidase	Large dimension of the monitor
	Sensor lifetime: 2 d		
	Sensor initialization period 1 h		
	Calibration minimum of 1 time point per 48 h, 2		
	if used in real-time		
	Monitor weight 245 g		
	Monitor size 11 × 2.5 × 7.5 cm		
	Data collected every 1 s, mean value reported		
	every 3 min		

Table 2
Summary of the main characteristics in terms of accuracy of the first-generation continuous glucose monitoring systems evaluated in dogs and cats

Device	Correlation Between BG and IG	Mean Difference (±SD) with the Reference Method[a,b]	Clinical Accuracy According to ISO Requirements (%IG Readings Zone A + B EGA)	Comments
MiniMed Gold (Medtronic)	Dog DM • r = 0.81[28] Cat DM • r = 0.93[29] Dog and cat DKA • r = 0.85[34]	CatDM: • 9.66 ± 6.8%[29,b]	Dog and cat DKA: • 99%[34]	Calibration frequency and ketosis, acidosis, hyperlactatemia, dehydration, and reduced blood pressure did not affect the accuracy of the device[34]
Guardian Real Time (Medtronic)	N.A.	Cat DM:[22,b] • 12.7 ± 70.5 mg/dL (hyperglycemic range) • 12.1 ± 141.5 mg/dL (euglycemic range) • 1.9 ± 40.9 mg/dL (hypoglycemic range) Healthy dog:[35,b] • −7 (−18.75 to 3 mg/dL) (euglycemic state) • 35 mg/dL (−74 to −15 mg/dL) (glycemic clamp)	Cat:[22] • 100% (hyperglycemic range) • 96% (euglycemic range) • 91% IG (hypoglycemic range) Dog:[35] • 99% (euglycemic state) • 86% (glycemic clamp)	In diabetic cats, the dorsal neck area provided superior results in terms of accuracy as compared with the lateral chest wall and knee fold[36] In dogs, values for the CGMS at the thorax site had the best correlation with BG concentrations; however, thorax sensors had the shortest functional life-span[35]
i-Pro (Medtronic)	Healthy cats:[31] • Sofsensor r = 0.67 • Enlitesensor r = 0.69	N.A.	Cat:[31] • 100%	Sof-sensor performance superior to Enlite-sensor[31]
GlucoDay (Menarini diagnostic)	Dog:[30] • r = 0.43 to 0.92	Dog:[30,a] • 5.3 mg/dL (±19.2 mg/dL, IR) • 11.7 mg/dL (±23.5 mg/dL, TR)	Dog:[30] • 99.3% (TR) • 99.7% (IR)	IR region associated with a higher incidence of fiber damage[30]

Abbreviations: BB, blood glucose; DKA, diabetic ketoacidosis; DM, diabetes mellitus; IG, interstitial glucose; IT, interscapular region; TR, thoracic region.
[a] Reference method = hexokinase method.
[b] Reference method = validated portable blood glucose meter.

and stored on the sensor (every 15 min) and displayed on the reader when scanned. The reader stores the data for 90 days. At the end of the recording period, the sensor is fully disposable; however, the reader can be re-used with a new sensor. A USB port on the reader can be used to charge it and to download all the data onto a computer, using the LibreView system. This is a free, secure, cloud-based diabetes management system provided by Abbott. The system generates summary glucose reports from the uploaded sensor data, including the AGP (see **Fig. 2**) and the Daily Log (**Fig. 3**), and provides a secure repository for data. Furthermore, using the FreeStyle LibreLink app, the glucose data can be easily shared with health care professionals using the same LibreView system. In this case, the data is automatically uploaded to LibreView when the phone is connected to the Internet.

The FreeStyle Libre is currently the most commonly used CGMS in veterinary medicine. Almost all the studies performed on dogs and cats have used FreeStyle Libre 1. The FreeStyle Libre 2 was developed some years later and a recent study has investigated its accuracy in cats.[38] The shape is identical to FreeStyle Libre 1 with which it shares the major part of its characteristics. The main difference and the most significant improvement is Bluetooth connectivity that means that the Libre 2 has the ability for optional alerts for high and low BG readings. The FreeStyle Libre 3 has recently received a European conformity mark (required for regulatory approval for use in human patients) for people with diabetes in Europe. This is the world's smallest, thinnest

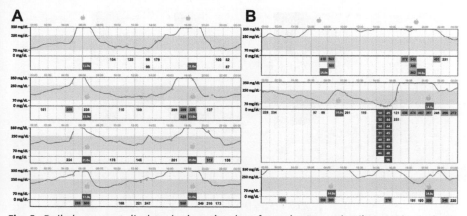

Fig. 3. Daily log report displayed when the data from the Freestyle Libre reader is downloaded to a computer or data automatically uploaded to the LibreView system when the sensor is scanned using the FreeStyle LibreLink app. IG fluctuations during 24-h periods are depicted. The IG values detected by the scans are reported as numbers and are identified by the empty circles. The red box highlights the IG values < 70 mg/dL, whereas the yellow box highlights IG values > 350 mg/dL. Using the reader or the mobile app, there is the possibility of adding notes to track food (*yellow apple*), insulin administration (*green box*), exercise, and other events (not shown in this figure). Examples of one dog with no inter-day GV (*A*) and one dog with marked inter-day GV (*B*). Both dogs received porcine Lente insulin (0.7 U/kg dog A and 0.9 U/kg dog B) and were fed a commercial diabetic diet twice daily. In the second case, a marked difference between interstitial glucose (IG) on days 1 and 2 is evident. On day 1, the IG was more than 250 mg/dL for the major part of the day. On day 2, the IG was within the ideal range for the major part of the day, and hypoglycemia was recorded between 2 PM and 4 PM This highlights the importance of not considering the IG profile for only 1 day when making therapeutic decisions. Instead, it is recommended to consider the IG traces of several consecutive days before deciding to change the insulin dose.

glucose sensor (70% smaller than the previous systems, about the size of two stacked US pennies). This next-generation system provides the same benefits as FreeStyle Libre 2, including 14-day accuracy and optional glucose alarms. However, it has been improved with new features, such as continuous real-time glucose readings automatically delivered to the smartphone every minute and a sensor that is easy to apply using a one-piece applicator (**Fig. 4**). The Authors of the present review have had a recent experience with the use of this device. The FreeStyle Libre 3 application, and the necessary materials and equipment, are shown in **Fig. 4** and in Video 1. To date no veterinary studies have evaluated the accuracy and the clinical use of the FreeStyle Libre 3 and only a small recent study has investigated the accuracy of FreeStyle Libre 2 in healthy cats.[38]

Accuracy of FreeStyle Libre 1 in Dogs

The device is usually well-tolerated in dogs,[32,39–42] even if a greater risk of sensor failure might occur in dogs weighing <10 kg.[42] A mild erythema at the site of the sensor application has been the only complication recorded.[32,39–42] In dogs with DM, the device has adequate clinical accuracy. There is a good correlation between the values obtained from the device and those obtained using the reference hexokinase method ($r = 0.94$[32] and $r = 0.98$[42]). The mean ± standard deviation (SD) differences from the reference hexokinase method were 2.3 ± 46.8 mg/dL[32] and 17.2 ± 39.3 mg/dL.[42]

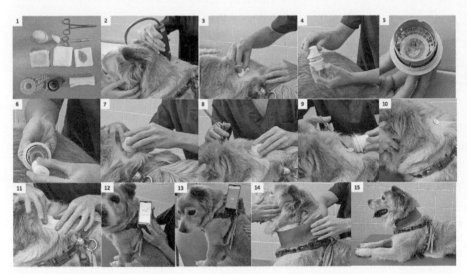

Fig. 4. FreeStyle Libre 3 application in a diabetic dog. (1) FreeStyle Libre one-piece Sensor Applicator with the necessary equipment: gauze (3 with chlorhexidine and 3 with alcohol), scissors and forceps, tissue glue, tape, cotton and elastic bandage; (2) the dorsal aspect of the neck is trichotomized; (3) the skin is cleaned with chlorhexidine and alcoholic wipes; (4) the cap is unscrewed from the Sensor Applicator and the cap is set aside; (5) the sensor applicator is ready; (6) a drop of tissue glue is added to the skin-surface of the sensor; (7) the sensor applicator is placed over the site and (8) pushed down firmly to apply the sensor; (9) it is ensured that the sensor is secure (if necessary, the forceps can be used to avoid the detachment of the sensor); (10) the sensor is correctly applied; (11) the sensor is additionally secured by covering it with a patch; (12) from the App Home Screen, touching "get started" and touching the sensor with the back of the phone, the sensor is scanned and (13) is ready to measure the glucose concentration after 60 min; (14) the sensor is secured with a cotton bandage and with an elastic bandage; (15) the dog is ready to go home.

However, the FGMS readings were less accurate for glucose concentrations <70 mg/dL (3.8 mmol/L).[32] Despite the lower accuracy in the hypoglycemic range, overall the results of the Consensus Error Grid Analysis (EGA) showed adequate clinical accuracy with 99% of the IG readings falling in zones A and B.[32] In the hypoglycemic range (reference method BG < 100 mg/dL), the mean absolute difference between the FGMS and the reference hexokinase method was 22.3 mg/dL.[43] The proportions of IG readings within ±15 mg/dL of the reference BG was only 39.1%; well below the >95% minimum mandated by the ISO 15197:2013 criteria.[44] The Consensus EGA showed that only 80.1% of paired glucose values were in zones A and B.[43] Moreover, although the IG changed rapidly after the IV bolus of regular insulin, the lowest median glucose concentration using the reference method occurred at 20 min, whereas the lowest IG concentration for the FGMS occurred at 50 min, indicating that the FGMS was not reliable in detecting rapid changes in the BG concentration.[43]

Changes in metabolic variables which occur in dogs with diabetic ketoacidosis (ketosis, acidosis, hyperlactatemia) did not affect the accuracy of the device[39]; however, in dehydrated animals, the FGMS was less accurate.[41] This was supported by the findings of another study in which a negative correlation between increased total proteins (a marker for subclinical dehydration) and a decreased IG concentration was found. In particular, for every 1 g/dL increase in TP, there is an expected decrease of 10.4 mg/dL in the FGMS-measured IG concentration.[42] Packed cell volume (PCV), hemolysis, icterus, or lipemia did not affect FGMS readings.[42] In contrast, skin thickness can affect FGMS accuracy because dogs with thinner skin showed less accurate measurements as compared with dogs with thicker skin (>5 mm).[45]

Accuracy of FreeStyle Libre 1 and 2 in Cats

The accuracy of the device has recently been studied in diabetic cats.[23,46–48] The correlation coefficient between the IG measured using the FGMS and the BG measured using the reference hexokinase method was 0.90[46] and 0.96[47]; similar results were obtained by comparing FGMS measurements with those obtained by a PBGM validated for use in veterinary species ($r = 0.90$[23] and $r = 0.88$[48]). The mean ± SD difference from the reference hexokinase method was 5.3 ± 31.6 mg/dL.[47] In another study, the relative deviation from the reference hexokinase method was 9.96%, with slightly higher median values in the hypoglycemic and normoglycemic ranges (12.3% and 12.6%, respectively).[46] In all the studies, the analytical accuracy was less than that stated by the ISO 15197:2013 criteria.[23,46,48] However, the clinical accuracy was acceptable, with 93% to 100% of the measurements in zones A and B of the EGA.[23,46,48] In the hypoglycemic range, the accuracy seemed to be lower.[23,46,48] However, in all of these studies the number of included cases was not enough to reach a statistical power sufficient to validate the device in hypoglycemic samples and therefore, additional validation is required. Changes in BG are rapidly detected (within few minutes) in the ISF by the FGMS.[23] However, the equilibration between BG and IG can take longer to occur (a lag of approximately 30 min was detected between the maximal IG and the maximal BG),[23] thus making the device less accurate during periods of rapidly changing BG levels. A recent study investigated the accuracy of FreeStyle Libre 2 in healthy cats that underwent a hyperinsulinemic-hypoglycemic clamp. Overall BG and IG concentrations strongly correlated ($r = 0.85$). Bias between IG and BG was positively correlated with level of glycemia. IG underestimated BG by 19.3 ± 11.4 mg/dL in the 80 to 120 mg/dL range, 9.9 ± 7.4 mg/dL in the 60 to 79 mg/dL range and 2.5 ± 5.6 mg/dL in the 50 to 59 mg/dL range. IG overestimated BG concentrations by 6.0 ± 6.8 mg/dL in the 38 to 49 mg/dL range.[38]

The most common complications encountered with the use of the FGMS in cats was the reduced sensor lifespan (5.5 to 10 days).[23,46–48] This limitation should be discussed with owners before considering the use of the FGMS in cats. Furthermore, additional fixation by adding glue on the skin-facing surface of the sensor is strongly advised in cats.[23,48] In cats no studies have evaluated whether the skin thickness could affect the accuracy of the device. However, a recent study has shown that the correlation between BG and IG was greater when the sensors were placed on the thorax rather than on the neck.[48] The dorsal neck location was also associated with a greater complication rate (early detachment, dermatologic changes, dysfunctional sensor) than the dorsolateral aspect of the thorax.[49] PCV and hemolysis can affect FGMS-measured IG concentration.[47] However, the interference of PCV is not clinically relevant (a predicted increase of 0.98 mg/dL on the FGMS-measured IG concentration for every 1% increase in PCV). In contrast, the effect of hemolysis could be clinically relevant in the context of a low IG concentration (predicted increase of 17.5 mg/dL on the FGMS-measured IG concentration compared with samples with no to mild hemolysis). Total protein, icterus, and lipemia did not affect FGMS readings.[47]

NEW TECHNOLOGIES

Eversense (Senseonics) is a novel long-term implantable CGMS consisting of a sensor implanted subcutaneously, a wearable transmitter, and a mobile application that displays glucose information on a handheld device.[50] Unlike the transcutaneous CGMSs, the sensor has to be implanted and removed from the skin by means of a minimally invasive surgical procedure performed by a health care professional.[50] The sensor is encased in biocompatible material and utilizes a unique fluorescent, glucose-indicating polymer. A light-emitting diode embedded in the sensor excites the polymer; the polymer then rapidly signals changes in glucose concentration via a change in light output. The measurement is then relayed to the smart transmitter. The sensor has a silicon collar containing dexamethasone that is slowly released to reduce the inflammation that could degrade sensor functioning. The transmitter is a reusable device worn externally over the implanted sensor that powers the sensor and sends glucose information to the mobile application via Bluetooth low-energy technology every 5 min. It is held in place with a mild silicone-based adhesive and is rechargeable via a micro-USB cable. The transmitter wirelessly powers the sensor to activate the transfer of glucose measurements. It receives the glucose data, calculates the glucose value, and sends it via Bluetooth to the Eversense mobile application. The mobile application needs to be run on a compatible handheld device to receive and display the sensor glucose data from the smart transmitter. The data are stored, for up to a year, on a cloud-based platform and are analyzed by dedicated software (Data Management System [DMS]) which is easily accessed by patients and health care providers, and generates summary glucose reports (AGP and other customized reports).[50–52] The detection limits of the sensor range from 40 to 400 mg/dL; when the IG concentration is < 40 mg/dL and >400 mg/dL, the mobile application indicates "LO" or "HI", respectively.

The main advantage of Eversense XL is the long-term sensor lifespan; it extends the possible average CGMS wear time of 7 to 14 days to up to 180 days.[50] A 365-day system is currently in development. The Eversense has additional advantages over transcutaneous CGMS: frequent sensor insertions through the skin are not needed and the transmitter can easily be removed without requiring sensor replacement.[52] However, unlike the transcutaneous CGMS, the Eversense XL sensor needs to be implanted and removed from the skin by means of a minimal surgical procedure performed by a health care professional under local anesthesia.[50]

To date, the clinical use of Eversense has been described only in three diabetic dogs.[33] The insertion and use of the device were straightforward and well tolerated by the dogs. The IG concentrations measured by Eversense XL were strongly correlated with the IG measured by FGMS ($r = 0.85$) as well as with the BG measured by a validated PBGM (rs = 0.81).[33] The mean $\pm$ SD difference between the BG and the IG was - 31.5 $\pm$ 54.5 mg/dL.[33] The device showed acceptable clinical accuracy with 95.5% of the IG reading in zona A and B of the EGA.[33] Analytical accuracy was not satisfied as only 44% of the measurements were within the limits established by ISO 15197:2013.[33] However, additional studies, with larger cohorts of dogs, are needed to determine the clinical and analytical accuracy of this device in diabetic dogs. During the wearing period, some device-related drawbacks, such as sensor migration and daily calibrations, were reported.[33] The dislocation of the sensor makes it difficult to carry out daily calibration tests as the connection between the sensor and the transmitter is possible only when the transmitter is positioned directly over the sensor. Furthermore, when daily calibration tests are not completed within a 24-h period, the system re-enters the initialization phase.[53] Based on the above, a constant commitment from the owner is required for the management of the device. Other disadvantages are the need for daily calibration, the high cost, and limited availability.

CONTINUOUS GLUCOSE MONITORING SYSTEMS IN ROUTINE CLINICAL PRACTICE: PUBLISHED EVIDENCE

The clinical use of CGMSs has been shown as advantageous in people with DM, improving glycemic control,[54,55] reducing hypoglycemic episodes[56] and glycemic variability,[57,58] and improving patient quality of life.[59] In veterinary medicine, only a few studies have investigated the clinical utility of these devices, and the results are promising.[28,40,42,60,61]

Insulin dose adjustments after evaluation of the glucose profiles generated by the CGMS do not significantly differ from those obtained by the PBGM.[28,40,60] When a disagreement between the insulin doses deduced from the two corresponding glucose profiles was observed, in most of the cases, the dose deduced from the CGMS profile was lower than the dose deduced from the PBGM profile.[60] A likely explanation is that the CGMS provides a more detailed glucose profile, allowing detection of the nadir that may not have been identified in the glucose profiles generated by a PBGM in which the BG concentration are determined every 2 h. In fact, most of the glucose nadirs identified by CGMSs were lower than those detected by the intermittent use of a PBGM.[60] Moreover, the interpretation of the BGCs seemed to be more subjective as compared with the interpretation of CGMS traces,[28] highlighting the variety of recommendations that could be made if important glucose fluctuations are missed. In support of these findings, another study showed that the use of an FGMS allowed more accurate identification of the glucose nadirs (79% vs 41%) and hypoglycemic episodes (60% vs 9%) as compared with the use of a PBGM.[40] Furthermore, it allowed detailed identification of the glycemic excursions occurring throughout the day, such as post-prandial hyperglycemia and circadian fluctuations in glucose concentrations.[42] Intra-day glycemic excursions, including episodes of hypoglycemia and hyperglycemia, are defined as glycemic variability (GV).[62] The causes of GV are reported in **Box 2**.[63] In people, GV is an indicator of glycemic control.[62,64] A high GV is considered to be a risk factor for hypoglycemia, microvascular complications, neuropathy, nephropathy, retinopathy, stroke and all-cause mortality.[64-69] In

---

Box 2
Causes of glycemic variability

Factors that can be improved:
    Poor owner compliance with insulin
    Poor owner compliance with dietary recommendations
    Application of interfering drugs (eg, steroids)
    Other diseases (eg, infection, pancreatitis, endocrinopathies, renal disease)
    Different levels of activity or stress

Intrinsic factors that cannot be identified:
    Variable amount of residual β-cell function
    Variable sensitivity to insulin
    Variable insulin absorption and degradation
    Defective counterregulation
    Impaired gastric emptying

Adapted from Reusch CE, Salesov E. Monitoring diabetes in cats. In: Feldman EC, Fracassi F, Peterson M. Feline endocrinology. 1st edition. Milano: Edra s.p.a.;2019; p. 522-539.

---

veterinary medicine, GV has just started to be explored.[70–72] Glycemic variability, assessed by standard deviation, is higher in diabetic cats experiencing posthypoglycemic hyperglycemia during insulin treatment as compared with diabetic cats without posthypoglycemic hyperglycemia.[70] Increased GV in cats with posthypoglycemic hyperglycemia is associated with a higher insulin dose, higher serum fructosamine concentrations, and decreased glycemic control.[70] Moreover, GV is higher in diabetic cats with hypersomatotropism as compared with cats not having hypersomatotropism,[72] supporting the existence of a connection between elevated GV and complicated glycemic control, which is common in cats with hypersomatotropism treated only with insulin and a low carbohydrate diet.[73] Finally, cats that achieve remission seem to have significantly lower GVs as compared with cats that did not achieve remission,[71,72] supporting the hypothesis that GV could be considered a potentially useful and simple index for predicting diabetic remission in feline patients. Future research into the modification of diabetic management which could mitigate these glucose concentration fluctuations is warranted. This might result in improved glycemic control, a higher rate of diabetic remission, and a lower risk of diabetic complications in small animal diabetic patients, as has been shown in human diabetic patients.[74]

Another important aspect highlighted by these studies was that there was an almost absent concordance between the IG concentration obtained on 2 consecutive days at home.[40] Between-day GV, expressed by means of daily differences in BG levels, has also been reported in 93% of human patients with DM,[75] and similarly high GV has been reported in dogs and cats with DM.[7,8] The use of CGMSs, allowing the assessment of GV on consecutive days, enables the clinician to make a more informed decision regarding the insulin dose, taking into account day-to-day variations in glycemic control.[40]

Some case examples highlighting the clinical utility of FGMSs are Reported in **Figs. 3, 5–8**. One drawback that authors have encountered when using the FGMS is that some owners become stressed with glycemic control (see **Fig. 8**). A recent study has investigated the impact of FGMS on pet owners' quality of life and the satisfaction related to its usability using an online survey.[76] This study reports that use of CGM increased anxiety in 12% of owners. In contrast, 88% of the owners reported a greater sense of control (88%) of the disease. Most of the diabetic pet owners considered the FGMS easier to use, and both less stressful, and painful for the animal, allowing them

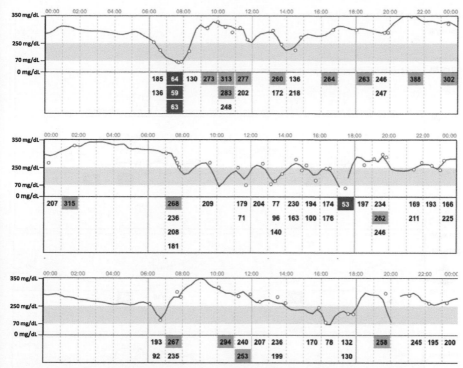

Fig. 5. Daily log report showing marked intra-day glycemic variability in a diabetic dog on porcine Lente insulin (1.2 U/Kg) administered twice daily (8:00 AM and 8 PM). The dog had concurrent hypercortisolism and was receiving trilostane twice daily.

to obtain more glucose data with less effort as compared with BGCs. Overall, 92% of owners reported that glycemic control of their pet was better when using an FGMS. The most challenging aspects of using the FGMS were ensuring proper sensor fixation during the wearing period, preventing premature detachment, and purchasing the

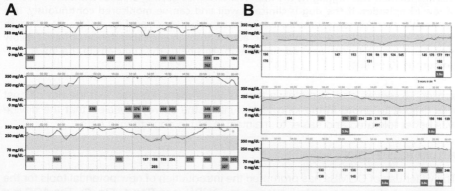

Fig. 6. (*A*) Daily log report showing intra-day GV in a diabetic cat with concurrent hyperso-matotropism. The cat was receiving 5 U (1.2 U/Kg) of glargine 300 U/mL twice daily. (*B*) The IG profile of the same cat after the introduction of exenatide extended-release. Notably, the intra-day GV was markedly decreased.

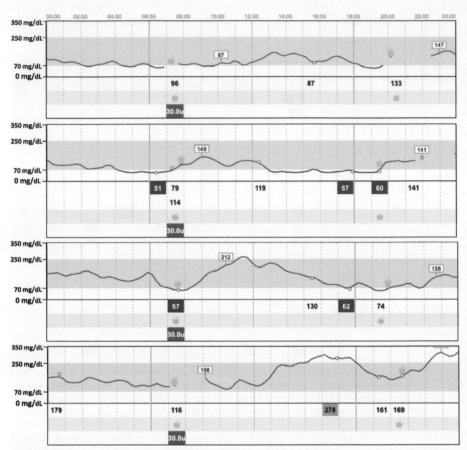

Fig. 7. Daily log report of a diabetic dog receiving 30 U (1.6 U/kg) of glargine 300U/ml once daily (7 AM). The IG profile showed low glucose values for several hours during consecutive days. However, the dog did not show any hypoglycemic signs. Thus, considering the poor accuracy of the device in the hypoglycemic range, the same insulin dose was maintained. This highlights the importance of not getting anxious from the evidence of low IG episodes. If the dog is clinically well and can be monitored continuously, it is reasonable to take some time to evaluate consecutive IG profiles before deciding to decrease the insulin dose. Of notes, the added notes in correspondence of food (*yellow apple*) and insulin (*green box*) administration. This helps the clinicians in the interpretation of the IG profile.

sensor. Moreover, approximately a third of the owners reported that the device cost was difficult to afford in the long term. Finally, the survey revealed that the device was better tolerated and easier to maintain in situ in dogs than in cats.

FUTURE PERSPECTIVE

The wider use of CGMSs has prompted the introduction of new potential tools for the assessment of glucose control, such as the AGP[77] (see **Box 1**, **Fig. 2**). The AGP is a visual report, an easy-to-interpret graph which converts the IG readings into a waveform based on pattern recognition. Although the waveform will start to develop after at least 5 days of data collection, 14 days of data collection has been deemed to be ideal

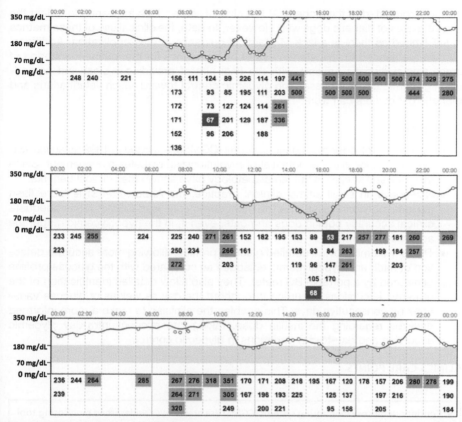

Fig. 8. Daily log report of a diabetic dog on porcine Lente insulin. The number of individual scans (reported as numbers and identified by empty circles) that this diabetic pet owner performed daily, even during the night hours, should be noted.

for most accurately reflecting glucose control.[10,13,78] The AGP is presented as a median glucose value which reflects "what usually happens" rather than the mean which might be more strongly affected by outlying values, alongside the 25 to 75th and 10 to 90th percentiles, as calculated from the range of IG values at each time point.[77] This graph reflects the changes in glucose levels, and displays the actual variability and stability over the period selected. Moreover, it provides novel metrics including time in range (TIR), time above range (TAR), time below range (TBR), and the glucose management indicator (GMI), along with mean glucose (MG) and glycemic variability (coefficient of variation [CV]%)[79,80] (see **Box 1**, **Fig. 2**). Currently, in human diabetology, the AGP provides a simple and informative method of analysis of complex glucose data, and thereby a more consistent and standardized approach to the reporting and interpretation of these data in routine clinical practice.[78] In 2019, an International Consensus statement provided recommendations for using the AGP and its metrics in clinical practice, with the aim of assessing glycemic status and guiding therapy.[79] These metrics have now emerged as additional glycemic targets and outcome measurements together with glycated hemoglobin (HbA1c).[79]

In veterinary medicine, a preliminary study has assessed the utility of different metrics of monitoring diabetic dogs which are readily available with the use of the FGMS.[81] The results of this study are promising as TIR%, TAR% and MG were strongly correlated to the diabetic ALIVE clinical score,[2] thus appearing to reflect the clinical status of diabetic dogs well. However, to date, the clinical use of these metrics is still limited as there is a lack of practical guidance in their application. Additional studies are needed to validate the use of these metrics for the routine monitoring of small animal diabetic patients with the final aim of providing a clear and agreed-upon glycemic target for assessing glycemic control toward which veterinarians and diabetic pet owners can work.

SUMMARY

- Continuous glucose monitoring systems (CGMSs) emerged in 1999 as an innovative technology with the potential of revolutionizing diabetes management. Since then, several studies in human diabetology have shown their clinical benefits.
- Nowadays, in small animal clinical practice, the Abbott FreeStyle Libre flash glucose monitoring system is the most commonly used CGMS. It has adequate clinical accuracy both in dogs and cats, even if, in the hypoglycemic range, the accuracy is lower.
- These systems provide detailed glucose profiles, allowing more accurate detection of nadir and hypoglycemic episodes as compared with the glucose profiles generated by a portable BG meter. They also allow detailed identification of the glycemic excursions occurring throughout the day as well as of glucose variations on consecutive days. This enables the clinician to make a more informed decision regarding the insulin dose, taking into account intra-day glycemic excursion and day-to-day variations in glycemic control.

CLINICS CARE POINTS

- Continuous glucose monitoring systems (CGMS) are nowadays a widespread monitoring tool for small animal diabetic patients. The FreeStyle Libre is the CGMS used most commonly.
- FreeStyle Libre has adequate clinical accuracy both in dogs and cats. However, the device is less accurate during periods of rapidly changing blood glucose levels and in the hypoglycemic range.
- The use of these systems allows an accurate identification of the glucose nadirs and hypoglycemic episodes. Furthermore, they allow detailed identification of the glycemic excursions occurring throughout the day as well as of glucose variations during consecutive days.
- When using these systems, it is recommended to consider the interstitial glucose (IG) traces of several consecutive days before deciding to change the insulin dose.
- Because of the poor accuracy of FreeStyle Libre in the hypoglycemic range, when a low IG episode is detected, if the dog is clinically well and can be monitored continuously, it is reasonable to take some time to evaluate consecutive IG profiles before deciding to decrease the insulin dose.

DISCLOSURE

The author has no conflicts of interest.

SUPPLEMENTARY DATA

Supplementary data related to this article can be found online at https://doi.org/10.1016/j.cvsm.2023.01.008.

REFERENCES

1. Behrend EN, Holford A, Lathan P, et al. 2018 AAHA diabetes management guidelines for dogs and cats. J Am Anim Hosp Assoc 2018;54:1–21.
2. European Society of Veterinary Endocrinolgy. ALIVE Project. Definition: treatment goals of diabetes mellitus 2021. Available at: https://www.esve.org/alive/search.aspx/. Accessed August 14, 2022.
3. Nelson RW. Canine diabetes mellitus. In: Feldman EC, Nelson RW, Reusch CE, et al, editors. Canine and feline endocrinology. 4th edition. St Louis, MO: Elsevier Saunders; 2015. p. 213–53.
4. Reusch CE. Feline diabetes mellitus. In: Feldman EC, Nelson RW, Reusch CE, et al, editors. Canine and feline endocrinology. 4th edition. St Louis, MO: Elsevier Saunders; 2015. p. 258–308.
5. Wiedmeyer CE, DeClue AE. Continuous glucose monitoring in dogs and cats. J Vet Intern Med 2008;22(1):2–8.
6. Reusch CE, Kley S, Casella M. Home monitoring of the diabetic cat. J Feline Med Surg 2006;8:119–27.
7. Alt N, Kley S, Haessig M, et al. Day-to-day variability of blood glucose concentration curves generated at home in cats with diabetes mellitus. J Am Vet Med Assoc 2007;230:1011–7.
8. Fleeman LM, Rand JS. Evaluation of day-to-day variability of serial blood glucose concentration curves in diabetic dogs. J Am Vet Med Assoc 2003;222:317–21.
9. Cook AK. Monitoring methods for dogs and cats with diabetes mellitus. J Diabetes Sci Technol 2012;6:491–5.
10. Mazze R. Advances in glucose monitoring: improving diabetes management through evidence-based medicine. Prim Care Diabetes 2020;14:515–21.
11. Cappon G, Vettoretti M, Sparacino G, et al. Continuous Glucose Monitoring Sensors for Diabetes Management: a review of technologies and applications. Diabetes Metab J 2019;43:383–97.
12. Didyuk O, Econom N, Guardia A, et al. Continuous Glucose Monitoring Devices: past, present, and future focus on the history and evolution of technological innovation. J Diabetes Sci Technol 2021;15(3):676–83.
13. Mazze RS, Strock E, Borgman S, et al. Evaluating the accuracy, reliability, and clinical applicability of continuous glucose monitoring (CGM): Is CGM ready for real time? Diabetes Technol Ther 2009;11:11–8.
14. Mazze RS, Strock E, Wesley D, et al. Characterizing glucose exposure for individuals with normal glucose tolerance using continuous glucose monitoring and ambulatory glucose profile (AGP) analysis. Diabetes Technol Ther 2008;10:149–59.
15. Aronson R, Abitbol A, Tweden KS. First assessment of the performance of an implantable continuous glucose monitoring system through 180 days in a primarily adolescent population with type 1 diabetes. Diabetes Obes Metab 2019;21(7):1689–94.
16. Cappon G, Acciaroli G, Vettoretti M, et al. Wearable continuous glucose monitoring sensors: a revolution in diabetes treatment. Electronics 2017;6:65.
17. Gerritsen M, Jansen JA, Kros A, et al. Influence of inflammatory cells and serum on the performance of implantable glucose sensors. J Biomed Mater Res 2001;54:69–75.
18. Heinemann L. on behalf of the Glucose Monitoring Group. Continuous glucose monitoring by means of the microdialysis technique: underlying fundamental aspects. Diabetes Technol Ther 2003;5:545–61.

19. Rebrin K, Steil GM. Can interstitial glucose assessment replace blood glucose measurements? Diabetes Technol Ther 2000;2(3):461–72.

20. Sternberg F, Meyerhoff C, Mennel FJ, et al. Subcutaneous glucose concentration in humans. Real estimation and continuous monitoring. Diabetes Care 1995; 18(9):1266–9.

21. Rebrin K, Steil GM, Van Antwerp WP, et al. Subcutaneous glucose predicts plasma glucose independent of insulin: implications for continuous monitoring. Am J Phys 1999;277:561–71.

22. Moretti S, Tschuor F, Osto M, et al. Evaluation of a novel real-time continuous glucose-monitoring system for use in cats. J Vet Intern Med 2010;24(1):120–6.

23. Del Baldo F, Fracassi F, Pires J, et al. Accuracy of a flash glucose monitoring system in cats and determination of the time lag between blood glucose and interstitial glucose concentrations. J Vet Intern Med 2021;35(3):1279–87.

24. Chen C, Zhao XL, Li ZH, et al. Current and emerging technology for continuous glucose monitoring. Sensors 2017;17(1):182.

25. Dehennis A, Mortellaro MA, Ioacara S. Multisite study of an implanted continuous glucose sensor over 90 days in patients with diabetes mellitus. J Diabetes Sci Technol 2015;9(5):951–96.

26. Wiedmeyer CE, Johnson PJ, Cohn LA, et al. Evaluation of a continuous glucose monitoring system for use in veterinary medicine. Diabetes Technol Ther 2005; 7(6):885–95.

27. Surman S, Fleeman L. Continuous glucose monitoring in small animals. Vet Clin North Am Small Anim Pract 2013;43(2):381–406.

28. Davison LJ, Slater LA, Herrtage ME, et al. Evaluation of a continuous glucose monitoring system in diabetic dogs. J Small Anim Pract 2003;44:435–42.

29. Ristic JM, Herrtage ME, Walti-Lauger SM, et al. Evaluation of a continuous glucose monitoring system in cats with diabetes mellitus. J Feline Med Surg 2005;7(3):153–62.

30. Affenzeller N, Benesch T, Thalhammer JG, et al. A pilot study to evaluate a novel subcutaneous continuous glucose monitoring system in healthy Beagle dogs. Vet J 2010;184(1):105–10.

31. Salesov E, Zini E, Riederer A, et al. Comparison of the pharmacodynamics of protamine zinc insulin and insulin degludec and validation of the continuous glucose monitoring system iPro2 in healthy cats. Res Vet Sci 2018;118:79–85.

32. Corradini S, Pilosio B, Dondi F, et al. Accuracy of flash glucose monitoring system in diabetic dogs. J Vet Intern Med 2016;30:983–8.

33. Tardo AM, Irace C, Del Baldo F, et al. Clinical use of a 180-day implantable glucose monitoring system in dogs with diabetes mellitus: a case series. Animals (Basel) 2022;12(7):860.

34. Reineke EL, Fletcher DJ, King LG, et al. Accuracy of a continuous glucose monitoring system in dogs and cats with diabetic ketoacidosis. J Vet Emerg Crit Care 2010;20(3):303–12.

35. Koenig A, Hoenig ME, Jimenez DA. Effect of sensor location in dogs on performance of an interstitial glucose monitor. Am J Vet Res 2016;77(8):805–17.

36. Hafner M, Lutz TA, Reusch CE, et al. Evaluation of sensor sites for continuous glucose monitoring in cats with diabetes mellitus. J Feline Med Surg 2013; 15(2):117–23.

37. Hoss U, Erwin SB, Hanqing L, et al. Feasibility of factory calibration for subcutaneous glucose sensors in subjects with diabetes. J Diabetes Sci Technol 2014;8(1):89–94.

38. Berg AS, Crews CD, Castro AA, et al. Assessment of the FreeStyle Libre 2 interstitial glucose monitor in hypo- and euglycemia in Cats. Paper presented at the 2022 ACVIM Congress; June 23–25 2022; Austin, Texas.

39. Malerba E, Cattani C, Del Baldo F, et al. Accuracy of flash glucose monitoring system in dogs with diabetic ketoacidosis. J Vet Intern Med 2020;34:83–91.

40. Del Baldo F, Canton C, Testa S, et al. Comparison between a flash glucose monitoring system and a portable blood glucose meter for monitoring dogs with diabetes mellitus. J Vet Intern Med 2020;34(6):2296–305.

41. Silva DD, Cecci GRM, Biz G, et al. Evaluation of a flash glucose monitoring system in dogs with diabetic ketoacidosis. Domest Anim Endocrinol 2021;74:106525.

42. Shea EK, Hess RS. Assessment of postprandial hyperglycemia and circadian fluctuation of glucose concentrations in diabetic dogs using a flash glucose monitoring system. J Vet Intern Med 2021;35(2):843–52.

43. Howard LA, Lidbury JA, Jeffery N, et al. Evaluation of a flash glucose monitoring system in nondiabetic dogs with rapidly changing blood glucose concentrations. J Vet Intern Med 2021;35(6):2628–35.

44. BSI Standards Publication, In vitro diagnostic test systems –Requirements for blood-glucose monitoring systems for self-testing in managing diabetes mellitus (EN ISO 15197:2013). Avaiable at: https://www.iso.org/standard/54976.html. Accessed February 18, 2023.

45. Del Baldo F, Diana A, Canton C, et al. The Influence of Skin Thickness on Flash Glucose Monitoring System Accuracy in Dogs with Diabetes Mellitus. Animals (Basel) 2021;11(2):408.

46. Deiting V, Mischke R. Use of the "FreeStyle Libre" glucose monitoring system in diabetic cats. Res Vet Sci 2021;135:253–9.

47. Shea EK, Hess RS. Validation of a flash glucose monitoring system in outpatient diabetic cats. J Vet Intern Med 2021;35(4):1703–12.

48. Knies M, Teske E, Kooistra H. Evaluation of the FreeStyle Libre, a flash glucose monitoring system, in client-owned cats with diabetes mellitus. J Feline Med Surg 2022;24(8):223–31.

49. Shoelson AM, Mahony OM, Pavlick M. Complications associated with a flash glucose monitoring system in diabetic cats. J Feline Med Surg 2021;23(6):557–62.

50. Deiss D, Szadkowska A, Gordon D, et al. Clinical practice recommendations on the routine use of Eversense, the first long-term implantable continuous glucose monitoring system. Diabetes Technol Ther 2019;21(5):254–64.

51. Irace C, Cutruzzolà A, Nuzzi A, et al. Clinical use of a 180-day implantable glucose sensor improves glycated hemoglobin and time in range in patients with type 1 diabetes. Diabetes Obes Metab 2020;22:1056–61.

52. Kropff J, Choudhary P, Neupane S, et al. Accuracy and longevity of an implantable continuous glucose sensor in the PRECISE study: a 180-day, prospective, multicenter, pivotal trial. Diabetes Care 2017;40:63–8.

53. Senseonics Inc. Eversense XL user guide. Available at. https://global.eversensediabetes.com/patient-education/eversense-user-guides. Accessed August 15, 2022.

54. Benkhadra K, Alahdab F, Tamhane S, et al. Real-time con- tinuous glucose monitoring in type 1 diabetes: a systematic review and individual patient data meta-analysis. Clin Endocrinol 2017;86(3):354–60.

55. Dicembrini I, Cosentino C, Monami M, et al. Effects of real-time continuous glucose monitoring in type 1 diabetes: a meta-analysis of randomized controlled trials. Acta Diabetol 2021;58(4):401–10.

56. Haak T, Hanaire H, Ajjan R, et al. Flash glucose-sensing technology as a replacement for blood glucose monitoring for the management of insulin-treated type 2 diabetes: a multicenter, open-label randomized controlled trial. Diabetes Ther 2017;8:55–73.

57. Jamiolkowska M, Jamiolkowska I, Luczynski W, et al. Impact of real-time continuous glucose monitoring use on glucose variability and endothelial function in adolescents with type 1 diabetes: new technology. New possibility to decrease cardiovascular risk? J Diabetes Res 2016;2016:4385312.

58. Tumminia A, Crimi S, Sciacca L, et al. Efficacy of real-time continuous glucose monitoring on glycaemic control and glucose variability in type 1 diabetic patients treated with either insulin pumps or multiple insulin injection therapy: a randomized controlled crossover trial. Diabetes Metab Res Rev 2015;31:61–8.

59. Rusak E, Ogarek N, Wolicka K, et al. The Quality of life and satisfaction with continuous glucose monitoring therapy in children under 7 years of age with T1D using the rtCGM system integrated with insulin pump-A caregivers point of view. Sensors 2021;21(11):3683.

60. Dietiker-Moretti S, Müller C, Sieber-Ruckstuhl N, et al. Comparison of a continuous glucose monitoring system with a portable blood glucose meter to determine insulin dose in cats with diabetes mellitus. J Vet Intern Med 2011;25(5):1084–8.

61. Mori A, Kurishima M, Oda H, et al. Comparison of glucose fluctuations between day- and night-time measured using a continuous glucose monitoring system in diabetic dogs. J Vet Med Sci 2013;75(1):113–7.

62. Suh S, Kim JH. Glycemic variability: how do we measure it why is it important? Diabetes Metab J 2015;39:273–382.

63. Reusch CE, Salesov E. Monitoring diabetes in cats. In: Feldman EC, Fracassi F, Peterson M, editors. Feline endocrinology. 1st edition. Milano: Edra s.p.a.; 2019. p. 522–39.

64. Frontoni S, Di Bartolo P, Avogaro A, et al. Glucose variability: an emerging target for the treatment of diabetes mellitus. Diabetes Res Clin Pract 2013;102:86–95.

65. Brownlee M, Hirsch IB. Glycemic variability: a hemoglobin A1c- independent risk factor for diabetic complications. JAMA 2006;295(14):1707–8.

66. Umpierrez GE, Kovatchev BP. Glycemic variability: how to measure and its clinical implication for type 2 diabetes. Am J Med Sci 2018;356(6):518–27.

67. Lachin JM, Genuth S, Nathan DM, et al. for the DCCT/EDIC Research Group. Effect of glycemic exposure on the risk of microvascular complications in the diabetes control and complications trial-revisited. Diabetes 2008;57(4):995–1001.

68. Zinman B, Marso SP, Christiansen E, et al. Day-today fasting glycemic variability in DEVOTE: associations with severe hypoglycemia and cardiovascular outcomes (DEVOTE 2). Diabetologia 2018;61:48–57.

69. Lin CC, Yang CP, Li CI, et al. Visit-to-visit variability of fasting plasma glucose as a predictor of ischemic stroke: competing risk analysis in a national cohort of Taiwan diabetes study. BMC Med 2014;26:165.

70. Zini E, Salesov E, Dupont P, et al. Glucose concentrations after insulin-induced hypoglycemia and glycemic variability in healthy and diabetic cats. J Vet Intern Med 2018;32(3):978–85.

71. Krämer AL, Riederer A, Fracassi F, et al. Glycemic variability in newly diagnosed diabetic cats treated with the glucagon-like peptide-1 analogue exenatide extended release. J Vet Intern Med 2020;34(6):2287–95.
72. Linari G, Fleeman L, Gilor C, et al. Insulin glargine 300 U/ml for the treatment of feline diabetes mellitus. J Feline Med Surg 2022;24(2):168–76.
73. Niessen SJ, Forcada Y, Mantis P, et al. Studying cat (*Felis catus*) diabetes: beware of the acromegalic imposter. PLoS One 2015;10:e0127794.
74. Evans M, Welsh Z, Ells S, et al. The impact of flash glucose monitoring on glycaemic control as measured by hba1c: a meta-analysis of clinical trials and real-world observational studies. Diabetes Ther 2020;11(1):83–95.
75. Mori H, Okada Y, Kurozumi A, et al. Factors influencing inter-day glycemic variability in diabetic outpatients receiving insulin therapy. J Diabetes Investig 2017;8:69–74.
76. Re M, Del Baldo F, Tardo AM, et al. Monitoring of diabetes mellitus with Flash Glucose Monitoring System: the owners' point of view. Paper presented at the 32nd ECVIM-CA Congress; September 1–3 2022; Gothenburg, Sweden.
77. Evans M, Cranston I, Bailey CJ. Ambulatory glucose profile (AGP): utility in UK clinical practice. Br J Diabetes 2017;17(1):28–33.
78. Bergenstal RM, Ahmann AJ, Bailey T, et al. Recommendations for standardizing glucose reporting and analysis to optimize clinical decision making in diabetes: the ambulatory glucose profile. J Diabetes Sci Technol 2013;7:562–78.
79. Battelino T, Danne T, Bergenstal RM, et al. Clinical targets for continuous glucose monitoring data interpretation: recommendations from the international consensus on time in range. Diabetes Care 2019;42:1593–603.
80. Bergenstal RM, Beck RW, Close KL, et al. Glucose management indicator (GMI): A new term for estimating A1C from continuous glucose monitoring. Diabetes Care 2018;41:2275–8220.
81. Del Baldo F, Tardo AM, Alessandrini F, et al. The usefulness of different freestyle libre-derived metrics in assessing glycemic control in diabetic dogs. J Vet Intern Med 2021;35:3115.

Insulin Therapy in Small Animals, Part 1: General Principles

Linda Fleeman, BVSc, PhD, MANZCVS[a],*, Chen Gilor, DVM, PhD, DACVIM[b]

KEYWORDS

• Detemir • Glargine • Protamine • Lente • Diabetes mellitus

KEY POINTS

• Ideally, insulin therapy in most dogs with diabetes should mimic a basal-bolus pattern. The intermediate-acting insulin formulations might provide a better approximation of bolus insulin secretion in many dogs than the rapid-acting formulations that are typically used for this purpose in people with diabetes.

• In patients with some residual beta cell function such as many diabetic cats, administering only a basal insulin might lead to complete normalization of blood glucose concentrations if postprandial endogenous insulin secretion is sufficient to make up for the bolus requirement and/or if bolus requirement is sustained and prolonged.

• No insulin formulation should be considered best by default. Rather, the choice of insulin formulation should be tailored to the specific clinical situation. Different goal-oriented treatment strategies should be considered, with pros and cons to each.

• Compared with insulin suspensions (NPH, lente, and PZI), insulin solutions (glargine, detemir, and degludec) are associated with less day-to-day variability.

• Compared with the traditional vial/syringe combination, insulin pens improve the quality of life of the caregiver, improve adherence, and allow better dosing accuracy and precision.

INTRODUCTION

Diabetes mellitus is a syndrome of relative or absolute insulin deficiency that leads to abnormal glucose homeostasis. Insulin therapy is required for the survival of most dogs and cats suffering from diabetes but it is associated with many inherent challenges that must be overcome for treatment to be safe, effective, and sustainable. These challenges develop from factors related to the complex nature of glycemic control, pharmacological limitations of available insulin formulations, and from life-long

[a] Animal Diabetes Australia, 5 Hood Street, Collingwood, Victoria 3066, Australia; [b] Small Animal Internal Medicine, Department of Small Animal Clinical Sciences, College of Veterinary Medicine, University of Florida, 2015 Southwest 16th Avenue, Gainesville, FL 32608, USA
* Corresponding author.
E-mail address: L.Fleeman@AnimalDiabetesAustralia.com.au

Vet Clin Small Anim 53 (2023) 615–633
https://doi.org/10.1016/j.cvsm.2023.02.002
0195-5616/23/© 2023 Elsevier Inc. All rights reserved.

burden on nonprofessional caregivers. These issues have been significantly diminished in human medicine with the movement away from traditional insulin suspensions that require the use of syringe and needles multiple times a day, toward the use of recombinant insulin analogs, and application methods such as injection pens and insulin pumps, and continuous glucose monitoring systems. On the horizon are further improvements in insulin therapy including formulations with ultralong duration (7 days and more), oral insulin, and "smart" glucose-responsive insulin formulations. Even with the use of the traditional tools, smarter understanding of the pharmacology of insulin and how it relates to the pathophysiology of diabetes can lead to better clinical outcomes.

Insulin has been used to treat diabetes for 100 years. During this time, a plethora of insulin formulations have been developed and carefully tested for human patients. In contrast, there is striking paucity of high-level evidence from direct comparison in clinical trials to suggest that any one insulin formulation is advantageous compared with any other in any veterinary clinical scenario. In this context, we provide a review of current understanding of insulin pharmacology and relevant diabetes pathophysiology, integrated with practical considerations and key monitoring principles for the application of insulin therapy.

THE CHOICE OF INSULIN DEPENDS ON THE SPECIFIC CLINICAL SCENARIO

Insulin formulations vary in their average time-action profiles, day-to-day variability, cost, methods of administration, and more. There are currently 2 "veterinary" insulin formulations labeled for use in dogs and cats but more than a dozen other "human" formulations are available on the market. Some of these "human" formulations are routinely used in dogs and cats. The choice between insulin formulations depends on interdependent factors that will differ between patients and between different times for the same patient: (1) disease pathophysiology (including concurrent diseases), (2) insulin-related factors (including insulin pharmacology, cost, regional prescribing regulations), (3) pet and owner compliance, (4) diet (composition and frequency), (5) monitoring strategy, and (6) goals of therapy for the specific patient (considering risk of hypoglycemia).

Therefore, no insulin formulation should be considered best by default. Rather, the choice of insulin formulation should be tailored to the specific clinical situation. Often, opposing needs will result in compromise. For example, for a fractious cat or for an owner who is struggling to give injections, minimizing the number of injections by using a long-acting insulin formulation once-daily might be a necessary compromise even if the glycemic control is not optimal. In contrast, a formulation that is shorter in duration but much less expensive might be ideal for an owner who can easily administer insulin but cannot afford expensive formulations.

PATHOPHYSIOLOGY: INSULIN REQUIREMENTS ON THE DIABETES SPECTRUM
Insulin Physiology in Health

Insulin is secreted by the beta cells of the islets of Langerhans in the pancreas. It reaches the liver through the portal circulation where about 50% of it is cleared. The remaining insulin enters the systemic circulation and is delivered to other target organs, mainly skeletal muscle and adipose tissue. Insulin synthesis and secretion are stimulated predominantly by increases in blood glucose concentrations but the degree to which beta cells respond to glucose is modified by a multitude of other factors including other nutrients, hormones, and neural input.[1]

Endogenous insulin secretion can be divided into 2 phases: the basal phase, in which insulin is secreted continuously at a relatively constant rate, and the bolus phase, in which insulin is secreted in response to nutrients digested and absorbed from the gut.[2] In health, insulin secretion is constantly adjusted in response to various signals to maintain euglycemia. The primary role of basal insulin secretion is to limit lipolysis and hepatic glucose production in the fasting state. Although basal insulin secretion is relatively constant throughout the day, it changes over time in response to changes in insulin sensitivity; it increases when insulin resistance develops (eg, with obesity or other diseases) and decreases when insulin sensitivity increases (eg, with exercise).[3] Bolus insulin primarily suppresses hepatic glucose output and stimulates glucose utilization by muscle and adipose tissue during the postprandial period, thus curbing hyperglycemia after meals.[2] Bolus insulin secretion is largely determined by factors such as the carbohydrate, fat, and protein contents of the meal, gastrointestinal transit time, and the effects of intestinal hormones.[2]

Insulin Physiology in Dogs and Cats Compared with People

In people, the bolus phase usually lasts only 2 to 4 hours with 5-fold increases from baseline in insulin peak concentrations.[4] However, this bolus phase depends on the type and quantity of food. In healthy dogs, the bolus phase also varies significantly in shape and magnitude with diet. Although insulin also increases within minutes after feeding and often peaks within 30 minutes at 5 to 7 times the baseline concentration, it can remain increased for 6 to 9 hours in dogs depending on the diet (**Table 1**).[5–7] In healthy cats, bolus insulin secretion typically has a longer duration (6–12 hours) and a later and much lower peak (peaking at 1–8 hours and reaching 1.5–3 times baseline concentrations) depending on the diet fed (see **Table 1**).[8–10] These data should be taken with a grain of salt however because in these studies, cats were fasted for a relatively long time before being fed a single meal during a 24 hour period. In a recent study, when once daily feeding was compared with 4 feedings per day in healthy cats, insulin increased as described above during the single meal. However, when the daily caloric intake was divided into 4 meals, the increase in plasma insulin was minimal and sustained throughout the 24-hour period.[11] This sustained insulin requirement with no clear bolus phase is likely more representative of insulin requirements of cats in the clinical setting.

Insulin Treatment: the Human Diabetes Model

Regardless of the type of diabetes, people are treated with insulin based on their residual beta cell capacity. Most patients with type 1 diabetes have little-to-no beta cells and are therefore treated with a more aggressive protocol. This often comprises a combination of a basal insulin (typically long-acting with a flat time-action profile and

Table 1		
Comparison of "bolus" insulin secretion in people, dogs, and cats		
	Duration of Bolus Insulin Secretion	Magnitude of Increase of Insulin During Bolus Insulin Secretion
Human	2–4 h	5-fold
Dog	6–9 h	5–7-fold
Cat	6 - >12 h	0–3-fold

Note that this is a rough guide only because there is large individual variability depending on meal composition, quantity consumed, and frequency of feeding.

administered once daily) and a bolus insulin (typically rapid and short-acting and administered at the time of the meals, with the number of injections depending on the number of meals) (**Fig. 1**). The dose of basal insulin depends on the interaction between residual beta cell function and background insulin resistance. The dose of bolus insulin is based on the premeal interstitial or blood glucose concentration, the carbohydrate content of the meal, and anticipated physical activity.[12]

Most type 2 diabetic human patients are treated with drugs supporting insulin secretion (insulin sensitizers, potentiators of insulin secretion, and so forth) and, at the later stages of disease, with basal insulin replacement. Even in these later stages, basal insulin replacement is typically sufficient for meeting glycemic goals because endogenous secretion can fill at least some of the gap in the postprandial phase despite the fact that incretin responses are reduced and therefore endogenous bolus insulin secretion is substantially diminished. Patients with type 2 diabetes are infrequently treated with a basal-bolus insulin combination.

Another option for mimicking the basal-bolus pattern is to use an insulin pump that can be programmed to deliver insulin at variable rates. Such insulin pumps are widely used in human medicine, and although they have been used in animals, cost and other practical considerations limit their use. For example, the Omnipod is a "patch-pump" that is small, adheres to the skin, and is "tangle-proof" because it has no external tubing that can be accidentally removed. Pet-specific pumps have been studied as well although currently none are commercially available.[13]

There are "smart" glucose-responsive insulin formulations under development that release insulin from the subcutaneous (SC) depot in response to changes in blood glucose concentrations.[14] These formulations should be ideal for mimicking the basal-bolus pattern; however, none is currently available outside of the research arena.

Although these strategies can effectively mimic the basal-bolus pattern of healthy insulin physiology, an important limitation of most insulin formulations that are administered SC is loss of normal liver-periphery insulin concentration gradient.[15] Inhibition of hepatic glucose output, a major factor in maintaining euglycemia, requires high insulin concentrations in hepatic portal blood, whereas inhibition of lipolysis requires much

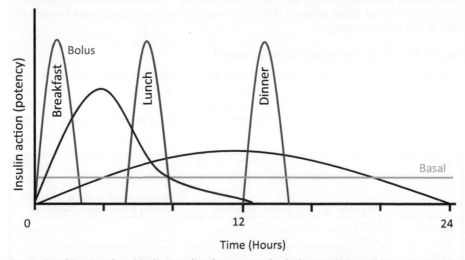

Fig. 1. Combination basal-bolus Insulin therapy: Red – bolus insulin requirement; Green – basal insulin requirement; Blue – Typical basal insulin kinetics; Black – Typical intermediate insulin kinetics.

lower concentrations in peripheral adipose tissue. More than half of the insulin secreted by the pancreas is removed from the bloodstream by the liver before the remainder is circulated to other target organs. When insulin is subcutaneously injected, equal concentrations are delivered to the liver, muscles, and adipose tissue. This skewed concentration ratio accomplishes either appropriate control of hepatic glucose output with inappropriately high concentrations of insulin in adipose tissue, which promotes weight gain, or appropriate concentrations in adipose tissue with insufficient control of hepatic glucose output leading to poor glycemic control. Synthetic insulin analogs that preferentially target the liver would likely decrease the magnitude of this problem.[15]

PRINCIPLES OF INSULIN PHARMACOLOGY
How Is Insulin Pharmacology Studied?

In veterinary medicine, blood glucose curves have been used traditionally to study the effect of exogenous insulin. However, blood glucose curves reflect not only the effect of exogenous insulin but also the effect of endogenous insulin, stress hormones, and the effects of feeding and exercise. Therefore, the validity of studies reporting insulin pharmacodynamics (PD) based on serial blood glucose measurements is limited. For example, if insulin action peaks at 16 hours after injection but the dog is fed a carbohydrate-rich meal every 12 hours, blood glucose concentrations will increase after feeding, creating a nadir just before the meal, giving the appearance that peak action of the insulin is at 12 hours. Similarly, an insulin injection that lowers blood glucose rapidly, might lead to the activation of stress hormones, leading to a nadir that is earlier than the peak action of the insulin. To measure insulin PD accurately, one must use the glucose clamp method in which blood glucose concentrations are maintained (clamped) at euglycemia. This is achieved by infusing glucose at a changing rate that is sufficient to counteract the glucose-lowering effects of insulin. Glucose clamps allow the study of the effect of injected insulin with minimum interference from confounding factors such as hypoglycemia, stress hormones, and endogenous insulin secretion.[16] Glucose clamps, however, are both labor intensive and expensive. Only a few insulin pharmacodynamic studies using the glucose clamp technique have been reported in cats and dogs. In this review, pharmacodynamic parameters, such as duration of action and time to peak action, will be presented when data from glucose clamps are available. These pharmacodynamic data will be supplemented with pharmacokinetic data when available. Otherwise, when only data from serial blood glucose curves are available, the effect of insulin will be described in more vague terms describing its perceived appropriateness for clinical use, such as recommended frequency of administration. The common terminology that assigns duration of action ("short-acting," "intermediate- acting," and "long-acting") will be used for convenience, considering the above caveat. In addition, it is important to note that this terminology is problematic because for most insulin formulations, the duration of action can be extended to some degree by increasing the insulin dose (**Fig. 2**A, **Table 2**).[2] Extended duration might be advantageous in terms allowing reduced frequency of administration but it also results in higher peak insulin concentration and increased risk of hypoglycemia. In contrast, reducing the dose and increasing the frequency of administration would decrease the risk of hypoglycemia (**Fig. 2**B).

The unique pharmacodynamic characteristics of all of the commercial formulations described in this review are only relevant to SC injections.[17] When administered intravenously, dilution in the blood leads to immediate dissociation of insulin hexamers resulting in the same ultrarapid action as intravenously administered regular insulin.[18]

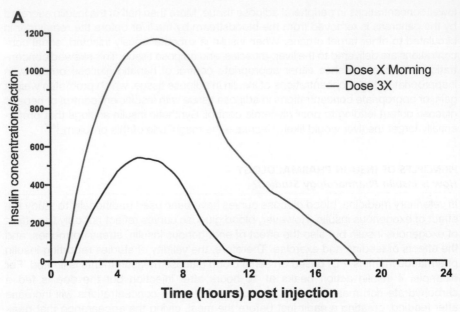

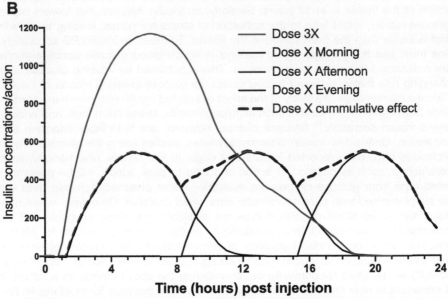

Fig. 2. Effects of changing the dose and frequency of administration of an intermediate-acting insulin. *(A)* A 3-fold dose increase of a typical intermediate-acting insulin formulation nearly doubles the duration of action but also doubles peak action and increases the risk of hypoglycemia. *(B)* Decreasing the dose and tripling the frequency of administration decreases the risk of hypoglycemia and achieves lesser intra-day variation.

Insulin Suspensions: Lente, NPH, PZI

Insulin has a natural tendency to precipitate and crystallize, especially in the presence of zinc. In the pancreatic beta cells, insulin is stored as hexamers surrounding molecules of zinc. Insulin hexamers are slow to penetrate capillaries but when released

Table 2
Comparison of insulin suspensions and insulin solutions

	Suspension	Solutions
Mixing before drawing	Required	Not required
Interday variability	High	Low
Dose-dependent duration	Substantial	Minimal

from the beta cells, the zinc is diluted and the hexamers break down to dimers and monomers that are absorbed into the bloodstream.[19] When administered subcutaneously, regular insulin hexamers quickly break down into dimers and monomers that are then released from the SC depot and are biologically active. After SC injection, regular insulin has a duration of action of about 5 to 8 hours.[20-22] To overcome this relatively short duration, the natural tendency of insulin to crystallize is enhanced in classic insulin formulations, causing precipitation in the vial and at the site of injection.[18] This is achieved by adding either zinc (lente formulations), or the basic, arginine-rich protein protamine (Neutral Protamine Hagedorn [NPH] formulations), or both zinc and protamine (Protamine Zinc Insulin [PZI] formulations). Once injected subcutaneously, the zinc slowly diffuses away from the injection site and protamine is slowly degraded, thus allowing insulin crystals to slowly deprecipitate, releasing insulin dimers and monomers into the blood more slowly compared with the release of insulin with no additives (regular insulin). This strategy of slowing the absorption of insulin by enhancing its crystallization leads to slower onset and longer duration of action but it has some consequential disadvantages. For one, insulin has to be resuspended evenly before each dose (see **Table 2**). The recommendation is to resuspend the insulin by gently rolling then inverting the vial or, in the case of Vetsulin/Caninsulin, to vigorously shake the vial until completely mixed. However, the process of resuspension is often inconsistent and leads to inaccuracy in dosing.[23] A second disadvantage is that the deprecipitation in the injection site is highly variable and unpredictable, which leads to considerable variation in insulin absorption.[2,19,24] Third, these formulations have time-action profiles that are usually not congruent with physiological insulin secretion patterns. The onsets of action may be too slow and durations of action too long to mimic the bolus phase; whereas, insulin action profiles are often too peaked and durations may not be long enough to mimic basal secretion.[18,19] Better congruency might be achieved with formulations that mix short-acting and intermediate-acting suspensions such as the premixed combinations of 30% regular and 70% NPH insulin, or porcine lente insulin, which is a mix of 35% amorphous semi-lente insulin and 65% crystalline ultra-lente insulin. However, absorption of the short-acting component might still sometimes be too slow in these formulations. In addition, there is inability with the commercial insulin mixes to separately fine-tune the short-acting and intermediate-acting components, a limitation that may be overcome by administering the short-acting and intermediate-acting insulins by separate injections.

PD, pharmacokinetics (PK), and guidelines for the frequency of administration of specific insulin suspensions can be found in Insulin Therapy parts 2 (canine) and 3 (feline) in this issue.

Insulin Solutions: Recombinant Analogs

Recombinant insulin analogs are designed to mimic physiologic insulin secretion as closely as possible and to have low day-to-day variability, which is an important feature in the prevention of hypoglycemic events.[18] Amino acid addition or substitutions in the B26-B30 region and other alterations increase or decrease the tendency of insulin to form hexamers and crystallize while retaining the ability to activate insulin receptors.[4,18] Insulin analogs with decreased tendency to form hexamers result in a rapid onset (30–60 minutes), a relatively high peak in activity, a short duration of action (2–3 hours), and greater predictability when compared with regular insulin.[4] Thus, when injected subcutaneously, these formulations are more suited to mimic postprandial bolus insulin secretion in people than regular insulin. Examples include lispro, aspart, and glulisine (**Table 3**).

Long-acting insulin analogs are altered so that they associate more strongly either as hexamers or through lipophilic interactions, and result in decreased rate of absorption and more flat (peakless) time-action profiles with low intraday variability. These are used as basal formulations in people. Examples (in people) include insulin degludec and insulin glargine U300. The combination of synthetic rapid-acting bolus insulin analogs and slow-release basal insulin analogs enables better mimicking of basal-bolus requirements and separate fine-tuning of each component in diabetic people (see **Fig. 1**). Bolus formulations are adjusted daily to food intake by the patient while basal formulations are adjusted periodically based on fasting glucose concentrations and long-term measures of glycemia such as hemoglobin A1c.

Recombinant insulin analog solutions are significantly more predictable than suspensions for 2 reasons (see **Table 2**): (1) They are provided as solutions that do not need to be resuspended, bypassing the unpredictable resuspension process and (2) Their absorption from the SC depot is less erratic. Because of superior predictability (low day-to-day variability), these formulations are associated with lower risk of hypoglycemia in people.

Insulin glargine is a human recombinant insulin with 2 arginine residues added to the C-terminus of the B chain at position 30. This modification increases the isoelectric pH of the molecule. Another modification is the replacement of asparagine in position A21 with glycine. This increases the stability of the molecule in acidic pH.[2] Insulin glargine is soluble at pH 4.0 (in which it is supplied) but in neutral pH (such as in SC tissue) it has a strong tendency to precipitate, thus slowing its absorption after injection.[25] Supplied as a solution, an insulin glargine vial or pen does not require rolling or shaking before drawing a dose, which increases the predictability of dosing. Yet, the precipitation–deprecipitation process in the SC introduces a component of variability in absorption. In total, this formulation is more predictable than NPH and likely other suspensions but is less predictable than other insulin analogs.[24,26] Insulin glargine U300 (Toujeo®, Sanofi, Paris, France) is biochemically identical to insulin glargine U100 (eg, Lantus®, Sanofi, Paris, France) but it is 3 times more concentrated.[27] Because the same number of units is delivered as a smaller droplet with smaller surface area, its absorption is slower, its duration is longer, its time-action profile is flatter, and it is associated with decreased day-to-day variability when compared with insulin glargine U100.[26–29] In people with diabetes, insulin glargine U300 is superior to insulin glargine U100 in maintaining glycemic control while also reducing the risk of hypoglycemia.[26,27,29]

Insulin detemir has a 14-carbon fatty acid residue replacing threonine at position B30. Instead of the natural, weaker, ionic interactions between insulin molecules, insulin detemir molecules associate through strong hydrophobic interactions between the fatty acids. These fatty acids also bind reversibly to albumin, which buffers the concentration of insulin detemir in the blood and tissues, adding to its protracted and more predictable effect. In contrast to insulin glargine U100 and insulin suspensions, PD of insulin detemir are considered highly predictable in people, with minimal intersubject and intrasubject variabilities,[30,31] which is key to minimizing hypoglycemic

Table 3
Pharmacodynamics and pharmacokinetics of short-acting insulin solutions

Brand Name	Formulation (hr = Human Recombinant)	Modification	Concentration Syringe/Pen	Feline and Canine Data PD (for XX U/Kg): T_{OA} (min) T_{DA} (min) T_{Peak} (min)
Novolog/Novo L	hr insulin aspart	Proline at B28 is replaced with aspartic acid	U100 Syringe/pen	In cats: 0.25 U/kg:[72] N = 8 $T_{OA} \approx 12$ $T_{DA} \approx 160$ $T_{Peak} \approx 45$
Humalog	hr insulin lispro	A reversal of proline at the B28 position and lysine at the B29 position	U100 Syringe/pen	PK data on 0.2 U/kg in dogs:[73] Onset: 10 min. Insulin concentrations still increased at 3 h, peaked at 45 min (N = 10) Improved postprandial glycemia with 0.1 U/kg added to NPH[74]
Apidra	hr insulin glulisine	Lysine at B29 is replaced by glutamic acid and on position B3 asparagine is replaced by lysine	U100 Syringe/pen	
Afrezza	hr regular insulin	Aerosolized	Inhaler	Inhaled human insulin effective in lowering blood glucose in cats (through a spacer) but PK/PD unknown and not commercially available.[75] Afrezza cannot be used with standard veterinary spacers

Abbreviations: hr, human recombinant; T_{DA}, duration of action; T_{OA}, onset of action; T_{Peak}, Time to peak.

events.[30,32–34] The interaction of insulin detemir with albumin also increases its availability to organs with fenestrated capillaries such as the liver. Relatively high concentrations of insulin detemir are achieved in the liver compared with other target tissues. Thus, this insulin formulation inhibits hepatic glucose output more effectively, lipogenesis in adipose tissue is decreased, and weight gain is minimized.[15,32–34] Preferential insulinization of the liver and low day-to-day variability have not been demonstrated in dogs and cats and so the duration of action of insulin detemir is generally insufficient for once-daily use as a basal insulin.[35–37]

A unit of insulin is defined not by volume or by number of insulin molecules but by its blood-glucose-lowering effect. The potency of insulin detemir varies between species. In people, the potency of insulin detemir is 4 times lower than most other insulins so it is formulated at a concentration that is 4 times higher (Levemir, 2400 nmol/mL, 100 U/mL) than most other insulin formulations (eg, Humulin N, 600 nmol/mL, 100 U/mL) in order to achieve unit-of-action equivalency. This low potency is likely related to the fact that most insulin detemir molecules are bound in plasma to albumin, allowing only a small fraction to be biologically active.[18] This is likely the case in cats as well but not in dogs. Therefore, dose recommendations for insulin determir vary significantly between species.

Insulin degludec is a recombinant human insulin analog in which B30 is replaced by a fatty acid (hexadecanedioic acid) that is bound to B29 via a glutamic spacer. These changes allow for multihexamers to form in SC tissues and results in a long-acting and completely peakless time-action profile. In people, the half-life of insulin degludec is approximately 24 hours and its duration of action is greater than 40 hours. Originally studied as an every-other-day formulation in people, it is now used as a once-daily injection with flexible time of injection. After a few days of daily administration, insulin degludec reaches steady state, with minimal interday fluctuation even when the time of injection is not constant.[38] This makes it an ideal basal insulin in people, with greater patient compliance. Compared with people, the pharmacology of insulin degludec seems to be similar in dogs but differs significantly in cats.[39,40]

Insulin-Fc fusion formulation

A novel method of extending the duration of action of insulin is the fusion of insulin with the Fc region of immunoglobulins. The resulting insulin-Fc fusion protein is a ligand to the insulin receptor but also binds to the host neonatal Fc Receptor (FcRn). In contrast to other SC formulations, the prolonged duration of action of insulin-Fc does not rely on slowing absorption of insulin from the SC tissue but rather on intracellular circulation.[41,42] Insulin-Fc is free to diffuse from the SC tissue into the blood where it is distributed throughout the body. The FcRn is ubiquitously expressed in epithelia, endothelia, cells of hematopoietic origin, and other cells.[41] On binding to the FcRn, insulin-Fc is pinocytosed and eventually exocytosed. While inside the cell, Insulin-Fc is protected from proteolysis like other ligands of the FcRn.[41] This intracellular recycling extends the half-life of the insulin-Fc to 5 to 7 days, allowing for once-weekly administration and minimal intraday variability, making it an ideal basal insulin. Preliminary data suggest that insulin-Fc is a promising formulation in both cats and dogs.[43,44]

Species Source: Similarities, Differences, and Clinical Importance

Animal-source insulin (bovine and porcine) predominated throughout most of the twentieth century until recombinant DNA technology was developed. Since the 1990s, animal-source formulations have become less and less available. Currently, all commercially available insulin formulations are of human-recombinant source except for one porcine lente formulation (Vetsulin/Can-insulin®, MSD Animal Health, NJ, USA). Hypothetically, using an insulin that is most similar in sequence and least immunogenic is a logical choice; however, the clinical importance of this is questionable. Canine insulin is 100% homologous to porcine insulin and differs from human insulin by only 1 amino acid. Feline insulin differs from bovine insulin by 1 amino acid, from canine/porcine insulin by 3 amino acids, and from human insulin by 4 amino acids. Therefore, hypothetically, choosing porcine (or canine if available) insulin for dogs and bovine (or feline if available) insulin for cats would be the most appropriate choice. However, insulin autoantibodies develop even if 100% homologous insulin is used as seen in people treated with human insulin and dogs treated with porcine insulin.[45] Moreover, there is currently no evidence that these autoantibodies interfere with glycemic control in dogs, cats, or people, and both dogs and cats are routinely and successfully treated with human recombinant insulin.[46] Therefore, species-source is probably not a major factor in the choice of an insulin formulation.

COMPLIANCE, ADHERENCE, CONVENIENCE, AND COST
General Principles

Compliance can be divided to adherence and persistence. Adherence is "the extent to which a patient acts in accordance with the prescribed interval and dose of a dosing regimen" while persistence refers to "the act of continuing the treatment for the prescribed duration."[47] In veterinary medicine, one might refer to adherence in the context of owner actions and inactions and compliance as a more general term that encompasses both pet and owner actions.

In human medicine, nonadherence to antidiabetic medications is common and results in poor long-term glycemic control and the development of diabetic complications.[48,49] Medication nonadherence and discontinuation have been shown to be particularly common among those taking injectable antidiabetic medications.[48] Human patients consider insulin injections to be a serious burden and have a negative impact on quality of life.[50] In contrast, surveys of owners of diabetic cats and dogs identified few concerns relating to administration of insulin injections.[51,52] The greatest concerns were associated with the owners' quality of life, rather than that of the animal, with worry about who would care for their animal when they were unavailable near the top of the list. Therefore, it may be surmised that it might be helpful for veterinarians to be flexible and offer insulin treatment options that are client-focused, particularly with respect to timing of injections. It is also unknown how the act of injection itself affects the animals' compliance and the owners' short-term and long-term decisions to treat. Although not exclusively associated with this problem, it is reasonable to assume that the high euthanasia rate (40%) on diagnosis of diabetes is associated with compliance.[53,54]

Studies in people show that adherence declines with increasing dosing frequency.[55] Other reasons for poor adherence include the pain of injection, forgetfulness and having other priorities, regimen complexity (more than one medication or the need to draw up insulin doses), and cost of medication.[49,50] Treatment strategies that minimize these barriers would likely result in greater treatment success, improved quality of life for patient and client, and increased patient survival. In this context, it is also important to consider not only the treatment choice per se but also how it affects monitoring intensity and cost. For example, using a human recombinant basal insulin has the potential to achieve reasonably good glycemic control, with q24 h dosing using a convenient and less stress-inducing insulin pen, resulting in minimal day-to-day variability allowing less monitoring, and simplifying recommendations regarding episodes of inappetence, while lessening the concern regarding hypoglycemia.

Cost and availability are also factors in adherence. For example, veterinary formulations are relatively more expensive than "human" formulations in most countries but the opposite is true in the United States. In the United Kingdom and parts of Europe, regulation requires that veterinary products are used first in the prescribing "cascade."

Syringe-Administration Versus Pen-Administration

Multiple studies have found various advantages to using insulin-dosing pens over the traditional combination of multidose vial and syringe-needle, including increased patient adherence,[56,57] a significant reduction in hypoglycemic events,[58,59] and overall health-care cost-savings.[59,60] Most people preferred pens over vial-syringe and considered pens easier to use. Insulin pens are especially easier to use by those with visual impairments or dexterity problems and overall they lead to better patient satisfaction and improved quality of life.[56,57] Moreover, injection pens are consistently shown to have better dosing accuracy and precision compared with insulin syringes.[61–63] This effect is most pronounced at lower dosages, up to 5 U. The relative imprecision of vial-syringe method can be critical in contributing to increased day-to-day variability, which subsequently makes monitoring more complicated and more expensive. When using a traditional insulin syringe, for a target dose of 1 U, 50% of actual drawn doses were more than 20% different than the target dose.[64] This frequency and magnitude of inaccuracy can have substantial consequences on the management of patients with diabetes. Importantly, most syringe-measured doses exceed the intended dose.[65]

There is currently one insulin-dosing pen for use in veterinary patients containing 40 U/mL of porcine zinc suspension (lente) (VetPen, MSD Animal Health, NJ, USA). Initial pilot studies on this device have shown that the device is easy to use in dogs, is well tolerated under real-life conditions and is more accurate compared with the traditional syringe-vial system[66] and is preferred over syringe use by many owners.[67]

Other currently available insulin-dosing pens were designed for use in human patients. Overall, less insulin is wasted when using insulin-dosing pens, compared with using vials and syringes. Still, used as directed by the manufacturer, these pens might be too expensive for routine use in some countries (eg, United States). However, clinical experience suggests that with some modifications, substantial cost reductions can be achieved without significant compromise to patient care. These modifications to address financial constraints should be practiced with caution however, considering the lack of clinical research to support them. "Human" insulin-dosing pens are tested for only short-term stability (<42 days) and for use when not refrigerated. However, keeping the pen refrigerated while in use would likely retard bacterial contamination and allows extended use. We routinely use these pens until the reservoir has been completely depleted, often for many months, substantially reducing the relative cost. In contrast to reports from people, injection of cold insulin does not seem to be associated with pain in cats and dogs. Priming of the needle (air shot) with 1 to 3 U is also recommended before every injection. This might also make the use of a pen less economical. After priming once when starting a new pen to verify that the pen works, one of the authors who is based in the United States (CG) does not recommend routine priming of pens. Without regular priming, air bubbles in the pen might interfere with accurate dosing, or it might not be noticed that a pen has become faulty, and so these potential issues must be considered and the pen checked when a patient does not respond to insulin treatment as expected. It is advisable to regularly visually check the insulin cartridge and eject any air bubbles. The problem of air bubbles can also be avoided by tilting the pen during injection so that the plunger is higher than the needle tip, allowing the air bubbles move away from the needle. In people, it is recommended to keep the needle of the pen under the skin after injection for at least 3 seconds to allow the dose to be completely delivered. This does not seem to be necessary when small doses are delivered, as is the case for most animals. Most pens are limited to delivery of 1 U increments with only a few insulin pens allowing the dialing of 0.5 U increments. Although this might seem like a disadvantage, compared with the traditional vial-syringe approach, one needs to consider the very low precision and accuracy of insulin syringes for administration of 0.5-U dose increments.[64]

A more comprehensive review of the use of insulin injection pens can be found elsewhere.[68]

Managing Inappetence and Gastrointestinal Signs

In health, about half of the daily insulin requirement is basal and the other half is bolus, leading to the recommendation to lower the dose of intermediate-acting insulin by 50% in a patient that skips a meal or in a patient that is vomiting. There are 2 potential problems with this strategy. First, the 50% basal-bolus ratio is a general estimate, and might lead to significant overdosing or underdosing in any particular patient. Second, it is common for diabetic pets to be "picky eaters" or to have concurrent gastrointestinal disease, pancreatitis, or other disease that affects their appetite. The need to adjust the dose of insulin in these instances can have a significant impact on glycemic control and on the owners' stress levels. Some of this might be alleviated by using a basal-bolus insulin combination in which the dose and frequency of the basal insulin are unaltered during episodes of decreased appetite and the bolus insulin is simply skipped.

GOALS OF THERAPY FOR THE SPECIFIC PATIENT

In people, it is well established that the magnitude and quality of long-term dysglycemia are associated with long-term outcome.[69,70] Maintaining tight glycemic control has been shown in numerous studies to reduce the long-term risk of macrovascular and microvascular diseases in both type 1 and type 2 diabetes. However, maintaining tight glycemic control also increases the risk of hypoglycemia and the balance between risk and benefit depends on the specific complication being studied.[71] In addition, increased glycemic variability (fluctuations between hypoglycemia and hyperglycemia) is a risk factor for hypoglycemia. Therefore, glycemic targets are not absolute, but rather are tailored to the patient, taking into account the disease, comorbidities, compliance, and so forth.[71] As an extension of that, a blanket statement on "best" insulin recommendation cannot be made either.

Different goal-oriented treatment strategies should also be considered for dogs and cats, with pros and cons to each (**Fig. 3**). It is currently unknown if the risk for diabetic complications such as cataract formation or inability to achieve diabetic remission are proportional to the level of hyperglycemia, related to a certain threshold of hyperglycemia, to glycemic variability, or other factors. Until that is resolved, it cannot be assumed that the risk of diabetic complications is reduced by lower glycemic targets and corresponding increased risk of hypoglycemia. In this context, it is important to consider the abundant evidence that over time, hyperglycemia, hypoglycemia (even when subclinical, and/or intermittent and sporadic), and high glycemic variability lead to impaired counterregulatory responses and increased the risk of fatal

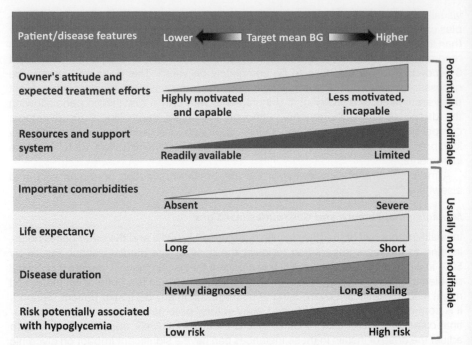

Fig. 3. Factors that influence clinical decisions regarding glycemic targets when treating diabetic dogs and cats.

insulin-induced hypoglycemia (See Mott J, and Gilor C, Hypoglycemia and Autonomic Failure in Dogs, *Vet Clin North Amer Small Anim Pract*, 2023 xx, xx). Because it is potentially fatal, avoidance of hypoglycemia is therefore a critically important treatment goal, although there are currently no guidelines in veterinary medicine regarding acceptable degree of hypoglycemia (both in terms of absolute glucose concentrations and of duration of hypoglycemia), and how they translate to low interstitial glucose.

The clinical decision on treatment and monitoring methods must also consider potential long-term attrition in client and animal compliance. What seems like an ideal treatment and monitoring scheme in the short term might backfire in the long-run if owners have maximized their financial capabilities, especially when concurrent diseases develop. In that respect, minimalist treatment and monitoring approaches might be better in the long-run.

CLINICS CARE POINTS

- No insulin formulation should be considered best by default. Rather, the choice of insulin should be tailored to the specific clinical situation.

- An effective and safe basal insulin has a flat time-action profile, which provides roughly the same action every hour of the day, with no distinct peak, and minimal day-to-day variability.

- The intermediate-acting insulin formulations are often an appropriate choice for bolus insulin treatment in diabetic dogs.

- Insulin pens improve the quality of life of the caregiver and allow better dosing accuracy and precision than syringe administration.

DECLARATION OF INTERESTS

L. Fleeman has received honoraria for educational seminars for MSD Animal Health, Zoetis, Royal Canin, Nestle Purina, and consulting fees from Dechra. C. Gilor has received research support or consulting fees from MSD Animal Health, Nestle Purina, Dechra, BiomEdit, Baycom Diagnostics, Edge Animal Health and Okava Pharmaceuticals.

REFERENCES

1.. Ahren B, Taborsky GJ. Beta-cell function and insulin secretion. In: Porte D, Sherwin R, Baron A, Ellenberg, editors. & rifkin's diabetes mellitus. New York: The McGrew-Hill Companies Inc; 2003.
2. Owens DR, Bolli GB. Beyond the era of NPH insulin–long-acting insulin analogs: chemistry, comparative pharmacology, and clinical application. Diabetes Technol Ther 2008;10:333–49.
3. Petersen MC, Shulman GI. Mechanisms of insulin action and insulin resistance. Physiol Rev 2018;98:2133–223.
4. Sheldon B, Russell-Jones D, Wright J. Insulin analogues: an example of applied medical science. Diabetes Obes Metabol 2009;11:5–19.
5.. Hill RC, Burrows CF, Bauer JE, et al. Texturized vegetable protein containing indigestible soy carbohydrate affects blood insulin concentrations in dogs fed high fat diets. J Nutr 2006;136:2024S–7S.
6. Carciofi AC, Takakura FS, de-Oliveira LD, et al., Effects of six carbohydrate sources on dog diet digestibility and post-prandial glucose and insulin response, J Anim Physiol Anim Nutr, 2008;92:326–336.
7. Elliott KF, Rand JS, Fleeman LM, et al. A diet lower in digestible carbohydrate results in lower postprandial glucose concentrations compared with a traditional canine diabetes diet and an adult maintenance diet in healthy dogs. Res Vet Sci 2012;93:288–95.
8. Appleton DJ, Rand JS, Sunvold GD. Insulin sensitivity decreases with obesity, and lean cats with low insulin sensitivity are at greatest risk of glucose intolerance with weight gain. J Feline Med Surg 2001;3:211–28.
9. Mori A, Sako T, Lee P, et al. Comparison of three commercially available prescription diet regimens on short-term post-prandial serum glucose and insulin concentrations in healthy cats. Vet Res Commun 2009;33:669–80.
10. de-Oliveira LD, Carciofi AC, Oliveira MC, et al. Effects of six carbohydrate sources on diet digestibility and postprandial glucose and insulin responses in cats. J Anim Sci 2008;86:2237–46.
11. Camara A, Verbrugghe A, Cargo-Froom C, et al. The daytime feeding frequency affects appetite-regulating hormones, amino acids, physical activity, and respiratory quotient, but not energy expenditure, in adult cats fed regimens for 21 days. PLoS One 2020;15:e0238522.
12. American Diabetes Association, 9. Pharmacologic approaches to glycemic treatment: standards of medical care in diabetes-2020. Diabetes Care 2020;43:S98–110.

13. Crinò C Iavazzo F, Ferri F,, et al. Diabetic remission in a cat treated with an implantable pump to deliver insulin. The Canadian veterinary journal = La revue veterinaire canadienne 2020;61:30–4.

14. Yang JF, Gong X, Bakh NA, et al. Connecting rodent and human pharmacokinetic models for the design and translation of glucose-responsive insulin. Diabetes 2020;69:1815–26.

15. Hermansen K, Davies M. Does insulin detemir have a role in reducing risk of insulin-associated weight gain? Diabetes Obes Metabol 2007;9:209–17.

16.. Heise T, Zijlstra E, Nosek L, et al. Euglycaemic glucose clamp: what it can and cannot do, and how to do it. Diabetes Obes Metabol 2016. https://doi.org/10.1111/dom.12703.

17. Horvath K, Bock G, Regittnig W, et al. Insulin glulisine, insulin lispro and regular human insulin show comparable end-organ metabolic effects: an exploratory study. Diabetes Obes Metabol 2008;10:484–91.

18. Hirsch IB, Juneja R, Beals JM, et al. The evolution of insulin and how it informs therapy and treatment choices. Endocr Rev 2020;41:733–55.

19. Havelund S, Plum A, Ribel U, et al. The mechanism of protraction of insulin detemir, a long-acting, acylated analog of human insulin. Pharm Res (N Y) 2004;21:1498–504.

20. Plum A, Agerso H, Andersen L. Pharmacokinetics of the rapid-acting insulin analog, insulin aspart, in rats, dogs, and pigs, and pharmacodynamics of insulin aspart in pigs. Drug Metab Dispos 2000;28:155–60.

21. Rave K, Potocka E, Heinemann L, et al. Pharmacokinetics and linear exposure of AFRESA compared with the subcutaneous injection of regular human insulin. Diabetes Obes Metabol 2009;11:715–20.

22. Gilor C, Keel T, Attermeier KJ, et al. Hyperinsulinemic-euglycemic clamps using insulin detemir and insulin glargine in healthy cats [abstract]. J Vet Intern Med 2008;22(3):729.

23. Jehle PM, Micheler C, Jehle DR, et al. Inadequate suspension of neutral protamine Hagendorn (NPH) insulin in pens. Lancet (London, England) 1999;354:1604–7.

24. Heise T, Nosek L, Rønn BB, et al. Lower within-subject variability of insulin detemir in comparison to NPH insulin and insulin glargine in people with type 1 diabetes. Diabetes 2004;53:1614–20.

25. Kohn WD, Micanovic R, Myers SL, et al. pI-shifted insulin analogs with extended in vivo time action and favorable receptor selectivity. Peptides 2007;28:935–48.

26. Becker RHA, Nowotny I, Teichert L, et al. Low within- and between-day variability in exposure to new insulin glargine 300 U/ml. Diabetes Obes Metabol 2015. https://doi.org/10.1111/dom.12416.

27. Steinstraesser A, Schmidt R, Bergmann K, et al. Investigational new insulin glargine 300 U/ml has the same metabolism as insulin glargine 100 U/ml. Diabetes Obes Metabol 2014. https://doi.org/10.1111/dom.12283.

28. Riddle MC, Bolli GB, Ziemen M, et al. New insulin glargine 300 units/mL versus glargine 100 units/mL in people with type 2 diabetes using basal and mealtime insulin: Glucose control and hypoglycemia in a 6-month randomized controlled trial (EDITION 1). Diabetes Care 2014. https://doi.org/10.2337/dc14-0991.

29. Ritzel R, Roussel R, Bolli GB, et al. Patient-level meta-analysis of the EDITION 1, 2 and 3 studies: Glycaemic control and hypoglycaemia with new insulin glargine 300 U/ml versus glargine 100 U/ml in people with type 2 diabetes. Diabetes Obes Metabol 2015. https://doi.org/10.1111/dom.12485.

30. Heise T, Pieber TR. Towards peakless, reproducible and long-acting insulins. An assessment of the basal analogues based on isoglycaemic clamp studies. Diabetes Obes Metabol 2007;9:648–59.
31. Soran H, Younis N. Insulin detemir: a new basal insulin analogue. Diabetes Obes Metabol 2006;8:26–30.
32. Danne T, Datz N, Endahl L, et al. Insulin detemir is characterized by a more reproducible pharmacokinetic profile than insulin glargine in children and adolescents with type 1 diabetes: results from a randomized, double-blind, controlled trial. Pediatr Diabetes 2008;9:554–60.
33. Fakhoury W, Lockhart I, Kotchie RW, et al. Indirect comparison of once daily insulin detemir and glargine in reducing weight gain and hypoglycaemic episodes when administered in addition to conventional oral anti-diabetic therapy in patients with type-2 diabetes. Pharmacology 2008;82:156–63.
34. Monami M, Marchionni N, Mannucci E. Long-acting insulin analogues versus NPH human insulin in type 2 diabetes: a meta-analysis. Diabetes Res Clin Pract 2008;81:184–9.
35. Gilor C, Ridge TK, Attermeier KJ, et al. Pharmacodynamics of insulin detemir and insulin glargine assessed by an isoglycemic clamp method in healthy cats. J Vet Intern Med 2010, 870-874;24.
36. Fink H, Herbert C, Gilor C. Pharmacodynamics and pharmacokinetics of insulin detemir and insulin glargine 300 U/mL in healthy dogs. Domest Anim Endocrinol 2018, 17-30;64.
37. Sako T, Mori A, Lee P, et al. Time-action profiles of insulin detemir in normal and diabetic dogs. Res Vet Sci 2011;90:396–403.
38. Heise T, Nørskov M, Nosek L, et al. Insulin degludec: Lower day-to-day and within-day variability in pharmacodynamic response compared with insulin glargine 300 U/mL in type 1 diabetes. Diabetes Obes Metabol 2017;19:1032–9.
39. Oda H, Mori A, Ishii S, et al. Time-action profiles of insulin degludec in healthy dogs and its effects on glycemic control in diabetic dogs. J Vet Med Sci 2018; 80:1720–3.
40. Gilor C, Culp W, Ghandi S, et al. Comparison of pharmacodynamics and pharmacokinetics of insulin degludec and insulin glargine 300 U/mL in healthy cats. Domest Anim Endocrinol 2019;69:19–29.
41. Pyzik M, Sand KMK, Hubbard JJ, et al. The Neonatal Fc Receptor (FcRn): A Misnomer? Front Immunol 2019;10:1540.
42. Roopenian DC, Akilesh S. FcRn: the neonatal Fc receptor comes of age. Nat Rev Immunol 2007;7:715–25.
43. Gilor C, Hulsebosch SE, Pires J, et al. An ultra-long-acting recombinant insulin for the treatment of diabetes mellitus in cats. J Vet Intern Med 2021;35:2123–30.
44. Hulsebosch SE, Pires J, Bannasch MJ, et al. Ultra-long-acting recombinant insulin for the treatment of diabetes mellitus in dogs. J Vet Intern Med 2022. https://doi.org/10.1111/jvim.16449.
45. Holder AL, Kennedy LJ, Ollier WER, et al. Breed differences in development of anti-insulin antibodies in diabetic dogs and investigation of the role of dog leukocyte antigen (DLA) genes. Vet Immunol Immunopathol 2015;167:130–8.
46. Hoenig M, Reusch C, Peterson ME. Beta cell and insulin antibodies in treated and untreated diabetic cats. Vet Immunol Immunopathol 2000;77:93–102.
47. Cramer JA, Roy A, Burrell A, et al. Medication compliance and persistence: terminology and definitions, *Value Heal.* J. Int. Soc. Pharmacoeconomics Outcomes Res. 2008;11:44–7.

48. Spain CV, Wright JJ, Hahn RM, et al. Self-reported barriers to adherence and persistence to treatment with injectable medications(for type 2 diabetes. Clin Therapeut 2016;38:1653–64.e1.
49. Giorgino F, Penfornis A, Pechtner V, et al. Adherence to antihyperglycemic medications and glucagon-like peptide 1-receptor agonists in type 2 diabetes: clinical consequences and strategies for improvement. Patient Prefer Adherence 2018; 12:707–19.
50. Rubin RR, Peyrot M, Kruger DF, et al. Barriers to insulin injection therapy: patient and health care provider perspectives. Diabetes Educat 2009;35:1014–22.
51. Niessen SJ, Powney S, Guitian J, et al. Evaluation of a quality-of-life tool for dogs with diabetes mellitus. J Vet Intern Med 2012;26:953–61.
52. Niessen SJ, Powney S, Guitian J, et al. Evaluation of a quality-of-life tool for cats with diabetes mellitus. J Vet Intern Med 2010;24:1098–105.
53. Niessen SJM, Hazuchova K, Powney SL, et al. The big pet diabetes survey: perceived frequency and triggers for euthanasia. Vet. Sci. 2017, 27;4.
54. Fall T, Hamlin HH, Hedhammar A, et al. Diabetes mellitus in a population of 180,000 insured dogs: incidence, survival, and breed distribution. J Vet Intern Med 2007;21:1209–16.
55. Osterberg L, Blaschke T. Adherence to medication. N Engl J Med 2005;353: 487–97.
56. Pfützner A, Asakura T, Sommavilla B, et al. Insulin delivery with FlexPen: dose accuracy, patient preference and adherence. Expet Opin Drug Deliv 2008;5: 915–25.
57. Dang DK, Lee J. Analysis of symposium articles on insulin pen devices and alternative insulin delivery methods. J. Diabetes Sci. Technol. 2010;4:558–61.
58. Asche CV, Shane-McWhorter L, Raparla S. Health economics and compliance of vials/syringes versus pen devices: a review of the evidence. Diabetes Technol Ther 2010;12(Suppl 1):S101–8.
59. Cobden D, Lee WC, Balu S, et al. Health outcomes and economic impact of therapy conversion to a biphasic insulin analog pen among privately insured patients with type 2 diabetes mellitus. Pharmacotherapy 2007;27:948–62.
60. Lee WC, Balu S, Cobden D, et al. Medication adherence and the associated health-economic impact among patients with type 2 diabetes mellitus converting to insulin pen therapy: an analysis of third-party managed care claims data. Clin Therapeut 2006;28:1711–2.
61. Gnanalingham MG, Newland P, Smith CP. Accuracy and reproducibility of low dose insulin administration using pen-injectors and syringes. Arch Dis Child 1998;79:59–62.
62. Luijf YM, DeVries JH. Dosing accuracy of insulin pens versus conventional syringes and vials. Diabetes Technol Ther 2010;12(Suppl 1):S73–7.
63. Keith K, Nicholson D, Rogers D. Accuracy and precision of low-dose insulin administration using syringes, pen injectors, and a pump. Clin Pediatr 2004;43: 69–74.
64. Borin-Crivellenti S, Bonagura J, Gilor C. Comparison of precision and accuracy of U100 and U40 insulin syringes [Abstract]. J Vet Intern Med 2014;28:1029.
65. Casella SJ, Mongilio MK, Plotnick LP, et al. Accuracy and precision of low-dose insulin administration. Pediatrics 1993;91:1155–7.
66. Burgaud S, Guillot R, Harnois-Milon G. Clinical evaluation of a veterinary insulin pen in diabetic dogs. In: Proceedings of the WSAVA/ FECAVA/BSAVA congress; 12-15 April 2012; Birmingham, UK. Abstract 122.

67. Del Baldo F, Colajanni L, Corradini S. Glycemic control and owner preference in insulin delivery in diabetic dogs (Abstract). J Vet Intern Med 2020;34:3134.
68. Thompson A, Lathan P, Fleeman L. Update on insulin treatment for dogs and cats: insulin dosing pens and more. Vet Med (Auckland, N.Z) 2015;6:129–42.
69. Holman RR, Paul SK, Bethel MA, et al. 10-year follow-up of intensive glucose control in type 2 diabetes. N Engl J Med 2008;359:1577–89.
70. Diabetes Control, Complications Trial Research Group, Nathan DM, Genuth S, Lachin J, et al. The effect of intensive treatment of diabetes on the development and progression of long-term complications in insulin-dependent diabetes mellitus. N Engl J Med 1993;329:977–86.
71. American Diabetes Association, 6. Glycemic Targets: Standards of Medical Care in Diabetes-2018. Diabetes Care 2018;41:S55–64.
72. Pipe-Martin HN, Fletcher JM, Gilor C, et al. Pharmacodynamics and pharmacokinetics of insulin aspart assessed by use of the isoglycemic clamp method in healthy cats. Domest Anim Endocrinol 2018;62.
73. Matsuo Y, Shimoda S, Sakakida M, et al. Strict glycemic control in diabetic dogs with closed-loop intraperitoneal insulin infusion algorithm designed for an artificial endocrine pancreas. J Artif Organs 2003;6:55–63.
74. Bertalan AV, Drobatz KJ, Hess RS. Effects of treatment with lispro and neutral protamine Hagedorn insulins on serum fructosamine and postprandial blood glucose concentrations in dogs with clinically well-controlled diabetes mellitus and postprandial hyperglycemia. Am J Vet Res 2020;81:153–8.
75. DeClue AE, Leverenz EF, Wiedmeyer CE, et al. Glucose lowering effects of inhaled insulin in healthy cats. J Feline Med Surg 2008;10:519–22.

Insulin Therapy in Small Animals, Part 2: Cats

Linda Fleeman, BVSc, PhD, MANZCVS[a],*, Chen Gilor, DVM, PhD, DACVIM[b]

KEYWORDS

- Basal insulin • Glargine U300 • Feline • Diabetes mellitus

KEY POINTS

- No insulin formulation should be considered best by default. Rather, the choice of insulin formulation should be tailored to the specific clinical situation. Different goal-oriented treatment strategies should be considered, with pros and cons to each.
- Postprandial endogenous bolus insulin secretion in cats is typically prolonged and unpredictable, regardless of the dietary carbohydrate content of the food. Therefore timing of meals does not need to be matched to insulin injections. Regardless, it is crucial that food intake is reliable and predictable to minimize the risk of insulin-induced hypoglycemia.
- In patients with some residual beta cell function (most cats), administering only a basal insulin might lead to complete normalization of blood glucose concentrations because bolus requirement is typically sustained and prolonged.
- Basal insulin requirements are relatively constant throughout the day. Therefore, for an insulin formulation to be effective and safe as a basal insulin, its action should be roughly the same every hour of the day. At present, only insulin glargine U300 (Toujeo) approaches this definition in cats.
- Currently available insulin suspensions (NPH, NPH/regular mixes, lente, and PZI) as well as insulin glargine U100, insulin detemir, and insulin degludec are intermediate-acting formulations that require twice-daily administration.

INTRODUCTION

The prevalence of diabetes mellitus (DM) varies with geographic region and is reported to affect 50 to 94 of 10,000 domestic cats.[1] Upon diagnosis, insulin therapy is most often required for the survival of cats suffering from DM, but in a proportion of cats, dependence on exogenous insulin is transient and they eventually experience remission, that is, their exogenous insulin requirement decreases to zero. The main clinical challenge of insulin therapy in cats is the potential for DM remission. If remission

a Animal Diabetes Australia, 5 Hood Street, Collingwood, Victoria 3066, Australia; b Small Animal Internal Medicine, Department of Small Animal Clinical Sciences, College of Veterinary Medicine, University of Florida, 2015 Southwest 16th Avenue, Gainesville, FL 32608, USA
* Corresponding author.
E-mail address: L.Fleeman@AnimalDiabetesAustralia.com.au

Vet Clin Small Anim 53 (2023) 635–644
https://doi.org/10.1016/j.cvsm.2023.02.004
0195-5616/23/© 2023 Elsevier Inc. All rights reserved.

cannot be achieved, the principles of insulin therapy in feline DM are generally the same as in dogs, although the pharmacology of specific insulin formulations varies between these species.

Despite a hundred years of veterinary experience and a plethora of available insulin formulations, there is striking paucity of high-level evidence from direct comparison in clinical trials to suggest that any one insulin formulation is advantageous compared with any other in any veterinary clinical scenario. In this context, this article provides a review of current understanding of insulin pharmacology and relevant pathophysiology, integrated with practical considerations and key monitoring principles for the application of insulin therapy.

No insulin formulation should be considered "best" by default. Rather, the choice of insulin formulation should be tailored to the specific clinical situation. Often, opposing needs will result in compromise. For example, for a fractious cat or for an owner who is struggling to give injections, minimizing the number of injections by using a long-acting insulin formulation once daily might be a necessary compromise even if the glycemic control is not optimal. In contrast, a formulation that is shorter in duration but much less expensive might be ideal for an owner who can easily administer insulin but cannot afford expensive formulations.

PATHOPHYSIOLOGY: INSULIN REQUIREMENTS ON THE DIABETES SPECTRUM
Insulin Therapy in the Context of Relative Insulin Deficiency and the Potential for Remission

Two factors contribute to DM remission: (1) recovery of beta cell function when glucose toxicity and lipotoxicity resolves and (2) reduction in insulin requirement. To achieve remission, a cat must have sufficient beta cells to release enough insulin to match daily requirements. Insulin requirements vary between cats and within individuals and depend on insulin sensitivity as well as the load of digested carbohydrates. Currently, residual beta cell mass and the potential to achieve remission cannot be predicted in an individual cat at any stage of DM. Because of the potential for ongoing beta cell loss as a result of glucose toxicity and lipotoxicity, it is recommended to initiate insulin therapy as soon as possible after diagnosis to maximize the chance of future remission.

Regardless of the potential for remission, it is thought that most diabetic cats have residual beta cell function,[2] even if that residual function is insufficient to meet daily insulin requirements and attain remission. In cats with residual beta cell function, endogenous insulin release could potentially close the gap between the amount of insulin that is required to maintain euglycemia at any given moment and the amount of exogenous insulin that is being delivered. Therefore, it is often unnecessary to mimic precisely the physiologic pattern of insulin secretion to achieve excellent glycemic control in these cats. In these cats, it is expected that glucose variability would be low (because functioning beta cells help control blood glucose), potentially explaining the observation that in cats experiencing low glucose variability the likelihood of remission is higher.[3] It is also possible, however, that low glucose variability confers an environment that is more conducive to the recovery of beta cells from glucose toxicity, therefore positively contributing to remission.

In cats with residual beta cell function, administering only a basal insulin formulation (see Linda Fleeman and Chen Gilor's article, "Insulin Therapy in Dogs and Cats, Part 1: General Principles" in this issue) might lead to complete normalization of blood glucose concentrations because the postprandial bolus requirement is typically sustained and prolonged, and because endogenous insulin secretion is often sufficient to make up for the bolus insulin requirement. This is especially true in cats in which the postprandial insulin requirement is peakless and unchanging throughout the day as a result of slow transit time, feeding multiple times a day, and/or feeding a diet that is low in carbohydrates.[4]

Insulin Therapy in Cats with No Functional Beta Cells (Absolute Insulin Deficiency)

In cats that have no functioning beta cells (whether a transient state of dysfunction secondary to glucose toxicity and lipotoxicity or a permanent state secondary to complete beta cell loss), insulin therapy will generally follow the same principles as in dogs, although the pharmacology of specific insulin formulations differs between species (see below), and there is typically no requirement for exogenous bolus insulin administration in cats.

Insulin Therapy in Hypersomatotropism

Extreme insulin resistance is certainly a contributor to the DM phenotype in feline hypersomatotropism, but the effect of growth hormone excess on beta cells is currently unclear. Cats with hypersomatotropism that are managed with only insulin without any treatment of their primary disease present a clinical picture that is most consistent with absolute insulin deficiency. However, beta cell function can recover once hypersomatotropism is treated, even if severe insulin resistance was previously present for years; this indicates that the effect of excess growth hormone on beta cell function might be different than for other causes of insulin resistance.

TIMING OF INSULIN INJECTION IN CONJUNCTION WITH FEEDING

Compared with dogs and people, postprandial endogenous bolus insulin secretion in cats is typically prolonged and unpredictable, regardless of the dietary carbohydrate content of the food (**Table 1**). Therefore timing of meals does not need to be matched with insulin injections and diabetic cats may be fed at any time, which allows more flexibility with the feeding of diabetic cats than for diabetic dogs. Nevertheless, reduced ingestion of food or subsequent vomiting of a meal after insulin administration is commonly reported in cats with neuroglycopenia at an emergency center. These signs might be either a consequence or a cause of insulin-induced hypoglycemia. Therefore it is crucial that food intake be reliable and predictable to minimize the risk of insulin-induced hypoglycemia. Any diet change should be introduced gradually when the cat is eating well at home and preferably after pathologic weight loss has been arrested. Prompt veterinary assessment is warranted when there is anorexia and/or vomiting in diabetic cats. Consumption of cat foods cannot be relied upon as a treatment of neuroglycopenia. A source of readily absorbed sugar such as glucose syrup or honey can be liberally applied to the oral mucosa or can be added to cat food.

Table 1		
Comparison of bolus insulin secretion in people, dogs, and cats		
	Duration of Bolus Insulin Secretion	Magnitude of Increase of Insulin During Bolus Insulin Secretion
Human	2–4 h	5-fold
Dog	6–9 h	5- to 7-fold
Cat	6–>12 h	0- to 3-fold

Note that this is a rough guide only because there is large individual variability depending on meal composition, quantity consumed, and frequency of feeding.

GLUCOSE VARIABILITY IN DIFFERENT STRATEGIES OF INSULIN THERAPY

When using an intermediate-acting insulin, incongruity between required and delivered insulin often results in frequent intra-day fluctuations in blood glucose concentrations. With residual beta cell function, endogenous insulin secretion might eliminate or minimize this incongruity, minimizing glucose variability. Cats with no residual beta cell function might be prone to greater glycemic variability than dogs because the renal threshold for glucose tends to be lower in dogs (180–200 mg/dL, 10–11 mmol/L)[5] than in cats (270 mg/dL, 15 mmol/L),[6,7] which allows dogs but not cats to reduce hyperglycemia in the 180 to 270 mg/dL (10–15 mmol/L) range by excreting glucose in urine. Providing a basal insulin might result in complete congruity with insulin requirement in cats that are fed a low carbohydrate diet, even in cats with little or no residual beta cell function.

Considering the intra-day blood glucose fluctuations and substantial inter-day variability in insulin action associated with intermediate-acting formulations, and aiming for resolution of clinical signs but not necessarily aiming for remission, it is usually recommended to aim for blood glucose concentrations that range above normal between a low end of 80 to 100 mg/dL (4.5–5.5 mmol/L) and a high end of 250 to 350 mg/dL (14–19 mmol/L). Although uncommonly realized,[8,9] the ideal blood glucose curve is typically expected to be at the high end of this range just before insulin administration and the nadir to occur at about 6 hours.[10,11] Because the renal threshold in cats is about 270 mg/dL (15 mmol/L), this blood glucose concentration target might result in complete alleviation of clinical signs. However, levels of glycated proteins are expected to remain above the reference interval. If glycated protein levels are normal, or if the blood glucose concentration nadir is less than 80 mg/dL (<4.5 mmol/L), it is assumed that the cat is overcontrolled and the insulin dose should be decreased.

GOALS OF THERAPY FOR THE SPECIFIC PATIENT

In people, it is well-established that the magnitude and quality of long-term dysglycemia are associated with long-term outcome.[12,13] Maintaining tight glycemic control has been shown in numerous studies to reduce the long-term risk of macrovascular and microvascular disease both in type 1 and type 2 DM. However, maintaining tight glycemic control also increases the risk of hypoglycemia and the balance between risk and benefit depends on the specific complication being studied.[14] In addition, increased glycemic variability is a risk factor for hypoglycemia. Therefore, glycemic targets are not absolute, but rather are tailored to the patient, taking into account the disease, comorbidities, compliance, and so on.[14] As an extension of that, a blanket statement on best insulin recommendation cannot be made either.

Different goal-oriented treatment strategies should also be considered for the specific patient, with pros and cons to each (see the Linda Fleeman and Chen Gilor's article, "Insulin Therapy in Dogs and Cats, Part 1: General Principles" in this issue). It is currently unknown if the likelihood of achieving diabetic remission is inversely correlated with the level of hyperglycemia, related to a certain threshold of hyperglycemia, to glycemic variability, or to other factors. In this context, it is important to consider the abundant evidence that over time, hyperglycemia, hypoglycemia (even when subclinical, and/or intermittent and sporadic), and high glycemic variability lead to impaired counterregulatory responses and increased risk of fatal insulin-induced hypoglycemia. Multiple well-established mechanisms that explain this phenomenon have been described in people and rodents with some recent, although still scarce, evidence in dogs.[15–18] There is currently no evidence to suggest that the same phenomenon exists in cats, but, because it is potentially fatal, avoidance of hypoglycemia is a critically important treatment goal. There are currently no guidelines in veterinary medicine regarding acceptable levels of low blood glucose concentrations (both in terms of absolute concentrations and of duration), and how they translate to low interstitial glucose levels as measured by continuous glucose monitors.

Clinical decisions on treatment and monitoring methods must also take into account potential long-term attrition in client and pet compliance. What seems like an ideal treatment and monitoring scheme in the short term might backfire in the long run if owners have maximized their financial capabilities, especially when concurrent diseases develop. In that respect, minimalist treatment and monitoring approaches might be better in the long run.

GUIDELINES FOR CHOOSING INSULIN FORMULATIONS

Details on commonly used insulin formulations are presented in **Table 2**.

Intermediate-Acting Insulin Formulations in Cats

In cats, porcine lente, and even more so Neutral Protamine Hagedorn (NPH), tends to have a shorter duration of action compared with Protamine Zinc Insulin (PZI), insulin glargine U100, insulin detemir, and insulin degludec, although all of them are most appropriately used in cats as intermediate-acting insulin formulations.[19–21]

Insulin detemir: Preferential insulinization of the liver and low day-to-day variability have not been demonstrated in cats yet, and the duration of action of insulin detemir is generally insufficient for once-daily use as a basal insulin.[21–23] Using the glucose clamp method, insulin detemir at a dose of 0.5 U/kg had a duration of action of about 12 hours in cats.[21] There was a distinct peak to the time-action profile, although some cats displayed a peakless time-action profile. As in people, and in contrast to dogs, the potency of detemir (on a molar basis) is reduced in cats. Therefore, the commercial formulation Levemir (2400 nmol/mL, 100 U/mL), which is 4 times more concentrated than most other formulations (eg, Lantus, 600 nmol/mL, 100 U/mL), has similar potency per unit as other insulin formulations. The dose range required for achieving good glycemic control is similar (median of about 2 U/cat every 12 hours) for insulin detemir and insulin glargine U100.[24,25] Therefore it is recommended to start insulin detemir at the same dose as other insulin formulations in cats.

Insulin degludec: The pharmacodynamics of insulin degludec in cats is more consistent with it being an intermediate-acting insulin than a basal insulin (in contrast to other species). The duration of action of insulin degludec was about 10 hours in cats with a very distinct peak at about 5 hours.[26] Therefore, this insulin should not be used as a once-daily treatment in cats.

Insulin glargine U100: Insulin glargine U100 has been touted as advantageous in inducing remission in cats based on uncontrolled and nonrandomized studies, but there is currently no compelling evidence to support this.[27] In a small clinical study in cats, once-daily administration of insulin glargine U100 was compared with twice daily porcine lente in cats fed a low-carbohydrate diet.[28] In that study both treatment groups experienced improvement in serum fructosamine concentrations, and glycemia assessed by 16-hour intermittent blood glucose curves was improved. Four of the 13 cats of this study experienced remission of diabetes, but only 1 of these was in the insulin glargine U100-treated group. In another study comparing insulin glargine U100 with PZI, both administered twice daily, there was no difference in remission

Table 2
Pharmacodynamics, pharmacokinetics, and guidelines for frequency of administration of specific insulin formulations

Brand Name	Formulation	Concentration	Syringe/Pen	Feline Data — Frequency PD	PD (For X U/Kg): DA (h), T_{PEAK} (h)	Comments
Humulin N, Novolion N	hr NPH suspension	U100	Syringe/pen	q 8		
Vetsulin/Caninsulin	Porcine Lente suspension	U40	Syringe/pen	q 8–12		PK data on 0.4 (0.2–0.9) U/kg in DM[19]: insulin peak at 1.6 ± 0.2 h, and returned to baseline in 8 ± 0.2 h (N = 25). PK data on 0.5 U/kg in healthy cats[32]: insulin peak at 2.9 ± 0.8 h (0.5–6), and returned to baseline in 8.4 ± 0.5 h (5.6–10.2) (N = 9)
Prozinc	hr PZI suspension	U40	Syringe	q 12→		PK data on 0.5 U/kg in healthy cats[32]: insulin peak at 3.4 ± 1h (1–10), and returned to baseline in 10.5 ± 1.3 h (5.3–16.4) (N = 9)
Tresiba	hr Insulin degludec solution	U100/U200	Pen	q 12	0.4U/kg:[26] N = 6 DA ≈ 10 ± 3 T_{Peak} ≈ 5	
Levemir	hr Insulin detemir solution	U100/U200	Syringe/pen	q12→	0.5U/Kg:[21] N = 10 DA ≈ 14 ± 4 T_{Peak} ≈7	

| Lantus/Optisulin/ Basaglar/ Semglee/ Abasria | hr Insulin glargine solution | U100 Syringe/pen | q12→ | 0.5U/kg:[21] N = 10 DA ≈11 ± 5 T_{Peak} ≈5 0.8U/kg:[30] N = 7 DA ≈13 ± 3 T_{Peak} ≈7 | In most cats, a distinct peak action is observed in isoglycemic clamps |
| Toujeo | hr Insulin glargine solution | U300 Pen | q 12–q 24 | 0.4U/kg:[26] N = 6 DA ≈15 ± 2 T_{Peak} ≈8 0.8U/kg:[30] N = 7 DA ≈17 ± 5 T_{Peak} ≈10 | Flatter time-action profile compared with glargine U100 |

Arrows represent potentially longer or shorter interval.

Abbreviations: DA, duration of action; hr, human recombinant; PD, pharmacodynamics; PK, pharmacokinetics; q, every; T_{Peak}, time to peak.

rates between treatments.[29] In similar clinical settings, insulin glargine U100 and detemir were associated with similarly high remission rates.[24,25]

Once- versus twice-daily administration of intermediate-acting insulin

Once-daily injection of a higher dose of PZI, insulin glagine U100, or insulin detemir in cats might result in acceptable level of clinical control, especially in cats that have residual beta cell function and therefore might not require a high dose. However, this approach will increase the risk of hypoglycemia; conversely, decreasing the dose and increasing the frequency of injections of an intermediate-acting insulin to 3 times daily will decrease the likelihood of hypoglycemia (see the Linda Fleeman and Chen Gilor's article, "Insulin Therapy in Dogs and Cats, Part 1: General Principles" in this issue).

Long-Acting Basal Insulin Formulations in Cats

Basal insulin requirements are constant throughout the day. Therefore, for an insulin formulation to be effective and safe as a basal insulin, its within-day variability of action should be low—its action should be roughly the same every hour of the day. Currently, insulin glargine U300 (Toujeo) comes the closest to meeting this standard in cats, although its duration of action is on average only 16 hours.[26,30] A basal-mimicking time-action profile has been observed infrequently in cats treated with insulin glargine U100 or insulin detemir.[21]

Insulin glargine U300 can only be accurately administered using the manufacturer's injection pen delivering 1 unit increments. Although this might appear to limit the ability to fine-tune treatment in cats, it is important to take into account the poor precision of insulin syringes that results in the inability to make safe incremental dose changes of less than 1 U.

Insulin glargine U300 is less potent on a unit-by-unit basis compared with other insulin formulations in people. There is currently no evidence that this is also the case in cats,[30,31] but larger studies might be required to detect a relatively small difference in potency.

CLINICS CARE POINTS

- Basal insulin treatment is an appropriate choice for most diabetic cats. Currently, only insulin glargine U300 approximates the criteria for a basal insulin in cats.

- In patients with some residual beta cell function (most cats), administering only a basal insulin might lead to complete normalization of blood glucose concentrations.

- Postprandial endogenous bolus insulin secretion in cats is typically prolonged and unpredictable, regardless of the dietary carbohydrate content of the food. Therefore timing of meals does not need to be matched to insulin injections. Regardless, it is crucial that food intake is reliable and predictable to minimize the risk of insulin-induced hypoglycemia.

DISCLOSURE

L. Fleeman has received honoraria for educational seminars for MSD Animal Health, Zoetis, Royal Canin, Nestle Purina, and consulting fees from Dechra. C. Gilor has received research support or consulting fees from MSD Animal Health, Nestle Purina, Dechra, BiomEdit, Baycom Diagnostics, Edge Animal Health, and Okava Pharmaceuticals.

REFERENCES

1. McAllister M. Feline and canine diabetes prevalence in the USA. Banfield State of Pet Health. 2020. Available at: https://www.banfield.com/state-of-pet-health.
2. Gilor C, Niessen SJ, Furrow E, et al. What's in a name? Classification of diabetes mellitus in veterinary medicine and why it matters. J Vet Intern Med 2016;30: 927–40.
3. Krämer AL, Riederer A, Fracassi F, et al. Glycemic variability in newly diagnosed diabetic cats treated with the glucagon-like peptide-1 analogue exenatide extended release. J Vet Intern Med 2020. https://doi.org/10.1111/jvim.15915.
4. Hewson-Hughes A.K., Gilham M.S., Upton S., et al., The effect of dietary starch level on postprandial glucose and insulin concentrations in cats and dogs, Br J Nutr, (106 Suppl), 2011, S105–S109.
5. Miki Y, Mori A, Hayakawa N, et al. Evaluation of serum and urine 1,5-anhydro-D-glucitol and myo-inositol concentrations in healthy dogs. J Vet Med Sci 2011;73: 1117–26.
6. EGGLETON MG, SHUSTER S. Glucose and phosphate excretion in the cat. J Physiol 1954;124:613–22.
7. Kruth S., Cowgill L., Renal glucose transport in the cat. (Abstract), Congress Proceedings ACVIM, Washington DC, 1982, 78.
8. Ward CR, Christiansen K, Li J, et al. Field efficacy and safety of protamine zinc recombinant human insulin in 276 dogs with diabetes mellitus. Domest Anim Endocrinol 2020;75:106575.
9. Maggiore A Della, Nelson RW, Dennis J, et al. Efficacy of protamine zinc recombinant human insulin for controlling hyperglycemia in dogs with diabetes mellitus. J Vet Intern Med 2012;26:109–15.
10. Clark M, Thomaseth K, Heit M, et al. Pharmacokinetics and pharmacodynamics of protamine zinc recombinant human insulin in healthy dogs. J Vet Pharmacol Ther 2012;35:342–50.
11. Graham PA, Nash AS, McKellar QA. Pharmacokinetics of a porcine insulin zinc suspension in diabetic dogs. J Small Anim Pract 1997;38:434–8.
12. Holman RR, Paul SK, Bethel MA, et al. 10-year follow-up of intensive glucose control in type 2 diabetes. N Engl J Med 2008;359:1577–89.
13. Diabetes Control and Complications Trial Research Group, Nathan DM, Genuth S, Lachin J, et al. The effect of intensive treatment of diabetes on the development and progression of long-term complications in insulin-dependent diabetes mellitus. N Engl J Med 1993;329:977–86.
14. 6. glycemic targets: standards of medical care in diabetes-2018. Diabetes Care 2018;41:S55–64.
15. Gilor C, Pires J, Greathouse R, et al. Loss of sympathetic innervation to islets of Langerhans in canine diabetes and pancreatitis is not associated with insulitis. Sci Rep 2020;10.
16. Taborsky GJJ, Mundinger TO. Minireview: the role of the autonomic nervous system in mediating the glucagon response to hypoglycemia. Endocrinology 2012; 153:1055–62.
17. Mundinger TO, Cooper E, Coleman MP, et al. Short-term diabetic hyperglycemia suppresses celiac ganglia neurotransmission, thereby impairing sympathetically mediated glucagon responses. Am J Physiol Endocrinol Metab 2015;309: E246–55.
18. Gilor C, Duesberg C, Elliott DA, et al. Co-impairment of autonomic and glucagon responses to insulin-induced hypoglycemia in dogs with naturally occurring

insulin-dependent diabetes mellitus. Am J Physiol Endocrinol Metab 2020;319: E1074–83.

19. Martin GJ, Rand JS. Pharmacology of a 40 IU/ml porcine lente insulin preparation in diabetic cats: findings during the first week and after 5 or 9 weeks of therapy. J Feline Med Surg 2001;3:23–30.

20. Marshall RD, Rand JS, Morton JM. Glargine and protamine zinc insulin have a longer duration of action and result in lower mean daily glucose concentrations than lente insulin in healthy cats. J Vet Pharmacol Ther 2008. https://doi.org/10.1111/j.1365-2885.2008.00947.x.

21. Gilor C, Ridge TK, Attermeier KJ, et al. Pharmacodynamics of insulin detemir and insulin glargine assessed by an isoglycemic clamp method in healthy cats. J Vet Intern Med 2010;24:870–4.

22. Fink H, Herbert C, Gilor C. Pharmacodynamics and pharmacokinetics of insulin detemir and insulin glargine 300 U/mL in healthy dogs. Domest Anim Endocrinol 2018;64.

23. Sako T, Mori A, Lee P, et al. Time-action profiles of insulin detemir in normal and diabetic dogs. Res Vet Sci 2011;90:396–403.

24. Roomp K, Rand J. Evaluation of detemir in diabetic cats managed with a protocol for intensive blood glucose control. J Feline Med Surg 2012;14:566–72.

25. Roomp K, Rand J. Intensive blood glucose control is safe and effective in diabetic cats using home monitoring and treatment with glargine. J Feline Med Surg 2009;11:668–82.

26. Gilor C, Culp W, Ghandi S, et al. Comparison of pharmacodynamics and pharmacokinetics of insulin degludec and insulin glargine 300 U/mL in healthy cats. Domest Anim Endocrinol 2019;69.

27. Gostelow R, Forcada Y, Graves T, et al. Systematic review of feline diabetic remission: Separating fact from opinion. Vet J 2014. https://doi.org/10.1016/j.tvjl.2014.08.014.

28. Weaver KE, Rozanski EA, Mahony OM, et al. Use of glargine and Lente insulins in cats with diabetes mellitus. J Vet Intern Med 2006. https://doi.org/10.1892/0891-6640(2006)20[234:UOGALI]2.0.CO;2.

29. Gostelow R, Scudder CK, Hazuchova Y, et al. One-Year Prospective Randomized Trial Comparing Efficacy of Glargine and Protamine Zinc Insulin in Diabetic Cats. J Vet Intern Med 2017;1273.

30. Saini NK, et al. Comparison of pharmacodynamics between insulin glargine 100 U/mL and insulin glargine 300 U/mL in healthy cats. Domest Anim Endocrinol 2020;75:106595.

31. Linari G, Fleeman L, Gilor C, et al. Insulin glargine 300 units/mL for treatment of feline diabetes mellitus. J Feline Med Surg 2022;168–76.

32. Marshall RD, Rand JS, Morton JM. Insulin glargine has a long duration of effect following administration either once daily or twice daily in divided doses in healthy cats. J Feline Med Surg 2008. https://doi.org/10.1016/j.jfms.2008.05.002.

Insulin Therapy in Small Animals, Part 3: Dogs

Linda Fleeman, BVSc, PhD, MANZCVS[a],*, Chen Gilor, DVM, PhD, DACVIM[b]

KEYWORDS

- Basal-bolus insulin • Glargine U300 • Degludec • Canine • Diabetes

KEY POINTS

- Ideally, insulin therapy in most diabetic dogs should mimic a basal-bolus pattern.
- The intermediate-acting insulin formulations might provide a better approximation of bolus insulin secretion in many dogs than the rapid-acting formulations that are typically used for this purpose in diabetic people.
- There is considerable day-to-day and inter-dog variability of both dietary carbohydrate absorption and the action of intermediate-acting insulin formulations, which often means there is marked incongruity between required and delivered insulin that results in fluctuations in blood glucose concentrations. To minimize the risk of hypoglycemia, protocols of twice daily administration of intermediate-acting insulin are therefore usually geared toward alleviating (but not eliminating) clinical signs of diabetes.
- Basal insulin requirements are relatively constant throughout the day. Therefore, for an insulin formulation to be effective and safe as a basal insulin, its action should be roughly the same every hour of the day. Currently, two formulations meet this standard in dogs: insulin glargine U300 (Toujeo) and insulin degludec (Tresiba).
- Goals regarding glycemic control are very different for protocols using basal insulin compared with those for intermediate-acting insulin. In most dogs, good control of clinical signs is achieved when using a basal insulin alone. In a small minority, bolus insulin at the time of at least one meal per day may be added to optimize glycemic control.

INTRODUCTION

The prevalence of diabetes mellitus (DM) varies with geographic region and is reported to affect 25 to 36 of 10,000 pet dogs.[1] Insulin therapy is required for the survival of affected dogs but is associated with many inherent challenges (Insulin Therapy in Small Animals, Part 1: General Principles).

Diabetic dogs were first treated with insulin in 1921, when Banting and Best extracted insulin from the surgically removed pancreata of beagle dogs and then

[a] Animal Diabetes Australia, 5 Hood Street, Collingwood, Victoria 3066, Australia; [b] Small Animal Internal Medicine, Department of Small Animal Clinical Sciences, College of Veterinary Medicine, University of Florida, 2015 Southwest 16th Avenue, Gainesville, FL 32608, USA
* Corresponding author.
E-mail address: L.Fleeman@AnimalDiabetesAustralia.com.au

Vet Clin Small Anim 53 (2023) 645–656
https://doi.org/10.1016/j.cvsm.2023.02.003
0195-5616/23/© 2023 Elsevier Inc. All rights reserved.

used these extracts to treat these beagles that became diabetic. One hundred years later, and after a plethora of insulin formulations have been developed and carefully tested for human beings, there is a striking paucity of high-level evidence from direct comparison in clinical trials to suggest that any one insulin formulation is advantageous compared with any other for management of canine diabetes. Currently, no insulin formulation should be considered best by default. Rather, the choice of insulin formulation should be tailored to the specific clinical situation.

INSULIN PHYSIOLOGY AND PATHOPHYSIOLOGY

Regardless of the specific etiology, at the time of clinical diagnosis, diabetic dogs are dependent on exogenous insulin administration to survive. It is estimated that signs of diabetes develop only when about 90% of beta cell mass has been lost.[2,3] This process is currently considered irreversible in dogs and that at the time of diagnosis, with few exceptions, life-long dependency on exogenous insulin therapy can be assumed. However, there is evidence for the ongoing loss of beta cells after diagnosis which could be one explanation for an increase in insulin requirement after initiation of insulin therapy.[3] Another explanation for this phenomenon could be the development or worsening of insulin resistance. Alternatively, insulin requirement might decrease with the resolution (or improvement) of glucose toxicity and resolution (or improvement) in insulin resistance.

Basal, Basal-Bolus, and Intermediate Treatment Strategies

Ideally, insulin therapy in most diabetic dogs should mimic a basal-bolus pattern to optimize glycemic control (**Fig. 1**),[4] although this will not always be a practical option because of cost and the need for multiple injections daily. This strategy entails using a long-acting insulin to control fasting hyperglycemia (basal insulin) combined with a rapid-acting insulin at mealtimes to control postprandial hyperglycemia (bolus insulin). The alternative is one of two compromises: (1) choose either a basal or bolus insulin, or (2) choose an intermediate-acting formulation that is long enough in duration to be

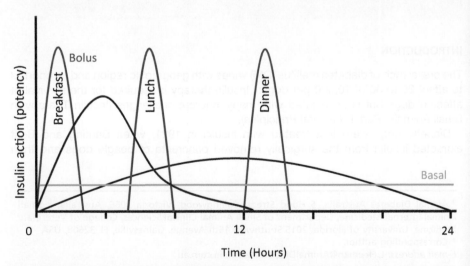

Fig. 1. Combination basal-bolus Insulin therapy: Red – bolus insulin requirement; Green – basal insulin requirement; Blue – Typical basal insulin kinetics; Black – Typical intermediate insulin kinetics.

administered only once or twice daily but also has a curved time-action profile with a peak that is somewhat congruent with peak insulin requirement postprandially.

Intermediate-Acting Insulin Strategy

This traditional treatment strategy is most commonly employed by veterinarians. With the currently available intermediate-acting formulations (eg, lente, neutral protamine Hagedorn [NPH], protamine zinc insulin [PZI], insulin detemir, and insulin glargine 100 U/mL) this strategy is associated with substantial limitations: 1. On average, these formulations peak at about 3 to 6 h post-injection,[5–7] which might not correlate well with the peak postprandial carbohydrate absorption if the meal is fed at the time of the insulin injection, creating incongruency between required and delivered insulin; and 2. These formulations (with the exception of insulin detemir) are typically associated with substantial day-to-day variability,[8–13] which further limits the congruence of required and delivered insulin, and also increases the risk of hypoglycemia. This results in a need to maintain wide safety margins of the target blood glucose concentrations.

To allow once- or twice-daily injection frequency, intermediate-acting insulin formulations are usually administered at a dose range that would cause hypoglycemia in the fasting dog. To avoid hypoglycemia, it is frequently recommended to administer the insulin only after a full meal has been consumed, which can result in a lot of anxiety for owners of dogs that have a finicky appetite.

When healthy dogs are fed half their daily calorie requirement every 12 h, the average duration of endogenous postprandial insulin secretion is about 6 to 9 h. It therefore might be surmised that administration of an intermediate-acting insulin to diabetic dogs at mealtimes would result in exogenous insulin action matching the expected postprandial period. However, there is considerable day-to-day and inter-dog variability of both dietary carbohydrate absorption and exogenous insulin action, which often means there is marked incongruity between required and delivered insulin that results in intra-day fluctuations in blood glucose concentrations.

Protocols of twice daily administration of intermediate-acting insulin are usually geared toward alleviating (but not eliminating) clinical signs of diabetes. Considering the intra-day blood glucose fluctuations and substantial inter-day variability in insulin action associated with these intermediate-acting formulations, it is usually recommended to aim for blood glucose concentrations that range above normal, between a low end of 80 to 100 mg/dL (4.4 to 5.5 mmol/L) and a high end of 250 to 350 mg/dL (14 to 20 mmol/L). Although uncommonly realized,[14,15] the ideal blood glucose profile after an injection of an intermediate-acting insulin is typically expected to be at the high end of this range just before insulin administration and nadir at about 6 h.[5,6] Considering the renal threshold for glucose reabsorption in dogs is about 180 to 200 mg/dL (10 to 11 mmol/L), it is expected that this treatment strategy would result in a substantial amount of time above that threshold, resulting in some degree of polyuria and polydipsia. A patient that presents with completely normal water intake and urine production is therefore likely to experience hypoglycemia at least intermittently, considering an expected decrease of about 200 mg/dL (11 mmol/L) when an intermediate-acting insulin is administered q12 h. If control of polyuria and polydipsia is achieved with q24 h injection frequency, the risk of hypoglycemia is greater because of the need to increase the total dose per injection (**Fig. 2**A). If control of polyuria and polydipsia is achieved with q8h injection frequency, the risk of hypoglycemia is lessened because the dose per injection is lower (**Fig. 2**B). Similarly, a q12 h approach with an intermediate-acting insulin is also expected to be associated with glycated protein test results (eg, fructosamine) above the reference interval. If glycated proteins are

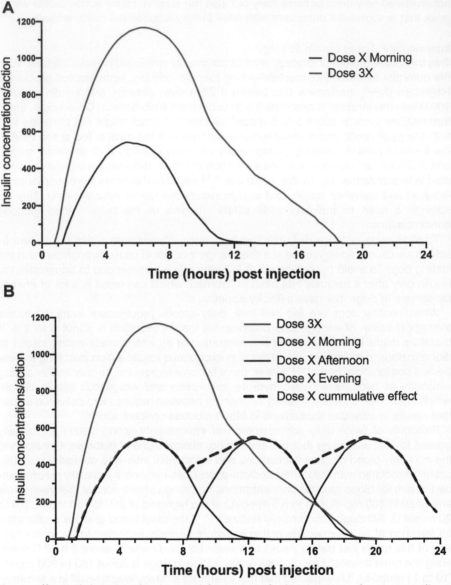

Fig. 2. Effects of changing the dose and frequency of administration of an intermediate-acting insulin. (A) threefold dose increase of a typical intermediate-acting insulin formulation nearly doubles the duration of action but also doubles peak action and increases the risk of hypoglycemia. (B) Decreasing the dose and tripling the frequency of administration decreases the risk of hypoglycemia and achieves lesser intra-day variation.

instead within the reference interval, it is assumed that the dog is over-controlled and experiencing hypoglycemia, at least intermittently.

Basal-Bolus or Basal Insulin Strategy

Goals regarding blood glucose control are very different for strategies using basal insulin compared with those for intermediate-acting insulin. When using basal insulin, the dose is increased gradually until the blood glucose nadir is about 80 mg/dL (4.4 mmol/L). It is highly recommended to monitor this dose escalation process with continuous glucose monitoring. A basal insulin is administered irrespective of food administration. Blood glucose is then expected to rise following the meals and decline back to baseline when carbohydrate digestion and absorption has subsided. The resulting blood glucose fluctuations might or might not remain below the renal threshold, depending on the type of food and the frequency of feeding. In most dogs, good control of clinical signs is achieved when using a basal insulin alone. In a small minority of dogs, a bolus insulin at the time of at least one meal per day may be added to optimize glycemic control.[16]

Unlike the traditional approach of using an intermediate-acting insulin as sole therapy, there is often no need to reduce the dose of basal insulin because of planned or unplanned fasting, and there is minimal risk of hypoglycemia if the dog has vomited food after eating. Although the risk of hypoglycemia is much lower when food is not consumed, there is individual variation and some dogs with very good glycemic control when treated with a basal insulin might benefit from a decrease of the dose when fasted.

If choosing to add a bolus insulin, the time-action profile of the exogenous bolus insulin should mimic the physiologic bolus insulin secretion required by the animal. Considering the differences in physiologic bolus insulin secretion in dogs and in people (Insulin Therapy in Small Animals, Part 1: General Principles), A mixture of 65% to 70% intermediate-acting insulin such as NPH and 30% to 35% regular insulin (eg, Vetsulin, Humulin 70/30, or Novolin 70/30) at starting dose of about 0.25 U/kg might provide a better approximation of bolus insulin secretion in many dogs than the rapid-acting formulations that are typically used for this purpose in people with diabetes.

The requirement for the addition of bolus insulin to a basal insulin regimen can be identified by reviewing continuous interstitial glucose data over several days while the dog is fed the usual diet with the usual feeding routine. Bolus insulin may be required with one or more of the daily meals. Alternatively the owner might opt to change the diet or the feeding routine to minimize postprandial hyperglycemia and so avoid the need for additional daily insulin injection(s).

Side-by-side clinical trials comparing the efficacy and safety of intermediate-acting formulations to basal or to bolus insulin formulations are rare in veterinary medicine. In one study in dogs, there was no difference in mean daily blood glucose concentrations or in the frequency of hypoglycemic events when an intermediate-acting insulin (porcine lente, Vetsulin/Caninsulin) was compared with basal formulations insulin degludec and insulin glargine U300.[11] In another study, the mean blood glucose concentrations were higher when four diabetic dogs were treated with intermediate-acting NPH insulin twice daily compared with basal insulin degludec twice daily, even though NPH was used at a higher dose, and postprandial hyperglycemia and lower prepran-dial glycemia were observed with insulin degludec.[17]

MANAGING INAPPETENCE AND GASTROINTESTINAL SIGNS

In health, about half of the daily insulin requirement is basal and the other half is bolus, leading to the recommendation to lower the dose of intermediate-acting insulin by 50% in a patient that skips a meal or is vomiting. There are two potential problems with this strategy. First, the 50% basal:bolus ratio is a general estimate, and might lead to significant over- or under-dosing in any particular patient. Second, it is common for dogs suffering from diabetes to be "picky eaters" or to have concurrent gastrointestinal disease, pancreatitis, or other diseases that affects their appetite. The need to adjust the dose of insulin in these instances can have a significant impact on glycemic control and on the owners' stress level. Some of this might be alleviated by using a basal-bolus insulin combination in which the dose and frequency of the basal insulin are unaltered during episodes of decreased appetite and the bolus insulin is simply skipped.

GOALS OF THERAPY FOR THE SPECIFIC PATIENT

While maintaining tight glycemic control reduces the risk of hyperglycemia-related complications, it also increases the risk of hypoglycemia. It is currently unknown if the risk for cataract formation is proportional to the level of hyperglycemia, related to a certain threshold of hyperglycemia, to glycemic variability, or other factors. However, it is likely that the risk of cataract formation would be substantially reduced if consistent euglycemia was achieved. Owners interested in pursuing such a goal should be counseled on the substantial cost (financial, emotional, time) involved in maintaining euglycemia in an insulin-dependent patient, the increased risk of hypoglycemia, and the possibility that the goal might not be attainable. If owners do not choose euglycemia as a target, the default goal should be the minimization (but not necessarily elimination) of clinical signs. There is currently no evidence to support choosing specific blood glucose targets, as long as hypoglycemia is avoided.

The clinical decision on treatment and monitoring methods must also take into account potential long-term attrition in client and pet compliance. What seems like an ideal treatment and monitoring scheme in the short term might fail in the long run if owners have maximized their financial capabilities, especially when concurrent diseases develop. In that respect, minimalist treatment and monitoring approaches might be better in the long run.

FORMULATION-SPECIFIC CONSIDERATIONS

Details on commonly used insulin formulations are presented in **Table 1**.

Intermediate-Acting Insulin Formulations

Currently, available insulin suspensions (NPH, NPH/regular mixes, lente, and PZI) as well as insulin glargine U100 and detemir are generally used as intermediate-acting formulations that are administered twice daily (see **Table 1**). Porcine lente, PZI, and insulin detemir tend to have a duration of action that is longer than observed with NPH.[5,6,18] For some dogs, once-daily injection of a higher dose of porcine lente or PZI (but not NPH) might, therefore, result in an acceptable level of clinical control.[14,19] Importantly, however, this generally increases the risk of hypoglycemia. On the contrary, decreasing the dose of insulin injections and increasing the frequency to three times daily, coupled with 3 meals per day, will decrease the likelihood of hypoglycemia and can lead to better glycemic control (see **Fig. 2**B).

The pharmacodynamics of insulin glargine U100 and detemir have been studied in dogs and compared with NPH in small experimental studies.[20,21] Using the isoglycemic clamp technique and with a dose of 0.5 U/kg, both insulin solutions had a duration of action of about 16 to 24 h. Importantly, these formulations should not be considered long-acting or basal in dogs because of pronounced peaks that were observed at 7 to 9 h with these doses. Like other intermediate-acting formulations, increasing the dose will result in a longer duration but a higher peak (see **Fig. 2**A).[8] Further, the 0.5 U/kg dose is too high as a starting dose for insulin detemir and so is potentially dangerous.[22] When studied with a more clinically applicable dose (0.1 U/kg), the duration of action

Table 1
Pharmacodynamics, pharmacokinetics, and guidelines for frequency of administration of specific insulin formulations

Brand Name Frequency PD	Formulation	Concentration Syringe/Pen Frequency	Canine Data PD (for X U/kg): T_{DA} (h) T_{Peak} (h)	Comments
Humulin N Novolion N	hr NPH Suspension	U100 Syringe/pen	q8 to 12	0.5 U/kg:[20] $N = 3$ DA ≈ 12 T_{Peak} ≈ 6	PK data on 0.6 U/kg in DM[18]: Insulin returned to baseline in 8 ± 2 h, peak at 1.5 h ($N = 10$)
Vetsulin/Caninsulin	Porcine Lente Suspension	U40 Syringe/pen	q12->		PK data on 1.0 to 2.8 U/kg in DM:[6] Insulin first peak at 4 to 6 h, second peak (half of the first peak) at 11 h (8 to 14 h) returned to baseline in 16 h (14 to 24), in 8/10 dogs ($N = 10$) PK data on 0.64 to 1.12 U/kg in DM[7] ($N = 8$) Peak at 3 and 9 h, return to baseline by 16 h
Prozinc	hr PZI Suspension	U40 Syringe	q12 to 24		PK data on 0.8 U/kg:[5] Insulin peak at 7 (1 to 22)h, returned to baseline in 22 (12->24)h, ($N = 10$). Time-action profile markedly variable between dogs
Levemir	hr insulin detemir Solution	U100/U200 Syringe/Pen	q12->	0.1 U/kg:[23] $N = 8$ DA ≈ 11 ± 2 T_{Peak} ≈ 5 0.5 U/kg:[21] $N = 3$ DA ≈ 17 T_{Peak} ≈ 9	

(continued on next page)

Table 1
(continued)

Brand Name		Concentration Syringe/Pen		Canine Data	Comments
	Formulation	Frequency	PD (for X U/kg): T_{DA} (h) T_{Peak} (h)		
Frequency PD					
Lantus/Optisulin/Basalglar/ Semglee/Abasria	hr insulin glargine Solution	U100 Syringe/pen	q12->	0.5 U/kg:[20] $N = 3$ $DA_\Delta \approx 21$ $T_{Peak\Delta} \approx 7$	
Toujeo	hr insulin glargine Solution	U300 Pen	q12-q24	0.4 U/kg:[23] $N = 8$ $DA \approx 15 \pm 5$ $T_{Peak} \approx 10$	PD estimated from clamp and lowering of endogenous insulin
Tresiba	hr insulin degludec Solution	U100/U200 Pen	<q24	0.5 U/kg:[17] $N = 5$ $DA > 20$ $T_{Peak} \approx 10$	Clamp discontinued at 20 h

Arrows represent potentially longer or shorter interval.
Abbreviations: DA, duration of action; hr, human recombinant; T_{Peak}, time to peak.

of insulin detemir in dogs was closer to 12 h.[23] In diabetic dogs, the dose range of insulin detemir that was associated with good glycemic control was 0.05 to 0.35 U/kg,[22] and, therefore, it is recommended to start this insulin in dogs at a dose of 0.05 to 0.1 U/kg q12 h. Insulin detemir is therefore not recommended for dogs <10 kg, unless substantial insulin resistance is present. It is not recommended to dilute insulin detemir (or any other insulin) because dilution decreases the lipophilic interactions between insulin detemir molecules and might dramatically change the pharmacodynamic profile in undesired ways.

Long-Acting Basal Insulin Formulations

For an insulin formulation to be effective and safe as a basal insulin, its within-day variability of action should be low, that is, its action should be roughly the same every hour of the day. Currently, two formulations meet this standard of a basal insulin in dogs: insulin glargine U300 (Toujeo) and insulin degludec (Tresiba).[17,23]

In a glucose clamp study of 8 healthy dogs, insulin glargine U300 (0.4 U/kg, 2.4 nmol/kg) was compared with an equimolar dose of insulin detemir (0.1 U/kg) and was found to have a much weaker glucose-lowering effect, both when considered on a molar basis and on a U basis.[23] At this dose, 4 out of 8 dogs treated with insulin glargine U300 did not need a glucose infusion to maintain euglycemia, although endogenous insulin was suppressed in these dogs for over 16 h. By comparison, an identical molar dose of insulin detemir (0.1 U/kg) necessitated glucose infusion to maintain euglycemia in all 8 dogs. In the 4 dogs that needed glucose infusions after both insulin injections, the glucose-lowering effect of insulin detemir was about 3-fold higher compared with insulin glargine U300. Clinically, the median (range) dose of insulin glargine U300 that is associated with good glycemic control is 1.9 U/kg (0.2 to 5.2 U/kg) whether administered once daily or divided to q12 h (with about half of the dogs being well controlled on q24 h).[16] This low potency of insulin glargine U300 is advantageous in small dogs, allowing small alterations in effective dose with every U change. Insulin glargine U300 can only be accurately administered using the manufacturer's injection pen delivering 1 U unit increments.

One study showed promising pharmacodynamic characteristics of insulin degludec with a duration of action >20 h and a flat-time action profile suitable for use as a basal insulin.[17] Glucose clamps were terminated at 20 h after insulin administration so that the duration of action could not be precisely calculated but based on the indistinct peak at about 10 h after injection, and the slow decline in glucose infusion rate that followed, the duration of action of insulin degludec in dogs was approximately 24 h. In the same study, insulin degludec was compared with NPH in diabetic dogs, with both formulations administered twice daily. On average, glucose excursions were more pronounced postprandially with insulin degludec compared with NPH, consistent with a flat time-action profile of the former and the expected peak of the latter. Despite this postprandial hyperglycemia, overall glycemic control was better with insulin degludec, as a result of lower blood glucose during time intervals preceding meals.[17]

In dogs with toxin-induced diabetes, insulin glargine U300 was compared with porcine lente and insulin degludec.[11] This study assessed the responses to insulin by measuring interstitial glucose continuously and not by using the glucose clamp method and therefore pharmacodynamics could not be accurately assessed. Surprisingly, inter-dog variability was higher with insulin degludec compared with insulin glargine U300. The inter-dog variability was also substantial in a previous study of insulin degludec, although a comparison was not made directly to another insulin.[17] Nevertheless, the comparison study showed that day-to-day variability was lower with insulin degludec compared with porcine lente and similar to insulin glargine U300.[11] Intra-day variability was lower with porcine lente compared with insulin glargine U300 as a result of less pronounced postprandial hyperglycemia with the porcine lente. This probably resulted from significant peak in the action of porcine lente during the postprandial period compared with the flat time-action profile of insulin glargine U300, highlighting the advantage of the former formulation when used as a bolus insulin and the latter when used as a basal insulin in dogs.

Combination Basal-Bolus Treatment in Dogs

Two clinical scenarios when combination basal-bolus insulin treatment may be indicated in dogs are as follows: (1) intermediate-acting insulin has achieved good control of postprandial hyperglycemia, but there is underlying insulin resistance causing short duration of action of injected insulin resulting in marked hyperglycemia 6 to 12 h after injections, or (2) basal insulin has achieved good glycemic control for most of the day, but substantial postprandial hyperglycemia is present 1 to 6 h after meals.

In the first scenario, basal insulin can be added to the existing insulin treatment. When making this change, it is recommended that the total insulin dose that the dog is currently receiving every 12 h is not changed. This requires that the dose of the intermediate-acting insulin be reduced (by about 50%) and the remainder of the 12-hourly dose delivered by the basal insulin. It is obviously crucial that there is very clear communication with owners regarding the dose of each of the insulin formulations. In the second scenario, it is recommended that the same dose of the basal insulin is continued and an intermediate-acting insulin is added at 0.25 U/kg at meal times.

KeyPoints

- *No insulin formulation should be considered best by default. Rather, the choice of insulin formulation should be tailored to the specific clinical situation. Different goal-oriented treatment strategies should be considered, with pros and cons to each.*
- *When referring to specific insulin formulations, "Intermediate-acting" and "long-acting" are potentially misleading terms because the duration of action is affected by dose and it differs between individuals. Therefore, these terms are used as conventional shortcuts, not as actual descriptors.*
- *Currently available insulin suspensions (NPH, NPH/regular mixes, lente, and PZI) as well as insulin glargine U100 and detemir are generally used as intermediate-acting formulations that are administered twice daily in dogs.*
- *Ideally, insulin therapy in most diabetic dogs should mimic a basal-bolus pattern.*
- *The intermediate-acting insulin formulations might provide a better approximation of bolus insulin secretion in many dogs than the rapid-acting formulations that are typically used for this purpose in diabetic people.*
- *There is considerable day-to-day and inter-dog variability of both dietary carbohydrate absorption and the action of intermediate-acting insulin formulations, which often means there is marked incongruity between required and delivered insulin that results in fluctuations in blood glucose concentrations. To minimize the risk of hypoglycemia, protocols of twice daily administration of intermediate-acting insulin are therefore usually geared toward alleviating (but not eliminating) clinical signs of diabetes.*
- *Basal insulin requirements are relatively constant throughout the day. Therefore, for an insulin formulation to be effective and safe as a basal insulin, its action should*

be roughly the same every hour of the day. Currently, two formulations meet this standard in dogs: insulin glargine U300 (Toujeo) and insulin degludec (Tresiba).

- Goals regarding glycemic control are very different for protocols using basal insulin compared with those for intermediate-acting insulin. In most dogs, good control of clinical signs is achieved when using a basal insulin alone. In a small minority, bolus insulin at the time of at least one meal per day may be added to optimize glycemic control.

CLINICS CARE POINTS

- Goals regarding glycemic control are very different for protocols using basal insulin compared with those for intermediate-acting insulin.

- In most dogs, good control of clinical signs is achieved when using a basal insulin alone. In a small minority, bolus insulin at the time of at least one meal per day may be added to optimize glycemic control. The intermediate-acting insulin formulations are often an appropriate choice for bolus insulin treatment.

- There is considerable day-to-day and inter-dog variability of both dietary carbohydrate absorption and the action of intermediate-acting insulin formulations, which often results in the marked incongruity between required and delivered insulin. To minimize the risk of hypoglycemia, protocols of twice daily administration of intermediate-acting insulin are therefore usually geared toward alleviating (but not eliminating) clinical signs of diabetes.

DISCLOSURE

L. Fleeman has received honoraria for educational seminars for MSD Animal Health, Zoetis, Royal Canin, Nestle Purina, and consulting fees from Dechra. C. Gilor has received research support or consulting fees from MSD Animal Health, Nestle Purina, Dechra, BiomEdit, Baycom Diagnostics, Edge Animal Health, and Okava Pharmaceuticals.

REFERENCES

1. McAllister M. Feline and canine diabetes prevalence in the USA. Banfield State of Pet Helath, 2020, Available at: https://www.banfield.com/state-of-pet-health, Accessed June 3, 2022.
2. Shields EJ, et al. Extreme Beta-Cell Deficiency in Pancreata of Dogs with Canine Diabetes. PLoS One 2015;10:e0129809.
3. Gilor C, Pires J, Greathouse R, et al. Loss of sympathetic innervation to islets of Langerhans in canine diabetes and pancreatitis is not associated with insulitis. Sci Rep 2020;10.
4. Gilor C, Graves TK. Synthetic Insulin Analogs and Their Use in Dogs and Cats. Vet Clin North Am Small Anim Pract 2010;40.
5. Clark M, Thomaseth K, Heit M, et al. Pharmacokinetics and pharmacodynamics of protamine zinc recombinant human insulin in healthy dogs. J Vet Pharmacol Ther 2012;35:342–50.
6. Graham PA, Nash AS, McKellar QA. Pharmacokinetics of a porcine insulin zinc suspension in diabetic dogs. J Small Anim Pract 1997;38:434–8.
7. Fleeman LM, Rand JS, Morton JM. Pharmacokinetics and pharmacodynamics of porcine insulin zinc suspension in eight diabetic dogs. Vet Rec 2009;164:232–7.

8. Owens DR, Bolli GB. Beyond the era of NPH insulin–long-acting insulin analogs: chemistry, comparative pharmacology, and clinical application. Diabetes Technol Ther 2008;10:333–49.

9. Havelund S, Plum A, Ribel U, et al. The mechanism of protraction of insulin detemir, a long-acting, acylated analog of human insulin. Pharm Res (N Y) 2004;21: 1498–504.

10. Heise T, Nosek L, Rønn BB, et al. Lower within-subject variability of insulin detemir in comparison to NPH insulin and insulin glargine in people with type 1 diabetes. Diabetes 2004;53:1614–20.

11. Miller M, Pires J, Crakes K, et al. Day-to-Day Variability of Porcine Lente, Insulin Glargine 300 U/mL and Insulin Degludec in Diabetic Dogs. J Vet Intern Med 2021;35(5):2131–9.

12. De Marco V, T G, Chen G. Day-to-day variability of serial blood glucose curves in diabetic dogs treated with twice daily NPH or insulin detemir. J Vet Intern Med 2015;29:1173.

13. Fleeman LM, Rand JS. Evaluation of day-to-day variability of serial blood glucose concentration curves in diabetic dogs. J Am Vet Med Assoc 2003;222:317–21.

14. Ward CR, Christiansen K, Li J, et al. Field efficacy and safety of protamine zinc recombinant human insulin in 276 dogs with diabetes mellitus. Domest Anim Endocrinol 2020;75:106575.

15. Maggiore A Della, Nelson RW, Dennis J, et al. Efficacy of protamine zinc recombinant human insulin for controlling hyperglycemia in dogs with diabetes mellitus. J Vet Intern Med 2012;26:109–15.

16. Gilor C, Fracassi F, Berg A, et al. Once-daily insulin glargine 300 U/ml for the treatment of canine diabetes mellitus [Abstract]. J Vet Intern Med 2022;36(6): 2277.

17. Oda H, Mori A, Ishii S, et al. Time-action profiles of insulin degludec in healthy dogs and its effects on glycemic control in diabetic dogs. J Vet Med Sci 2018; 80:1720–3.

18. Palm CA, Boston RC, Refsal KR, et al. An investigation of the action of Neutral Protamine Hagedorn human analogue insulin in dogs with naturally occurring diabetes mellitus. J Vet Intern Med 2009;23:50–5.

19. Monroe WE, Laxton D, Fallin EA, et al. Efficacy and safety of a purified porcine insulin zinc suspension for managing diabetes mellitus in dogs. J Vet Intern Med 2005;19:675–82.

20. Mori A, Sako T, Lee P, et al. Comparison of time-action profiles of insulin glargine and NPH insulin in normal and diabetic dogs. Vet Res Commun 2008;32:563–73.

21. Sako T, Mori A, Lee P, et al. Time-action profiles of insulin detemir in normal and diabetic dogs. Res Vet Sci 2011;90:396–403.

22. Fracassi F, Corradini S, Hafner M, et al. Detemir insulin for the treatment of diabetes mellitus in dogs. J Am Vet Med Assoc 2015;247:73–8.

23. Fink H, Herbert C, Gilor C. Pharmacodynamics and pharmacokinetics of insulin detemir and insulin glargine 300 U/mL in healthy dogs. Domest Anim Endocrinol 2018, 17-30;64.

Nutritional Management of Cats and Dogs with Diabetes Mellitus

Valerie J. Parker, DVM[a], Richard C. Hill, MA, VetMB, PhD, MRCVS[b],*

KEYWORDS

- Body composition • Macronutrients • Micronutrients • Fiber • Carbohydrates
- Protein • Fat • Energy

KEY POINTS

- A long-term goal of nutritional management is to achieve an ideal body condition score.
- Each diabetic dog or cat should be assessed and managed as an individual patient.
- Diets marketed for "diabetic management" do not necessarily convey an advantage.
- Many animals do not require a change in diet, and sudden changes in diet in a sick patient may cause aversion.
- Modification of nutrient profile may facilitate glycemic control, especially if diabetic remission in cats is the goal.

INTRODUCTION

The main tenets of nutritional management of diabetes mellitus (DM) for dogs and cats include the following: (1) consistently consuming a complete and balanced diet and timing of meals relative to insulin administration when using an intermediate acting insulin and (2) maintaining an appropriate caloric intake to either achieve or maintain an optimal body weight (BW) and body composition. For most dogs and cats, any good quality adult maintenance diet will suffice. Dietary modification may improve glycemic control but any change should be undertaken with specific nutritional goals in mind, considering the individual animal's baseline diet and nutritional status. If necessary, diets should be changed ideally during a few days, and not when the patient is nauseous, to avoid aversion. This article will focus on how to provide initial recommendations for dogs and cats with uncomplicated DM as well as a few examples of more complicated comorbid conditions.

---

[a] The Ohio State University Veterinary Medical Center, 601 Vernon L. Tharp Street, Columbus, OH 43210, USA; [b] University of Florida College of Veterinary Medicine, 2015 Southwest 16th Avenue, Gainesville, FL 32608, USA
* Corresponding author.
E-mail address: parker.888@osu.edu

Vet Clin Small Anim 53 (2023) 657–674
https://doi.org/10.1016/j.cvsm.2023.01.007
0195-5616/23/© 2023 Elsevier Inc. All rights reserved.
vetsmall.theclinics.com

Nutritional Assessment and Energy Requirements

Nutritional management should be tailored to the individual patient. The first step is to assess body composition (BW, body condition score [BCS], and muscle condition score).[1] Dogs and cats with absolute or relative insulin insufficiency tend to lose weight. Maintaining food intake and avoiding further weight loss is a priority initially. Nevertheless, many dogs and cats remain overweight (ie, BCS > 5/9) at the time of diagnosis.[2,3] Obesity increases insulin requirements in dogs and cats,[4,5] and some obese cats with noninsulin-dependent DM might not require insulin if they lose weight. Therefore, long-term calorie intake may need to be reduced by 10% to 20% or more to achieve and maintain an ideal BCS. Animals with some comorbid conditions (eg, chronic kidney disease, heart disease) might benefit from some additional weight as a protective mechanism,[6–9] and cachectic animals with better muscle condition survive longer.[9–11]

The animal's BCS may dictate whether the caloric density of the diet should be adjusted. Thin animals should not be transitioned to low-calorie diets, just as overweight animals should not be transitioned to high-calorie diets without considering intake. A thorough diet history is an essential starting point before determining how to adjust a diet plan. It should include the brand of food fed, flavor(s), frequency and amount fed daily, information about treats, including rawhides and chew toys, and medications, and how and when they are administered.[1] The diet might not need to change if 90% of calories are from a complete and balanced diet, and the timing and amount fed can be standardized relative to the administration of an intermediate-acting suspension insulin. Specific daily caloric goals should ideally be made based on the animal's known caloric intake. If that is unknown, then veterinarians can estimate daily energy requirements using resting energy requirement and maintenance energy requirement calculations.[1]

Assessing the Macronutrient Composition of a Diet

In order to accurately compare one diet to another, pet food nutrient profiles should be compared in grams per 100 or 1,000 kilocalories (Mcal), *not* on a percent as fed or dry matter basis, because pet foods vary widely in energy density. The guaranteed analysis (GA) can be used to estimate the macronutrient composition of a diet but it is better to evaluate a diet's typical nutrient analysis (TNA) when available from the manufacturer. The carbohydrate content is never included on a GA but it can be estimated using the kilocalories per kilogram diet that is also required on the label (**Box 1**).

Nutrients provided on a percent as fed basis can then to converted to a grams per Mcal basis using the following equation (**Box 2**).

Macronutrient Composition

Evidence for the benefit of specific changes in macronutrient composition in the management of DM in dogs and cats is lacking because most studies have involved weight loss as well as a change in diet composition. Studies have also changed more than one nutrient, have not defined changes in ingredients or the amount of food or nutrient consumed, have often changed to meal feeding from free choice feeding, and have sometimes changed from dry to canned foods.[12–15] Some changes to macronutrient content might improve glycemic control and promote weight gain or loss but hormonal responses in dogs and cats sometimes differ from those in other species.

Incretin hormone responses to nutrients

The incretin hormones, glucose-dependent insulinotropic peptide and glucagon-like peptide 1 (GLP1), modulate insulin and glucose responses.[16] Studies using GLP1

Box 1
Estimating carbohydrate concentration from guaranteed analysis

The digestible carbohydrate fraction of a diet can be estimated by subtracting moisture, crude protein, crude fat, crude fiber ± ash (if provided) from 100%. Minimum and maximum nutrient concentrations reported on a GA may vary from TNA. Correction factors[a] have been published to attempt to more closely represent the TNA; however, these correction factors may not be accurate in all instances.

Here is an example estimating the carbohydrate concentration of a commercial dry cat food:

Nutrients on GA.

- Crude protein (min): 32%

- Crude fat (min): 12%

- Crude fiber (max): 3%

- Moisture (max): 12%

- Ash (calcium and phosphorus; max): 2%

Estimated carbohydrates = 100% − 32 − 12 − 3 − 12 − 2 = 39%

[a]Correction factors for estimating the TNA from a GA are as follows:

- Add 1.5% to protein minimum.

- Add 1% to fat minimums.

- Subtract 0.7% from crude fiber.

- Subtract 4% from moisture maximum.

---

receptor agonists suggest that increased secretion of GLP1 might be beneficial in diabetic dogs and cats.[16,17] Glucose, amino acids, and volatile fatty acids from carbohydrate fermentation in the intestinal lumen stimulate secretion of GLP1.[16]

Water
Water should be available at all times to compensate for diuresis caused by glycosuria. A hyperosmolar crisis can develop rapidly if access to water is curtailed. Changing from a dry to a canned diet provides more water and can facilitate weight loss because canned diets contain fewer kilocalories per kilogram as fed than dry diets and seem to the owner as a larger amount of food.[18]

Protein
Protein and amino acid requirements could be increased when diabetic patients are unregulated and in a catabolic state. Minimum and maximum requirements of diabetic dogs and cats with good glycemic control are probably similar, however, to those of nondiabetic animals and will be similarly affected by body composition and

---

Box 2
Converting nutrient from percent as fed basis to grams per Mcal basis

The nutrient concentration of a diet can be determined using the following equation:

Nutrient concentration (g/1,000 kcal) = % nutrient as fed ÷ kcal per kg diet × 10,000.

Using the diet example above, if the carbohydrate concentration is 39% as fed, and the kilocalories per kilogram of the diet is 3,900 kcal/kg, then the carbohydrate concentration on a grams per 1000 kcal is as follows:

39 ÷ 3,900 × 10,000 = 100 g carbohydrates per 1,000 kcal (10.0 g/100 kcal)

---

comorbidities. Higher protein diets help obese dogs and cats maintain muscle mass while preferentially losing fat.[19–21] High-protein intake may also contribute to satiety as caloric intake is decreased.[22] Obese dogs should be fed more than 6 g protein/100 kcal and obese cats more than 9 g protein/100 kcal.[1] Most veterinary therapeutic diets designed for obesity management typically provide at least 8 g protein/100 kcal and 10 g protein/100 kcal for dogs and cats, respectively. Nutrient profiles for veterinary therapeutic dry and canned diets marketed for dogs with DM are in **Table 1**.

This need to feed more protein to obese animals must be balanced against the need for protein restriction in patients with proteinuria. Proteinuria has been reported in 60% of dogs with DM,[23–25] and reducing dietary protein might decrease proteinuria and progression of kidney disease.[26–28] Veterinary therapeutic renal diets contain less protein but most contain more fat and more kilocalories per gram diet as fed, which may not be ideal in an obese patient. It may be possible, however, to achieve a 25% to 50% reduction in dietary protein intake without needing to feed a renal diet.[28,29] The protein concentrations in commercial diets varies widely: from 1.6 to 4.7 g protein per 100 kcal in "low" (or controlled) protein therapeutic dog diets, to about 4.5 to 5 g protein/100 kcal in the lowest over-the-counter (OTC) commercial diets for healthy dogs and some novel protein diets for dogs, to about 6 g protein/100 kcal in "low protein" cat diets, and more than 15 g protein/100 kcal in some OTC diets. It is important also to consider how much a patient is eating. Simply reducing the amount of commercial food reduces the protein as well as calories consumed. Any human food, treats, raw hide, and dental chews consumed should be considered also because they vary widely in protein and often provide many nonprotein calories.

Fat

The fat content of the diet might not need to be changed in many diabetic animals. Fat is more potent than fiber in slowing gastric emptying and reduces the amount of carbohydrate required as a source of calories. Fat also increases GLP1 release in dogs and cats.[16,30] Fat restriction might be necessary in patients with hypertriglyceridemia and, temporarily but not necessarily indefinitely, in patients recovering from severe, acute pancreatitis.[31–34] Acute necrotizing pancreatitis is a rare disease in cats but fat restriction may benefit these patients because fat stimulates cholecystokinin in cats as in other species.[35] Fat restriction is not necessary in most pets with DM because inflammation of the pancreas is often chronic and not necessarily associated with clinical signs.[36] Signs in cats when they do occur may be associated with inflammation of the bowel disease and/or liver.[37] These cats with concurrent chronic enteropathies may benefit from feeding a limited antigen or hydrolyzed diet a fiber-enriched diet instead.[38]

Dietary fat in commercially available diets for dogs and cats ranges from about 2 to more than 8 g fat/100 kcal. There is no ideal amount of fat for patients with DM but a lower or moderate fat diet (<2.5 or < 5 g fat/100 kcal, respectively) can be recommended where fat restriction is considered beneficial.

Carbohydrates

Carbohydrate can be divided into 4 types: (1) absorbable, such as sugars; (2) digestible, such as digestible sugars and starch; (3) indigestible but fermentable oligosaccharides and fiber; and (4) indigestible but poorly fermented fiber.[39] A minimum requirement for digestible or indigestible carbohydrate has not been established for either dogs or cats. Indigestible fermentable carbohydrate and protein are beneficial, however, because they support the intestinal microbiome and volatile fatty acids generated by fermentation maintain large intestinal enterocytes.[40,41]

Table 1
Comparison of metabolizable energy (kcal per can or cup and per gram) and selected nutrients of concern (gram per 100 kcal) for currently available veterinary therapeutic diets marketed for canine diabetes mellitus and/or obesity

Diet	Kcal per Cup/Can	Kcal/g	Crude Protein	Crude Fat	Carb	Crude Fiber	TDF
Hill's Prescription Diet w/d Vegetable and Chicken Stew (12.5 oz can)	201	0.57	6.5	3.1	14.9	4.3	7.9
Royal Canin Satiety Support Loaf (13.4 oz can)	241	0.63	10.6	3.2	9.4	2.0	5.4
Purina Pro Plan Veterinary Diets OM (13.3 oz can)	249	0.66	13.0	3.5	6.6	5.9	9.4
Royal Canin Glycobalance Loaf in Sauce (13.4 oz can)	307	0.81	11.0	4.9	5.4	1.7	4.6
Hill's Prescription Diet w/d (13 oz can)	305	0.82	5.7	3.3	14.8	4.0	7.4
Hill's Prescription Diet r/d (12.3 oz can)	299	0.85	10.1	2.6	12.1	3.8	7.4
BLUE Natural Veterinary Diet W + U (12.5 oz)	303	0.85	9.7	4.8	6.1	3.5	4.5
Hill's Prescription Diet Metabolic Chicken Flavor (13 oz can)	328	0.89	8.1	3.8	11.4	4.3	7.0
BLUE Natural Veterinary Diet W + M (12.5 oz can)	331	0.93	9.4	4.5	8.1	3.0	5.2
Royal Canin Satiety Support (dry)	214	2.89	11.5	3.6	11.3	6.4	10.8
Purina Pro Plan Veterinary Diets OM Select Blend (dry)	219	2.94	10.0	2.2	13.2	3.3	8.8
Hill's Prescription Diet r/d Chicken Flavor (dry)	242	2.94	10.6	2.7	11.6	4.5	8.2
Purina Pro Plan Veterinary Diets OM (dry)	260	2.95	9.3	2.2	14.1	3.5	7.5
BLUE Natural Veterinary Diet W + U (dry)	309	3.07	10.1	3.6	9.7	4.4	6.5
Hill's Prescription Diet w/d (dry)	255	3.10	6.1	3.8	13.3	4.7	8.1
Hill's Prescription Diet Metabolic Chicken Flavor (dry)	257	3.12	8.2	3.5	11.9	4.0	7.7
BLUE Natural Veterinary Diet W + M (dry)	325	3.23	9.5	4.1	9.3	3.7	5.6
Royal Canin Glycobalance (dry)	307	3.33	11.0	3.6	8.7	2.4	5.1
Purina Pro Plan Veterinary Diets EN Fiber Balance (dry)	324	3.39	6.5	3.5	13.2	1.8	5.8

Diets are listed by ascending caloric concentrations.
Note that nutrient profiles should be checked because they change over time (approximately every 6–12 mo).
Abbreviations: Carb, carbohydrate; TDF, total dietary fiber.

Dry and wet (canned or pouch) commercial pet foods contain very little sugar. Cats cannot taste sugar and although sugar enhances diet acceptance by dogs, amino acids and peptides, not sugars, are primarily used to stimulate appetite in dog and cat foods.[39] "Soft-moist" foods or treats with a spongy or flexible texture are not recommended for patient with DM. They are characterized by a guaranteed moisture content between 12% and 70% and must include appreciable quantities of sugar or sugar alcohols that chemically bind water to prevent spoilage.[42] Soft-moist treats containing the sugar alcohol, sorbitol, may be suitable for patients with DM, however, because sorbitol has been reported not to increase blood glucose.[43]

Dry foods do not need to contain sugars because they contain little water and are slow to spoil. Canned foods do not spoil because they are not exposed to air until they are opened. All dry pet foods and most wet pet foods contain digestible "complex" carbohydrate (starch) from grains, such as wheat and rice, from roots such as potato and carrots, and pulses such as peas and lentils. Digestible carbohydrate sources are included as an inexpensive source of calories and are required to form extruded dry kibble. The digestibility of starch can vary considerably, however, depending on the degree of processing/cooking, source, relative amounts of amylose and amylopectin in the starch, and size of granules.[44] "Slowly digested starch" may reduce postprandial hyperglycemia compared with "rapidly digested starch," whereas "resistant starch" is not digested and acts like soluble fiber. "Modified starch" may be included in some canned foods, for example, to thicken gravy.[43]

There is evidence that feeding a diet containing very little digestible carbohydrate to cats may increase the rate of diabetic remission in cats,[12,45,46] and this represents an ideal goal in the management of diabetic cats with type 2 diabetes. It is less clear that reducing the digestible carbohydrate content of dogs or cats with insulin-dependent DM is beneficial. There is no evidence that specifically feeding a high carbohydrate diet increases the risk of development of DM in cats.[47] Any calorically dense diet can increase the risk of obesity, which is a major risk factor for the development of DM in cats; obese cats are up to 4 times more likely than cats of ideal BCS to be diagnosed with DM.[48,49] Specific details regarding obesity management can be found elsewhere.[1]

Nutrient profiles for veterinary therapeutic dry diets marketed for cats with DM vary tremendously (**Table 2**). Some lower carbohydrate dry diets provide upward of 500 kcal per cup. Thus, it may be preferable to prioritize feeding a higher carbohydrate diet designed for obesity management (ie, less calorie dense ± high fiber) to an obese animal with DM if food intake cannot be safely limited to promote weight loss.

The range of digestible carbohydrate in commercial pet foods is quite large: the GA of some canned cat foods suggest they contain none (<1 g/100 kcal), whereas some dry diets contain more than 11 g/100 kcal. In general, a diet with < 4 g/100 kcal would be considered a relatively low carbohydrate diet; however, the lowest carbohydrate diets provide less than 1 to 2 g/100 kcal. Canned low carbohydrate diets also vary greatly in nutrient profiles (**Table 3**). In general, most canned diets contain fewer carbohydrates than their dry counterparts but not all canned diets are low in carbohydrates. **Table 4** provides some additional OTC low carbohydrate diets.

Fiber

Fiber varies in solubility, fermentability, and viscosity.[50] Carboxymethyl cellulose, for example, is soluble and viscous but not fermented by canine intestinal flora.[51] Both pectin and psyllium are viscous but the former is much more readily fermented.[52] Some viscous fibers, such as psyllium, may reduce postprandial hyperglycemia by slowing gastric emptying, slowing small intestinal transit, binding glucose and water,

Table 2
Comparison of metabolizable energy (kcal per cup and per gram) and selected nutrients of concern (per 100 kcal) for currently available veterinary therapeutic dry diets marketed for feline diabetes mellitus

Diet	Kcal/ cup	Kcal/ g	Crude Protein (g)	Crude Fat (g)	Carb (g)	Crude Fiber (g)	TDF (g)	Phos (mg)
Hill's Prescription Diet r/d	268	2.96	11.2	2.8	10.6	4.5	6.4	226
Hill's Prescription Diet w/d	293	3.23	11.6	2.7	10.4	1.7	3.2	239
Purina Pro Plan Veterinary Diets OM	285	3.23	15.9	2.8	5.9	1.8	4.6	390
BLUE Natural Veterinary Diet W + U	352	3.26	12.0	3.7	7.6	3.2	4.4	250
Hill's Prescription Diet Metabolic Chicken Flavor	299	3.40	10.7	3.7	8.8	2.7	4.5	210
Royal Canin Glycobalance	320	3.52	12.1	3.2	6.7	1.2	3.0	230
Purina Pro Plan Veterinary Diets DM	544	3.79	13.8	4.4	4.0	0.3	1.8	290
Hill's Prescription Diet m/d	463	3.98	12.5	5.2	3.6	1.0	1.8	189

Diets are listed by ascending caloric concentrations.
Note that nutrient profiles should be checked because they change over time (approximately every 6–12 mo).
Abbreviations: Carb, carbohydrate; Phos, phosphorus; TDF, total dietary fiber.

Table 3
Comparison of metabolizable energy (kcal per can and per gram) and selected nutrients of concern (per 100 kcal) for currently available veterinary therapeutic canned diets marketed for feline diabetes mellitus

Diet	Kcal/can	Kcal/g	Crude Protein (g)	Crude Fat (g)	Carb (g)	Crude Fiber (g)	TDF (g)	Phos (mg)
Royal Canin Glycobalance thin slices in gravy (3 oz)	57	0.67	12.4	4.1	3.7	1.0	2.3	300
Purina Pro Plan Veterinary Diets OM Savory Selects w/Chicken (5.5 oz)	113	0.73	14.2	3.9	5.0	2.3	3.5	260
Purina Pro Plan Veterinary Diets OM (5.5 oz)	115	0.74	13.6	3.5	6.4	3.5	3.8	240
Hill's Prescription Diet r/d Chicken Flavor (5.5 oz)	122	0.78	11.0	3.6	8.7	4.9	7.5	241
Hill's Prescription Diet Metabolic Chicken and Vegetable Stew (2.9 oz)	64	0.78	10.6	3.6	9.3	2.5	5.0	197
Hill's Prescription Diet w/d with Chicken (5.5 oz)	128	0.82	11.4	4.0	7.6	4.0	6.5	191
BLUE Natural Veterinary Diet W + U (5.5 oz)	134	0.86	12.0	5.7	4.4	2.3	4.1	440
Hill's Prescription Diet Metabolic Chicken Flavor (5.5 oz)	136	0.87	10.7	3.9	8.6	2.9	4.9	218
Hill's Prescription Diet m/d Chicken & Liver Stew (2.9 oz)	78	0.95	11.8	5.7	3.6	0.2	1.0	179
Purina Pro Plan Veterinary Diets DM Savory Selects (5.5 oz)	158	1.01	14.0	4.1	3.1	0.2	1.3	260
Purina Pro Plan Veterinary Diets DM (5.5 oz)	163	1.05	13.3	5.4	1.5	0.7	1.8	260
Hill's Prescription Diet m/d with Liver (5.5 oz)	173	1.11	11.9	5.7	3.0	0.6	1.1	151

Diets are listed by ascending caloric concentrations.
Note that nutrient profiles should be checked because they change over time (approximately every 6–12 mo) and values are for only some of the available flavors.
Abbreviations: Carb, carbohydrate; Phos, phosphorus; TDF, total dietary fiber.

Table 4
Comparison of metabolizable energy (kcal per can and per gram) and selected nutrients of concern (per 100 kcal) for selected over-the-counter low carbohydrate canned diets for cats

Diet	Kcal/can	Kcal/g	Crude Protein (g)	Crude Fat (g)	Carb (g)	Crude Fiber (g)	Phos (mg)
Purina Pro Plan Development Chicken & Liver Entree (3 oz)	99	1.17	11.1	7.1	0.7	0.1	366
Purina Pro Plan PRIME PLUS Adult 7+ Salmon & Tuna Entree (3 oz)	107	1.27	9.6	7.4	1.1	0.1	322
Purina ONE Urinary Tract Health Beef & Liver Recipe (3 oz)	101	1.19	9.3	7.5	1.1	0.1	246
Purina Friskies Pate Turkey & Giblets Dinner (5.5 oz)	181	1.16	9.9	7.0	1.4	0.2	333
Purina Friskies Pate Ocean Whitefish & Tuna Dinner (5.5 oz)	179	1.15	11.0	6.6	1.4	0.1	356
Purina Fancy Feast Flaked Trout Gourmet (3 oz)	104	1.23	14.1	5.3	1.4	0.3	266
Purina Friskies Pate Poultry Platter (5.5 oz)	184	1.18	10.0	7.5	1.5	0.1	338
Purina Friskies Pate Country Style Dinner Adult (5.5 oz)	182	1.17	9.9	7.0	1.5	0.2	339

Diets are listed by ascending carbohydrate (Carb) concentrations.
Note that nutrient profiles should be checked because they change over time (approximately every 6–12 mo) and values are for only some of the available flavors.
Abbreviation: Phos, phosphorus.

and thus, reducing intestinal absorption.[15] Fermentation metabolizes otherwise indigestible carbohydrates to short-chain fatty acids, which are then absorbed, facilitating water absorption. Fermentation in the ileum also stimulates the release of GLP1 in dogs and probably cats.

The GA on pet food labels is only required to report a maximum amount of crude fiber. Crude fiber is a poor measure of all the fiber in pet food because it includes no soluble fiber. Some TNAs report total dietary fiber (TDF), which includes soluble fiber but not oligosaccharides or resistant starch.[53] The crude fiber in commercial pet foods (and TDF when it is reported) varies from less than 1 g in some canned and liquid foods to about 6 g crude fiber and 11 g TDF per 100 kcal.

Insoluble fiber, which is largely measured as crude fiber, undergoes little or no fermentation in the large intestine of dogs and cats, is not viscous. It improves fecal form and reduces the likelihood of soft feces or diarrhea by absorbing additional water retained in the large intestine. Soluble fiber content is not reported for most pet foods but can be inferred from the crude fiber content because insoluble fiber is usually increased in proportion to soluble fiber in many commercial diets to reduce the risk of increased production of volatile fatty acids from fermentation causing diarrhea.

There is some evidence that increasing dietary fiber intake may be useful in dogs with DM.[13,14] Dietary fiber is proposed to slow digestion and absorption of dietary carbohydrates, and reduce postprandial hyperglycemia. The glycemic index, measured as the increase in blood glucose, when starch is fed as the only component of a meal to healthy animals, varies slightly among sources of starch. Glycemic index is not necessarily a good indicator of the physiologic response to mixed meals, however, because hyperglycemia is modest when the addition of fat to mixed meals slows gastric emptying.[54] Composition of a meal influences changes in postprandial incremental glucose and insulin in healthy dogs.[55] The effects of different starches on postprandial glucose and insulin responses in mixed meals has been studied in healthy dogs and dogs with DM but many of these studies have been performed with lower fat diets (<3 g fat/100 kcal).[15,56,57] In one study, diabetic dogs had better glycemic control when fed a sorghum-based diet compared with a rice-based diet, despite similar TDF concentrations.[15] These results may not apply to all insulin formulations.

Most "high" fiber diets are low in caloric density. In thin (or even ideal BCS) diabetic dogs, these diets may promote further undesirable weight loss. For an obese diabetic dog, feeding a veterinary therapeutic weight loss diet that is also high in fiber may be a good option. There are also some OTC and veterinary therapeutic diets that are slightly higher in caloric density but contain moderate to high amounts of fiber, which might help modulate postprandial glycemia in lean dogs (**Table 5**).

Minerals and Vitamins

There is currently no evidence that vitamin or mineral requirements differ between regulated diabetic and nondiabetic dogs or cats. Feeding a complete and balanced diet should provide all the micronutrients a well-managed patient with DM requires. Micronutrient deficiencies may occur, however, if unbalanced treats provide more than 10% of calories. Some trace nutrients, such as chromium, might beneficially affect glucose metabolism but evidence for supplementation at concentrations above that currently found in pet and human foods is poor.[58] Chromium supplementation of food fed to diabetic dogs and obese cats, at microgram per kilogram BW greater than that consumed by people eating standard diets, did not affect glucose tolerance.[59] The chromium concentrations of commercial pet foods have not been reported because chromium is difficult to measure and is not listed as being essential by the National Research Council or the Association of American Feed Control Officials.

Table 5
Comparison of metabolizable energy (kcal per cup and per gram) and selected nutrients of concern (gram per 100 kcal) for selected veterinary therapeutic and over-the-counter moderate-to-high fiber dry diets for dogs

Diet	Kcal/cup	Kcal/g	Crude Protein	Crude Fat	Carb	Crude Fiber	TDF
Royal Canin Labrador Retriever Adult 5+	277	3.38	8.5	3.1	11.3	1.3	3.1
Royal Canin Large Joint Care	314	3.53	7.2	4.2	10.7	1.6	3.6
Hill's Science Diet Adult Oral Care	274	3.45	6.7	4.3	11.7	2.7	4.8
Hill's Prescription Diet Gastrointestinal Biome	330	3.33	5.8	3.5	14.3	2.1	4.9
Purina Pro Plan Veterinary Diets EN Fiber Balance	324	3.39	6.5	3.5	13.2	1.8	5.8
Royal Canin Gastrointestinal High Fiber	290	3.37	7.1	4.9	10.6	3.2	6.3
Hill's Science Diet Adult Perfect Weight	299	3.19	8.2	3.2	12.5	3.0	6.6
Royal Canin Medium Weight Care	256	3.20	8.7	3.5	12.1	3.4	7.4
Hill's Science Diet Adult Light	271	2.99	7.7	2.5	14.7	3.8	7.6

Diets are listed by ascending total dietary fiber concentrations.
Note that nutrient profiles should be checked because they change over time (approximately every 6-12 mo) and values are for only some of the available flavors.

Chromium concentrations are likely to be similar to or greater than those in human diets because pet foods are made from similar ingredient types.

Low concentrations of vitamin D and calcium have been documented in human patients with noninsulin dependent (type 2) DM but evidence for the benefit of supplementation in these patients is poor.[60] Low ionized calcium has been documented in almost half of canine patients with DM.[61] The type of DM in dogs in that study was not documented, however, and most diabetic dogs have insulin-dependent DM. Additionally, concurrent diseases (eg, hyperadrenocorticism, pancreatitis) may have affected calcium concentrations. Hypocalcemia is often associated with hypomagnesemia and hypokalemia. Better documentation of blood concentrations of calcium and 25-hydroxyvitamin D is needed, therefore, *after* correction of potassium and magnesium deficiencies, together with clarification of the benefits/risks, type of supplementation and dose of vitamin D, before either calcium or vitamin D supplementation of the diet can be recommended in dogs or cats with DM.

Additional Feeding Strategies

Meal feeding

Meal feeding twice daily immediately before insulin administration (at approximately 12-hour intervals) is usually recommended when using an intermediate acting insulin that is expected to substantially peak a few hours after injection. This strategy seeks to control postprandial hyperglycemia and allows the insulin dose to be adjusted (ie, reduced, typically by half) if a patient does not eat. A study found no difference in total insulin dose per day, however, when diabetic dogs were fed either 2 or 3 times daily.[15] Newer insulin management protocols involving administration of basal insulins once daily, or even once weekly, that do not require consistent twice daily meal feeding, have also effectively managed hyperglycemia.[62,63] The pairing of insulin injection to the meal is also not important when an animal is fed a diet with a very low glycemic index. Thus, the emphasis on the importance of feeding consistent meals twice daily may not be necessary depending on the type of insulin, consistency of appetite, and type of food consumed.

Treats

Treats are often an important part of the human–animal bond. Nevertheless, treats are often not complete and balanced, contain primarily carbohydrate, some of which may be sugar (eg, soft-moist treats), and provide more calories than pet owners appreciate. Any dry balanced kibble can be given as a treat but unbalanced treats should provide 10% or less of calories to avoid unbalancing the diet. Vegetables and fruits make excellent treats provided the sugar, carbohydrate, fiber, *and* calories they provide are considered. A medium baby carrot may be a useful treat, for example, because it only provides 3.5 kcal even though about 90% of those calories are from carbohydrate and more than half are from sugar.

Acute Management of Diabetic Ketoacidosis

Managing a sick animal with DKA has its own nutritional challenges. These animals can be mildly to severely dehydrated on presentation and often require aggressive intravenous fluid support as well as supplementation of potassium and phosphate, sometimes magnesium, to correct electrolyte derangements. Liquid diets designed for human beings containing increased dextrins have the potential to cause life-threatening decreases in blood concentrations of potassium and phosphorus, and intravenous potassium phosphate supplementation may be required to maintain adequate serum concentrations.

Table 6
Comparison of metabolizable energy (kcal/can or bottle and per mL) and selected nutrients of concern (per 100 kcal) for selected liquid and canned diets for tube feeding

Diet	Kcal/can or Bottle	Kcal/mL	Crude Protein (g)	Crude Fat (g)	Carb (g)	Potassium (mg)	Phos (mg)
Royal Canin Recovery Liquid (8 fL oz bottle)	217	0.9	9.1	5.7	5.7	230	180
Royal Canin Renal Support Liquid Feline (8 fL oz bottle)	217	0.9	7.5	5.9	6.9	180	80
Royal Canin Renal Support Liquid Canine (8 fL oz bottle)	319	1.3	3.7	6.0	10.4	160	90
Royal Canin GI Low Fat Liquid Canine (8 fL oz bottle)	209	0.9	10.1	2.2	13.1	240	200
Emeraid Intensive Care HDN (1 mL powder:2 mL water)	42/scoop	1.1	8.6	6.0	2.8	160	220
Abbott Nutrition Jevity 1.5	355	1.5	4.3	3.3	14.2	145	83
Abbott Nutrition Ensure High Protein	160	0.7	10	1.2	11.9	294	156
Purina Pro Plan Veterinary Diets CN (5.5 oz can + 20 mL water)	206	1.3	8.2	7.4	2.4	250	260
Hill's Prescription Diet a/d (5.5 oz can + 30 mL water)[a]	183	1.0	9.0	6.7	2.7	242	237
Royal Canin Recovery Ultra Soft Mousse (5.1 oz can + 30 mL water)[a]	149	0.9	10.1	6.2	2.0	210	250

[a] Note that nutrient profiles should be checked because they change over time (approximately every 6–12 mo).

Animals with DKA often are hyporexic to anorexic and in a state of catabolism, which can contribute to weight loss and cachexia. Deleterious effects of anorexia (eg, enterocyte atrophy, decreased immune function) will occur within just a few days of anorexia.[64] Once vomiting, nausea, and pain are controlled, it is imperative to maintain a positive energy balance. Any complete and balanced diet should be considered acceptable in this acute setting. It is generally recommended to avoid transitioning ill animals to new, long-term diets during the hospitalization to reduce the risk of inducing a food aversion. Appetite stimulants can be useful in some animals to encourage voluntary food intake. Capromorelin acts on the growth hormone receptor in pancreatic delta cells and has been shown to increase post-prandial glucose concentrations in healthy dogs and cats by suppressing insulin secretion.[65] However, patients in DKA already secrete little or no insulin and likely would not respond negatively to a short course of capromorelin administration.

Assisted nutritional support should be provided to animals that have received fluid and electrolyte resuscitation and that remain hyporexic for more than 2 to 3 days. This can be achieved either with short-term nasoesophageal or nasogastric tube support or with longer-term esophagostomy or gastrostomy tubes. The decision to place a short-term versus a long-term tube should be made based on the animal's overall nutritional status and likelihood of short-term (<7 days) vs long-term (>7 days) assisted nutritional support. For example, animals that present with either concurrent acute necrotizing pancreatitis, hepatic lipidosis, or acute-on-chronic kidney disease are more likely to require long-term support.

Liquid enteral diets can be fed via small bore nasoenteral tubes, whereas canned diets can be made into slurries to be fed via larger bore esophagostomy or gastrostomy tubes (**Table 6**). Liquid foods increase blood glucose soon after a meal even in healthy animals because liquid empties from the stomach rapidly and all liquid foods contain dextrins (hydrolyzed starch that is readily hydrolyzed to sugar in the intestine) or sugar. Only a few contain indigestible carbohydrate. Additional details about assisted enteral nutrition can be found elsewhere.[64,66] Regarding specific nutritional profiles for the sick with DKA, priority should be ensuring that adequate energy and protein requirements are met to maintain BW and lean muscle mass. Nearly any liquid enteral diet can be fed safely to a DKA patient for 5 to 7 days. If longer term assisted enteral nutritional support is required beyond 1 week, a longer term feeding tube should be placed.

Diabetic Patients with Comorbid Conditions

Other features of a diet's nutrient profile may take precedence for a middle-aged or older patient with diabetes and a comorbid condition. For example, it would be prudent to choose a diet that limits phosphorus intake in a diabetic cat with chronic kidney disease.[29] Similarly, feeding a limited antigen diet or modifying dietary fat and/or fiber intake may be important for a diabetic pet with a chronic enteropathy such as inflammatory bowel disease.[38] Conversely, a juvenile patient with diabetes should be fed a diet that meets its requirements for growth (mainly higher protein, fat, calcium, and phosphorus requirements).

SUMMARY

In conclusion, there is no single best nutritional approach that should be applied to every dog or cat with diabetes. When presented with a patient with diabetes, veterinarians should start by assessing the animal, its nutritional status, including body composition and a complete diet history, and any comorbid conditions. With those essential pieces of information, specific nutritional goals can be applied to each individual patient. It is also important to include pet owners in discussions about changes in diet to gather their perspectives and to increase client compliance. Pending the animal's response to the nutritional and medical management plan implemented, some adjustments may be required.

DECLARATION OF INTERESTS

Dr V.J. Parker has received research support and honoraria from Nestle Purina, Royal Canin, and Hill's. Dr R.C. Hill has received stipend, research support, and honoraria from Alpo, Nestle Purina, Mars.

REFERENCES

1. Cline MG, Burns KM, Coe JB, et al. 2021 AAHA Nutrition and Weight Management Guidelines for Dogs and Cats. J Am Anim Hosp Assoc 2021;57:153–78.
2. Lund EM, Armstrong P, Kirk CA, et al. Prevalence and risk factors for obesity in adult cats from private US veterinary practices 2005;3:88–96.
3. Lund EM, Armstrong PJ, Kirk CA, et al. Prevalence and risk factors for obesity in adult dogs from private US veterinary practices 2006;4:177.
4. Mattheeuws D, Rottiers R, Kaneko JJ, et al. Diabetes mellitus in dogs: relationship of obesity to glucose tolerance and insulin response. Am J Vet Res 1984;45:98–103.
5. Appleton DJ, Rand JS, Sunvold GD. Insulin sensitivity decreases with obesity, and lean cats with low insulin sensitivity are at greatest risk of glucose intolerance with weight gain. J Feline Med Surg 2001;3:211–28.
6. Slupe JL, Freeman LM, Rush JE. Association of body weight and body condition with survival in dogs with heart failure. J Vet Intern Med 2008;22:561–5.
7. Finn E, Freeman LM, Rush JE, et al. The Relationship Between Body Weight, Body Condition, and Survival in Cats with Heart Failure. J Vet Intern Med 2010;24:1369–74.
8. Parker VJ, Freeman LM. Association between Body Condition and Survival in Dogs with Acquired Chronic Kidney Disease. J Vet Intern Med 2011;25:1306–11.
9. Pedrinelli V, Lima DM, Duarte CN, et al. Nutritional and laboratory parameters affect the survival of dogs with chronic kidney disease. PLoS One 2020;15:e0234712.
10. Ineson DL, Freeman LM, Rush JE. Clinical and laboratory findings and survival time associated with cardiac cachexia in dogs with congestive heart failure. J Vet Intern Med 2019;33:1902–8.
11. Santiago SL, Freeman LM, Rush JE. Cardiac cachexia in cats with congestive heart failure: Prevalence and clinical, laboratory, and survival findings. J Vet Intern Med 2020;34:35–44.
12. Bennett N, Greco DS, Peterson ME, et al. Comparison of a low carbohydrate-low fiber diet and a moderate carbohydrate-high fiber diet in the management of feline diabetes mellitus. J Feline Med Surg 2006;8:73–84.
13. Nelson RW, Duesberg CA, Ford SL, et al. Effect of dietary insoluble fiber on control of glycemia in dogs with naturally acquired diabetes mellitus. J Am Vet Med Assoc 1998;212:380–6.
14. Kimmel SE, Michel KE, Hess RS, et al. Effects of insoluble and soluble dietary fiber on glycemic control in dogs with naturally occurring insulin-dependent diabetes mellitus. J Am Vet Med Assoc 2000;216:1076–81.

15. Teshima E, Brunetto MA, Teixeira FA, et al. Influence of type of starch and feeding management on glycaemic control in diabetic dogs. J Anim Physiol Anim Nutr 2021;105:1192–202.

16. Model JFA, Rocha DS, Fagundes AdC, et al. Physiological and pharmacological actions of glucagon like peptide-1 (GLP-1) in domestic animals. Vet Anim Sci 2022;16:100245.

17. Massimino SP, McBurney MI, Field CJ, et al. Fermentable Dietary Fiber Increases GLP-1 Secretion and Improves Glucose Homeostasis Despite Increased Intestinal Glucose Transport Capacity in Healthy Dogs. J Nutr 1998;128:1786–93.

18. Wei A, Fascetti AJ, Villaverde C, et al. Effect of water content in a canned food on voluntary food intake and body weight in cats. Am J Vet Res 2011;72:918–23.

19. Laflamme DP, Hannah SS. Increased dietary protein promotes fat loss and reduces loss of lean body mass during weight loss in cats. Intern J Appl Res Vet Med 2005;3:62–8.

20. German AJ, Holden SL, Bissot T, et al. A high protein high fibre diet improves weight loss in obese dogs. Vet J 2010;183:294–7.

21. Linder DE, Parker VJ. Dietary Aspects of Weight Management in Cats and Dogs. Vet Clin North Am Small Anim Pract 2016;46:869–82.

22. Weber M, Bissot T, Servet E, et al. A high-protein, high-fiber diet designed for weight loss improves satiety in dogs. J Vet Intern Med 2007;21:1203–8.

23. Struble AL, Feldman EC, Nelson RW, et al. Systemic hypertension and proteinuria in dogs with diabetes mellitus. J Am Vet Med Assoc 1998;213:822–5.

24. Herring IP, Panciera DL, Werre SR. Longitudinal prevalence of hypertension, proteinuria, and retinopathy in dogs with spontaneous diabetes mellitus. J Vet Intern Med 2014;28:488–95.

25. Priyanka M, Jeyaraja K, Thirunavakkarasu P. Abnormal renovascular resistance in dogs with diabetes mellitus: correlation with glycemic status and proteinuria. Iran J Vet Res 2018;19:304.

26. Burkholder WJ, Lees GE, LeBlanc AK, et al. Diet modulates proteinuria in heterozygous female dogs with X-linked hereditary nephropathy. J Vet Intern Med 2004; 18:165–75.

27. Cortadellas O, Talavera J, Fernández del Palacio MJ. Evaluation of the Effects of a Therapeutic Renal Diet to Control Proteinuria in Proteinuric Non-Azotemic Dogs Treated with Benazepril. J Vet Intern Med 2014;28:30–7.

28. Parker VJ, Freeman LM. Nutritional Management of Protein-Losing Nephropathy in Dogs. Compendium 2012;July:E1–5.

29. Parker VJ. Nutritional Management for Dogs and Cats with Chronic Kidney Disease. Vet Clin North Am Small Anim Pract 2021;51:685–710.

30. Gilor C, Graves TK, Gilor S, et al. The incretin effect in cats: comparison between oral glucose, lipids, and amino acids. Domest Anim Endocrinol 2011;40:205–12.

31. Xenoulis PG, Steiner JM. Canine hyperlipidaemia. J Small Anim Pract 2015;56: 595–605.

32. Xenoulis PG, Cammarata PJ, Walzem RL, et al. Effect of a low-fat diet on serum triglyceride and cholesterol concentrations and lipoprotein profiles in Miniature Schnauzers with hypertriglyceridemia. J Vet Intern Med 2020;34:2605–16.

33. James FE, Mansfield CS, Steiner JM, et al. Pancreatic response in healthy dogs fed diets of various fat compositions. Am J Vet Res 2009;70:614–8.

34. Mansfield C, Beths T. Management of acute pancreatitis in dogs: a critical appraisal with focus on feeding and analgesia. J Small Anim Pract 2015;56: 27–39.

35. Hill RC, Van Winkle TJ. Acute necrotizing pancreatitis and acute suppurative pancreatitis in the cat. A retrospective study of 40 cases (1976-1989). J Vet Intern Med 1993;7:25–33.

36. Newman S, Steiner J, Woosley K, et al. Localization of pancreatic inflammation and necrosis in dogs. J Vet Intern Med 2004;18:488–93.

37. Fragkou FC, Adamama-Moraitou KK, Poutahidis T, et al. Prevalence and Clinico-pathological Features of Triaditis in a Prospective Case Series of Symptomatic and Asymptomatic Cats. J Vet Intern Med 2016;30:1031–45.

38. Rudinsky AJ, Rowe JC, Parker VJ. Nutritional management of chronic enteropathies in dogs and cats. J Am Vet Med Assoc 2018;253:570–8.

39. National Research Council. Nutrient requirements of dogs and cats. Washington DC, USA: National Academies Press; 2006.

40. Fischer MM, Kessler AM, de Sá LRM, et al. Fiber fermentability effects on energy and macronutrient digestibility, fecal traits, postprandial metabolite responses, and colon histology of overweight cats. J Anim Sci 2012;90:2233–45.

41. de Oliveira Matheus LF, Risolia LW, Ernandes MC, et al. Effects of Saccharomyces cerevisiae cell wall addition on feed digestibility, fecal fermentation and microbiota and immunological parameters in adult cats. BMC Vet Res 2021; 17:351.

42. Dzanis DA. Petfood types, quality assessment and feeding management. In: Kyamme J.L.P.T., Petfood technology. 1st edition. Malta: Watt Publishing Co; 2003. p. 68–73.

43. Hill DA. Specialty ingredients: considerations and use. In: Kyamme J.L.P.T., Petfood technology. 1st edition. Malta: Watt Publishing Co; 2003. p. 85–100.

44. Zhang G, Hamaker BR. Slowly Digestible Starch: Concept, Mechanism, and Proposed Extended Glycemic Index. Crit Rev Food Sci Nutr 2009;49:852–67.

45. Frank G, Anderson W, Pazak H, et al. Use of a high-protein diet in the management of feline diabetes mellitus. Vet Therapeut 2001;2:238–46.

46. Mazzaferro E. Treatment of feline diabetes mellitus using an α-glucosidase inhibitor and a low-carbohydrate diet. J Feline Med Surg 2003;5:183–9.

47. Verbrugghe A, Hesta M, Daminet S, et al. Nutritional modulation of insulin resistance in the true carnivorous cat: a review. Crit Rev Food Sci Nutr 2012;52: 172-82.

48. Scarlett JM, Donoghue S. Associations between body condition and disease in cats. J Am Vet Med Assoc 1998;212:1725–31.

49. O'Neill DG, Gostelow R, Orme C, et al. Epidemiology of Diabetes Mellitus among 193,435 Cats Attending Primary-Care Veterinary Practices in England. J Vet Intern Med 2016;30:964–72.

50. Moreno AA, Parker VJ, Winston JA, Rudinsky AJ. Dietary fiber aids in the management of canine and feline gastrointestinal disease. J Am Vet Med Assoc 2022;260:S33–45.

51. Calabrò S, Carciofi AC, Musco N, et al. Fermentation Characteristics of Several Carbohydrate Sources for Dog Diets Using the In Vitro Gas Production Technique. Ital J Anim Sci 2013;12:e4.

52. Swanson KS, Grieshop CM, Clapper GM, et al. Fruit and vegetable fiber fermentation by gut microflora from canines. J Anim Sci 2001;79:919–26.

53. de-Oliveira LD, Takakura FS, Kienzle E, et al. Fibre analysis and fibre digestibility in pet foods–a comparison of total dietary fibre, neutral and acid detergent fibre and crude fibre. J Anim Physiol Anim Nutr 2012;96:895–906.

54. Holste LC, Nelson RW, Feldman EC, et al. Effect of dry, soft moist, and canned dog foods on postprandial blood glucose and insulin concentrations in healthy dogs. Am J Vet Res 1989;50:984–9.
55. Hill RC, Burrows CF, Bauer JE, et al. Texturized vegetable protein containing indigestible soy carbohydrate affects blood insulin concentrations in dogs fed high fat diets. J Nutr 2006;136:2024s–7s.
56. Carciofi AC, Takakura FS, de-Oliveira LD, et al. Effects of six carbohydrate sources on dog diet digestibility and post-prandial glucose and insulin response. J Anim Physiol Anim Nutr 2008;92:326–36.
57. Adolphe JL, Drew MD, Silver TI, et al. Effect of an extruded pea or rice diet on postprandial insulin and cardiovascular responses in dogs. J Anim Physiol Anim Nutr 2014;99(4):767–76.
58. Balk EM, Tatsioni A, Lichtenstein AH, et al. Effect of chromium supplementation on glucose metabolism and lipids: a systematic review of randomized controlled trials. Diabetes Care 2007;30:2154–63.
59. Minerals. In National Research Council, Nutrient requirements of dogs and cats. National Academies Press; 2006. p. 145–92.
60. Pittas AG, Lau J, Hu FB, et al. The role of vitamin D and calcium in type 2 diabetes. A systematic review and meta-analysis. J Clin Endocrinol Metab 2007; 92:2017–29.
61. Hess RS, Saunders HM, Van Winkle TJ, et al. Concurrent disorders in dogs with diabetes mellitus: 221 cases (1993-1998). J Am Vet Med Assoc 2000;217: 1166–73.
62. Gilor C, Hulsebosch SE, Pires J, et al. An ultra-long-acting recombinant insulin for the treatment of diabetes mellitus in cats. J Vet Intern Med 2021;35:2123–30.
63. Hulsebosch SE, Pires J, Bannasch MJ, et al. Ultra-long-acting recombinant insulin for the treatment of diabetes mellitus in dogs. J Vet Intern Med 2022;36: 1211–9.
64. Chan DL. Nutritional Support of the Critically Ill Small Animal Patient. Vet Clin North Am Small Anim Pract 2020;50:1411–22.
65. Pascutti KM, O'Kell AL, Hill RC, et al. The effect of capromorelin on glycemic control in healthy dogs. Domest Anim Endocrinol 2022;81:106732.
66. Taylor S, Chan DL, Villaverde C, et al. 2022 ISFM Consensus Guidelines on Management of the Inappetent Hospitalised Cat. J Feline Med Surg 2022;24:614–40.

The Future of Diabetes Therapies

New Insulins and Insulin Delivery Systems, Glucagon-Like Peptide 1 Analogs, Sodium-Glucose Cotransporter Type 2 Inhibitors, and Beta Cell Replacement Therapy

Jennifer M. Reinhart, DVM, PhD[a],*, Thomas K. Graves, DVM, MS, PhD[b]

KEYWORDS

- Ultra-long-acting insulin analogs • GLP-1 analogs • SGLT-2 inhibitors
- Insulin infusion pump • Smart insulin • Beta cell replacement therapy

KEY POINTS

- Veterinarians should be aware of advances in diabetic therapy and how they may be translated to canine and feline patients.
- Species differences in pathophysiology, management practices and goals, and lifestyle may affect the translation of novel diabetic therapies for veterinary use.
- Therapies to watch include new ultra-long-acting insulin analogs, oral sodium-glucose cotransporter type 2 inhibitors, and oral insulins.
- Other therapies could provide tight glycemic control and a hands-off approach (eg, closed-loop insulin delivery systems) but implementation would represent a major paradigm shift in the veterinary approach to diabetes management.

INTRODUCTION

Given the increasing prevalence of diabetes mellitus (DM) in the human population, it is not surprising that antidiabetic pharmaceuticals are a multibillion-dollar industry with new treatments constantly in development. Many novel therapies are designed not only to improve glycemic control but also to reduce insulin injection frequency and

[a] Department of Veterinary Clinical Medicine, College of Veterinary Medicine, University of Illinois Urbana-Champaign, 1008 West Hazelwood Drive, Urbana, IL 61802, USA; [b] College of Veterinary Medicine, Midwestern University, 19555 North 59th Avenue, Glendale, AZ 85308, USA
* Corresponding author.
E-mail address: jreinha2@illinois.edu

Vet Clin Small Anim 53 (2023) 675–690
https://doi.org/10.1016/j.cvsm.2023.01.003
0195-5616/23/© 2023 Elsevier Inc. All rights reserved.

vetsmall.theclinics.com

risk of hypoglycemic events. Some of these therapies may hold promise in the management of small animal DM and veterinarians should be aware of potential treatments on the horizon (**Table 1**). Furthermore, as DM has become more prevalent in people, pet owners have become savvier about the disease and therapeutic options available to human diabetic patients. Thus, it is prudent for veterinarians to know about these options and their possible use in dogs and cats. However, it is also important to consider how species differences in pathophysiology, management practices, and goals, and lifestyle may affect the translation of novel diabetic therapies for veterinary use.

ULTRA-LONG-ACTING INSULINS

Ultra-long-acting insulins are insulin analog preparations with a duration of action greater than 24 h. In human patients, not only do they require less frequent dosing, but they also show activity profiles with less intra- and inter-dose variability. These properties allow tighter glycemic regulation and decrease the risk of hypoglycemia.[1] Ultra-long-acting insulins are commonly used in human DM patients for basal-bolus protocols. In these regimens, the ultra-long-acting insulin is administered daily to control fasting glucose concentrations (basal insulin) and is paired with a rapid- or ultra-rapid-acting insulin at mealtimes to control postprandial hyperglycemia (bolus insulin).[2] Because of the need for frequent blood glucose measurements and multiple daily injections, such treatment strategies may not be practical in many dogs and cats. However, ultra-long-acting insulins might still be useful as a single-agent therapy in small animal DM patients, and with the added potential to decrease dosing frequency.

Currently, there are two ultra-long-acting insulins that have been investigated in dogs and cats: insulin glargine U300 (Toujeo, Sanofi) and insulin degludec (Tresiba, Novo Nordisk). Insulin glargine U300 contains the same insulin analog as insulin glargine U100 (eg, Lantus, Semglee), but in a threefold more concentrated solution, forming a denser subcutaneous depot, which slows insulin release.[3] Insulin degludec is a human insulin analog with a fatty acid moiety, which facilitates the formation of subcutaneous depots and increases protein binding. These features delay absorption, provide a flatter time-action profile, and reduce day-to-day variability in glucose concentrations.[4–7] Information about veterinary use of insulin glargine U300 and insulin degludec can be found in "Insulin Therapy 1: General Principles", "Insulin Therapy 2: Dogs", and "Insulin Therapy 3: Cats" in this issue.

Decreasing insulin dosing frequency to daily or even less frequent administration could significantly improve treatment compliance and quality of life of diabetic pets and their owners. New insulins are in development that could function as ultra-long-acting insulins in dogs and cats. Insulin icodec is a once-weekly, ultra-long-acting, basal insulin currently in phase 3 trials in human patients. Its extremely long half-life (196 h in people) and duration of action are attributable to strong, reversible albumin binding, reduced enzymatic degradation, and slow receptor-mediated clearance.[8] In preclinical trials, insulin icodec had an average half-life of 60 h in dogs so, although weekly administration seems unlikely, alternate or every third-day administration might be a possibility.[9] Insulin icodec has not been evaluated in cats so, given the large species differences in pharmacokinetic properties (rat $t_{1/2} = 26$ h), it is impossible to predict how this insulin will behave in feline patients.

Another approach is the development of synthetic polypeptides in which insulin is expressed as a fusion protein with the Fc portion of immunoglobulin.[10] The Fc region binds to the neonatal Fc receptor allowing intracellular trafficking and recycling of the

Table 1
Overview of current and investigational diabetes mellitus therapies in human medicine, which may have future applications for veterinary patients

Therapeutic Approach	Specific Therapies	Mechanism of Action and Clinical Information
Ultra-long-acting insulin analogs	Currently approved: Insulin glargine U300 (Toujeo) Insulin degludec (Tresiba) Investigational therapies: Insulin icodec Insulin-Fc fusion proteins	• Basal insulin analogs with a duration of action >24 h (species-dependent), allowing once daily or less frequent injections. • Extended duration of action facilitated by prolonged absorption from subcutaneous depot, enhanced protein binding, or altered insulin clearance.
Incretin therapies	GLP-1 analogs: Exenatide (Byetta) Exenatide ER (Byureon) Liraglutide (Victoza) Lixisenatide (Adlyxin) Albiglutide (Tanzeum) Semaglutide, injection (Ozempic) Semaglutide, oral (Rybelsus) DPP-1 inhibitors (gliptins) Alogliptin Linagliptin Saxagliptin Sitagliptin Investigational therapies: GLP-1 receptor agonists	• GLP-1 analogs mimic GLP-1 action: ○ Increase insulin secretion by sensitizing beta cells to glucose stimulation ○ Decrease glucagon secretion ○ Increase satiety and decrease appetite ○ Promote beta cell differentiation/proliferation and inhibit apoptosis • GLP-1 analogs enhance weight loss and improve cardiovascular outcomes in human patients • Increase endogenous GLP-1 and other incretin concentrations by decreased degradation by dipeptidyl-peptidase-4 • Non-peptide, small-molecule drugs that mimic the action of GLP-1 • Improved oral bioavailability over GLP-1 analogs
SGLT-2 inhibitors	Currently approved: Canagliflozin (Invokana) Dapagliflozin (Farxiga) Empagliflozin (Jardiance) Ertugloflozin (Steglatro) Investigational therapies: Several	• Prevent glucose reabsorption in proximal tubules • Enhance renal glucose elimination and lower blood glucose • Orally administered • Improve cardiac and renal outcomes in human patients

(continued on next page)

Table 1
(continued)

Therapeutic Approach	Specific Therapies	Mechanism of Action and Clinical Information
Non-injectable insulins	Inhaled insulin (Afrezza) Oral insulin (investigational)	• Rapid acting, regular insulin for prandial/bolus use • Administered in a metered-dose inhaler • Co-formulated with digestive enzyme inhibitors and/or excipients to improve paracellular absorption, increasing bioavailability
Continuous insulin infusion	Insulin infusion pumps Insulin patches	• Provide continuous subcutaneous infusion of rapid- or ultra-rapid-acting insulin • Basal infusion rate delivers insulin throughout the day • Intermittent boluses administered at mealtimes
Smart insulins	Smart pens and pen caps Closed-loop systems Glucose-responsive insulin approaches (investigational)	• Assist in dose tracking and timing; measure residual insulin in pen • Insulin infusion pump and continuous glucose monitor communicate directly to adjust the basal rate and prandial boluses • Insulin is embedded in a glucose-responsive matrix, which releases insulin in response to surrounding glucose concentrations • Insulin molecule contains a glucose-sensing element that alters insulin kinetics or function based on blood glucose concentrations
Beta cell replacement therapies	Traditional transplantation Cell-culture approaches (investigational)	• Restores endogenous insulin secretion • Pancreatic islet transplants currently performed in human patients with variable success • Differentiation of mesenchymal or induced pluripotent stem cells into insulin-secreting cells appears promising, but is in early phases of development

molecule, which significantly extends the insulin's half-life. An insulin-feline Fc fusion protein was recently evaluated in five diabetic cats, administered subcutaneously once weekly for 7 weeks. In this pilot study, cats showed adequate glycemic control without significant clinical signs of DM, clinical hypoglycemia, or adverse effects.[11] In a similar study, of an insulin-canine Fc fusion protein, 4/5 diabetic dogs treated a once weekly insulin-canine Fc fusion protein achieved adequate diabetic control over an 8-week period.[12] Further study is needed, and insulin fusion proteins are not commercially available. However, this and other novel approaches represent possibilities for future use of ultra-long-acting insulin analogs in veterinary medicine to reduce injection frequency, improve compliance, and enhance patient outcomes.

GLUCAGON-LIKE PEPTIDE 1-BASED THERAPIES

Glucagon-like peptide 1 (GLP-1) is an incretin hormone secreted by L cells in the intestines in response to luminal nutrients, bacterial products, and secondary bile acids. Following a meal, GLP-1 acts as an "early warning system," preparing the rest of the body for the nutrient load, particularly glucose, about to arrive via the portal circulation. In the pancreas, GLP-1 increases insulin secretion by sensitizing beta cells to glucose stimulation and decreases glucagon release by alpha cells. It also increases satiety by delaying gastric emptying and suppressing appetite.[13] These features make GLP-1 an attractive strategy for diabetic therapies.

Thus far, the most successful and widely used incretin-based therapies are the GLP-1 analogs. Because their primary mechanism of action is dependent on residual beta cell function, GLP-1 analogs are used to treat type 2 DM (T2DM) in human patients. Similarly, GLP-1 analogs have the highest therapeutic potential in diabetic cats, although dogs might benefit from other, non-beta-cell-dependent effects.[14] Glucotoxicity and beta cell dysfunction are key features of feline DM. GLP-1 both inhibits beta cell apoptosis and promotes beta cell differentiation and proliferation.[15] These effects have primarily been documented in rodent models so whether GLP-1 analogs have a protective effect on the feline endocrine pancreas is still unknown. One possible reason these drugs are so effective in people is that treatment of T2DM is generally initiated early in the course of the disease, when significant beta cell mass still exists. In cats, DM is usually detected with the onset of clinical signs, after widespread beta cell loss has occurred. Although GLP-1 analogs help maximize the function of the remaining tissue, optimal use might only be achieved when paired with early detection strategies, which have yet to be implemented in cats. Another important consequence of this difference in management is that, in human patients, GLP-1 analogs can be used as a single agent or in combination with other noninsulin glucose-lowering drugs.[16] However, based on current experience, these drugs need to be combined with insulin to achieve appropriate glycemic control in cats.[17,18]

Native GLP-1 has too short a half-life to be clinically useful, due to rapid degradation by dipeptidyl-peptidase-4 (DPP-4) and other tissue proteases. Thus, GLP-1 analogs have modifications aimed at prolonging duration of action. Exenatide (Byetta, AstraZeneca) is a synthetic version of a peptide originally isolated from Gila monster venom with a high affinity for the GLP-1 receptor and intrinsic resistance to proteolysis by DPP-4.[13] Subcutaneous exenatide lowers blood glucose and increases insulin secretion in healthy cats in a dose-dependent manner.[19–21] An extended-release, depot formulation (exenatide ER; Bydureon, AstraZeneca) is available that allows for once weekly administration, which results in fewer gastrointestinal side effects in both people and cats compared with the twice daily immediate-release formulation.[22,23] Three small randomized, controlled, clinical trials have evaluated exenatide or exenatide ER in diabetic cats in combination with insulin and dietary therapy.[17,18,24] From these, the major effect of exenatide appears to be on body weight rather than glycemic control. Cats treated with exenatide either lost weight or did not gain weight compared with placebo, but there were no statistically significant differences in glycemic control or diabetic remission rate. These trials could have been underpowered to detect a difference. When treated with immediate-release exenatide, cats did have a lower median daily insulin requirement and exenatide ER lowered glycemic variability, which could reduce the risk for hypoglycemia.[17,25] Thus, despite its lack of impact on primary diabetic outcomes, exenatide may still have certain benefits for feline patients. Recently, two novel exenatide delivery systems have been developed for cats: a once-monthly, microsphere-based, subcutaneous injection and a subcutaneous implantable device that could last up to 6 months.[26,27] These systems could have the potential to enhance diabetic regulation while minimally impacting owner treatment burden, but they require further study.

Two other GLP-1 analogs have also been evaluated in small animals, both administered once daily. Liraglutide (Victoza, Novo Nordisk) is a GLP-1 analog with a fatty acid residue that increases plasma protein binding and extends duration of action.[28] In healthy cats, liraglutide increases insulin secretion and decreases body weight, but its effects have not been evaluated in diseased animals.[29] A single dose of liraglutide also showed glucose-lowering effects in a small cohort of diabetic dogs but multidose studies are needed.[14] Lixisenatide (Adlyxin, Sandofi), which is structurally related to exenatide, decreased glucose concentrations in a single-dose study in healthy dogs.[30,31]

Other GLP-1 analogs have not been evaluated in small animals but represent therapeutic possibilities. Dulaglutide (Trulicity, Lilly) and albiglutide (Tanzeum, GSK) are GLP-1 analogs linked to the immunoglobulin Fc portion and albumin, respectively. These fusion proteins greatly extend the duration of action and are administered as a once weekly subcutaneous injection in people.[32,33] Semaglutide is structurally related to liraglutide but with enhanced albumin binding and DPP-4 resistance. It is available as a once weekly subcutaneous injection (Ozempic, Novo Nordisk) and was recently approved as a once daily, oral tablet (Rybelsus, Novo Nordisk) making it the first oral GLP-1 analog on the market.[34,] Oral semaglutide is co-formulated with an absorption enhancer, which protects it from degradation and facilitates transport across the gastric mucosa. Despite having only 1% oral bioavailability, the enhancer combined with a higher dose and dosing frequency achieves therapeutic plasma semaglutide concentrations.[35] Oral delivery of peptide-based therapeutics is a major hurdle in drug development, so oral semaglutide represents quite the achievement and brings hope that similar strides can be made with other biologics, including insulin.

GLP-1 analogs have been commercially available in the United States for over 15 years and, through their use as antidiabetic agents, other health benefits have been discovered. GLP-1 analogs facilitate weight loss, and several have been approved for that indication in overweight, nondiabetic people.[36] Similar antiobesity effects have been documented for exenatide in cats with diabetes and may also be present for otherwise healthy, obese cats.[17,18,24] GLP-1 analogs improve cardiovascular and renal outcomes in people with T2DM and are considered a first-line therapy for diabetic patients with high risk for or established heart disease.[16] GLP-1 analogs are also documented to improve liver enzyme values and reduce hepatic fat accumulation in T2DM patients with nonalcoholic fatty liver disease.[38] These indications have not been evaluated in small animals but, if similar benefits exist, GLP-1 analogs could become an attractive therapeutic adjunct for feline diabetic patients with comorbidities.

Although GLP-1 analogs are the most widely used GLP-1-based therapy, others exist or are in development. DPP-4 inhibitors ("gliptins") are orally administered drugs that block the enzyme that degrades endogenous GLP-1, increasing its plasma concentrations and effect. Compared with GLP-1 analogs, DPP-4 inhibitors have less potent insulin-secreting and glucose-lowering effects, and they do not promote weight loss, likely because these drugs also increase glucose-dependent insulinotropic polypeptide (GIP), which promotes weight gain.[37] Several DPP-4 inhibitors have been evaluated in healthy cats and dogs, but none in clinical trials.[20,38,39–42] Given the current efficacy concerns for GLP-1 analogs in cats, a less potent incretin therapy seems unlikely to take hold in small animal medicine.

Although not yet an option for veterinary patients, bariatric surgery is a fascinating and highly effective therapy for T2DM in obese human patients due to decreased ghrelin secretion, increased nutrient delivery to the distal small intestine, and augmented incretin secretion.[43] A recent feasibility study showed that laparoscopic sleeve gastrectomy may be safe in cats, but efficacy has not yet been assessed.[44] Finally, non-peptide, small-molecule GLP-1 receptor agonists are currently in development. These compounds are intended to mimic the action of GLP-1 but have good bioavailability, allowing oral administration.[45] Whether such drugs will become a viable treatment option for veterinary diabetes remains to be seen.

SODIUM-GLUCOSE COTRANSPORTER TYPE 2 INHIBITORS

The sodium-glucose cotransporter type 2 (SGLT-2) inhibitors are the newest family of commercially available antidiabetic drugs. They exert their glucose-lowering effect by preventing glucose resorption in the proximal renal tubule, causing significant glucose elimination in the urine.[38] As such, this is the only family of antidiabetic drugs that exerts its glucose-lowering effect in an insulin-independent manner. SGLT-2 inhibitors are primarily used for treating human T2DM, alone or in combination; however, these drugs can also aid in the treatment of type 1 diabetes mellitus (T1DM), in insulin-dependent patients, when glycemic control is poor with insulin monotherapy.[38] SGLT-2 inhibitors currently approved by the United States Food and Drug Administration (FDA) include canagliflozin (Invokana, Janssen), dapagliflozin (Farxiga, AstraZenica), empagliflozin (Jardiance, Boehringer Ingelheim), and ertugloflozin (Steglatro, Merck). All are administered orally, once daily.

In addition to their effects on glycemic control, SGLT-2 inhibitors have significant health benefits for patients with cardiac and renal disease.[38] They facilitate both weight and blood pressure reduction in human patients. SLGT-2 inhibitors slow the progression of diabetic nephropathy by increasing distal tubule sodium delivery, normalizing glomerulotubular balance, and decreasing glomerular hyperfiltration. They also have a positive impact on cardiovascular outcomes. A variety of mechanisms likely contribute to this effect including increased diuresis and natriuresis, weight and blood pressure reduction, improved cardiac energy metabolism, and altered autonomic nervous outflow.[46] These benefits are supported by several, large, randomized controlled clinical trials, which have led to the recommendation that SGLT-2 inhibitors be used as first-line agents in T2DM human patients with heart failure or chronic kidney disease.[16]

Not much is known about SGLT-2 inhibitors in dogs beyond safety and pharmacokinetic/pharmacodynamic preclinical investigations.[47] However, both dapagliflozin and an investigational drug, velagliflozin, induce significant glucosuria without causing hypoglycemia in healthy cats.[48–51] Metabolic evaluation of these cats suggested that SGLT-2 inhibitors increase insulin sensitivity and fat metabolism, which could improve glycemic regulation in clinical patients.[48] To date, two studies have investigated SGLT-2 inhibitors in diabetic cats. A single-arm trial evaluated bexaglifloxin, which was recently approved for cats by the FDA, as an add-on therapy in 5 cats with poorly controlled DM. Mean blood glucose and insulin dose significantly decreased over 4 weeks of treatment and clinical signs were improved or resolved in all 5 cats.[52] A recent randomized, clinical trial compared once-daily oral velagliflozin to twice-daily insulin injection in diabetic cats (n = 13 per group). Cats in both groups showed similar improvement in clinical and biochemical outcomes.[53] Larger trials are needed, but these preliminary results are quite promising. The renal effects of SGLT-2 inhibitors in cats are also under investigation.[49] Whether or not diabetic nephropathy occurs in small animals is unclear but, regardless, chronic kidney disease is very common in elderly animals. If SGLT-2 inhibitors have renoprotective effects in feline DM, as they do in human DM, this could be an additional benefit for cats with comorbid chronic kidney disease.

An important consideration for the potential use of SGLT-2 inhibitors in cats and dogs is the adverse effect profile. Although multiple adverse effects have been attributed to these drugs, the ones supported by large clinical trials and meta-analyses in people are fungal genital infections and increased risk for diabetic ketoacidosis, the latter more commonly occurring in insulin-dependent patients.[38,54] SGLT-2 inhibitors also induce diuresis, which can lead to clinical polyuria. This is often transient, but some patients do require drug discontinuation.[38] If SGLT-2 inhibitors induce significant polyuria and polydipsia in diabetic animals, it may limit their therapeutic potential, particularly because resolution of clinical signs is a major indicator of diabetic regulation. Investigators disagree on whether SGLT-2 inhibitors induce polyuria and polydipsia in healthy cats.[48,50,51] The discordance may be explained by study differences in drug, drug dose, population characteristics, or other methodological disparities. Water consumption and urine output were not explicitly reported in the clinical diabetic cat studies, but polyuria and polydipsia were not reported as overt adverse effects.[52] In the second clinical trial, 8/13 cats treated with velagliflozin developed soft stools, half of which resolved without intervention.[53] Thus, gastrointestinal signs may be an important adverse effect of SGLT-2 inhibitors in this species, potentially due to off-target inhibition of the SGLT-1 isoform expressed in the intestines. Larger studies are needed to evaluate these and other potential adverse effects of SGLT-2 inhibitors in cats and dogs.

NON-INJECTABLE INSULINS

The need for frequent injections significantly and negatively impacts the quality of life for both people with DM and owners of diabetic pets.[55–57] Therefore, administering insulin by alternate routes is an active area of research. Currently, the only FDA-approved, non-injectable insulin product is Afrezza (MannKind Corp.). Afrezza is an inhalable, ultra-rapid-acting, recombinant human regular insulin.[58] Following administration with an inhaler, Afrezza passes through the thin alveolar lining and is rapidly absorbed through pulmonary circulation. By this mechanism, it quickly reaches peak effect, comparable to injectable ultra-rapid-acting insulin analogs.[58] Afrezza is a prandial insulin and, in people, must be paired with a long- or ultra-long-acting insulin to achieve glycemic control throughout the day, similar to a basal-bolus protocol. Such a protocol might be feasible for some veterinary patients and insulin is absorbed by the inhaled route, at least in cats.[59] However, the Afrezza inhaler device does not contain an actuator and functions solely on passive inhalation, so cannot be used with spacers that allow traditional inhalers to be adapted for veterinary patients (eg,

AeroKat, Trudell Animal Health); thus, a new device would need to be developed. Alternately, if an inhaled, long-acting insulin preparation were developed, it might be useful for small animals, but this seems unlikely given that the major benefit of inhaled systemic medications is their rapid absorption and onset of action. Buccally administered, rapid-acting, prandial insulins have also been developed, although are not commercially available in the United States.[60]

Oral insulin has been called the "holy grail" of diabetic therapies and, although hurdles still exist, the possibility seems closer than ever before. Two major barriers exist to insulin administration via the oral route. First, insulin is a polypeptide susceptible to degradation by gastric acid and digestive enzymes. Second, insulin is much larger than typical non-peptide drugs and so is relatively impermeant through mucosal surfaces. Strategies to overcome these barriers include co-formulation with enzyme inhibitors and/or absorption enhancers, which target the tight junctions of the intestinal epithelium to facilitate paracellular drug uptake. Microsphere and nanocapsule technologies have also been used to protect insulin molecules from degradation in the gastrointestinal tract.[60] An important consideration is that, despite these approaches, oral insulin bioavailability is currently very low compared with parenteral insulin, which increases dose requirements and cost. For example, OI338 (NovoNordisk) was a once-daily, long-acting oral insulin that showed glucose-lowering effects and low risk of hypoglycemia, comparable to insulin glargine in human phase 2 clinical trials. However, this product was subsequently reformulated into an injectable form and is in phase 3 clinical trials (see insulin icodec above), possibly because effective oral doses were too high.[9,61] Thus, if oral insulin formulations do come to market, cost could be an impediment to veterinary use. Another oral insulin, ORMD-0801 (Oramed Ltd) is currently in phase 3 clinical trials and similar technologies have successfully facilitated oral absorption of GLP-1 analogs in dogs.[62,63] However, whether oral insulin will be a viable option for dogs and cats remains to be seen.

CONTINUOUS INSULIN INFUSION

Insulin infusion pumps are commonly used in human diabetic patients, particularly those with T1DM. These devices contain a reservoir of rapid- or ultra-rapid-acting insulin that is administered at an adjustable rate and through a subcutaneous cannula, either connected by an infusion line or with the pump attached directly to the body. A basal infusion rate is set to deliver insulin throughout the day and intermittent boluses can be administered through the same infusion set at mealtimes. When used correctly, these devices eliminate the need for multiple daily insulin injections. In addition, the basal rate can be adjusted as needed, allowing improved glycemic control and decreasing the risk for hypoglycemia.[64] Insulin pumps have been available since the 1980s but have not been adopted by veterinarians because the pump and infusion set are too cumbersome for a dog or cat to wear without risking disconnection. Infusion sets require frequent changing and rotation of sites on the body to prevent the development of fibrotic tissue, which could block insulin absorption at the insertion site.[65] Species differences in skin thickness and composition might further complicate the adaptation of insulin pumps for dogs and cats. However, because infusions sets come with varying insertion cannula lengths and angles, and made of either steel or soft Teflon, it is possible that an infusion set could be found that would work well for a given veterinary patient.

Newer options for continuous insulin administration are the insulin patches and pods (eg, OmniPod, Insulet Corp.). These devices are similar to insulin pumps but have a smaller profile and the reservoir attaches directly to the skin with an adhesive, eliminating the need for an infusion line. They can also deliver insulin at very low rates, which might be beneficial for very small patients that could not otherwise benefit from insulin infusions. Given these features, insulin patches and pods seem a viable strategy for small animals; however, tampering with the device (eg, chewing, rubbing) could cause inadvertent insulin boluses and hypoglycemia, so safety should be carefully evaluated before adaptation for veterinary use.

SMART INSULIN

"Smart" insulin is a broadly applied term but generally refers to therapies in which a technology regulates insulin release or effect.[66] Currently available smart technologies include smart insulin pens, smart pen caps, and open- and closed-loop systems. Smart insulin pens are pens with an electronic component built-in, whereas pen caps are electronically-enabled devices that can be added onto a standard insulin pen. Features include tracking dose amount and dose timing as well as measuring remaining insulin in the pen. These devices help reduce missed doses and could be readily applied in veterinary medicine to improve owner compliance.[67] Some insulin pens also integrate with continuous glucose monitors (CGMs) to suggest dose adjustments. These systems would require a close evaluation and probable modification for canine and feline diabetics because the algorithms that derive the dose recommendations are specific to human physiology.

The integrated smart pen is an example of an open-loop system in which a CGM tracks glucose concentrations and calculates a new insulin dose, which the patient then administers.[67] Continuous insulin infusion pumps are also commonly integrated into open-loop systems, in which the operator manually adjusts the infusion rate based on CGM recommendations. The next advancement in smart insulin technologies is the closed-loop system in which a CGM communicates directly with the insulin pump to adjust the infusion rate. The basal rate is adjusted automatically based on measurements from the CGM, and prandial insulin doses are calculated by the pump based on user input of carbohydrate amounts consumed in a given meal. Fully automated, closed-loop systems (ie, the artificial pancreas) that do not require direct user input are in development. However, accurately delivering prandial insulin is more complicated than basal insulin because it requires predicting blood glucose based on interstitial glucose concentrations and accounting for the time to onset of subcutaneously administered insulin.[68] A fascinating innovation in this technology is the bi-hormonal system, which delivers both insulin and glucagon in response to CGM measurements. In experimental trials, these devices reduce the incidence of hypoglycemia, particularly during exercise or sleep.[69,70] Closed-loop systems compound the translational concerns of dosing algorithms and infusion pumps for use in cats and dogs. However, if these hurdles are overcome, such systems may become a treatment option, especially for clients interested in intensive diabetic management.

A highly innovative strategy in smart insulin technology is the development of glucose-responsive insulin formulations, which intrinsically sense glucose concentrations and alter the release or action of insulin.[71] In the matrix-based approach, insulin molecules are embedded in a resin or polymer, usually administered as a subcutaneous depot or transdermal patch. The matrix has glucose-responsive chemicals or enzymes that release insulin proportionately to the glucose concentration in the surrounding milieu. In the molecular approach, the insulin molecule itself contains a glucose-responsive element. Some compounds change their pharmacokinetics based on blood glucose concentrations, particularly by altering plasma protein binding or by changing drug clearance. Others smart analogs undergo a conformational change to expose the insulin receptor binding site in the presence of hyperglycemia. These technologies are still in their infancy and their commercial viability is untested. However, if they do eventually come to market, they could be an attractive "smart" option for dogs and cats because they eliminate the need for external devices.

BETA CELL REPLACEMENT THERAPY

Standard therapy for T1DM assumes that, once beta cell mass is gone, it cannot be replaced, and exogenous insulin must be supplemented life-long. In contrast, beta cell replacement therapy attempts to restore endogenous insulin secretion. Transplanted beta cells can sense glucose and respond appropriately, sometimes in concert with other secretory islet cells, leading to tighter and more natural glycemic regulation. Practical considerations and complications have thus far limited widespread beta cell replacement therapy in human diabetic patients, let alone veterinary species.

Traditional beta cell replacement involves transplantation of either whole pancreas or isolated pancreatic islets from an organ donor. Preclinical canine models played a large role in the development of these procedures so translation to clinical diabetic dogs is biologically feasible.[72] In human patients, insulin-independence rates are as high as 60% to 80% at 10 years post-transplantation. However, serious complications can occur including technical failures and acute rejection.[73] Immunosuppression is generally required to prevent transplant rejection, which increases the risk for opportunistic infections, although novel techniques are in development that may reduce or eliminate this requirement.[74] Donor sourcing would also be a particular problem for small animal patients because, although cadaveric isolation techniques have been developed for dogs, the large infrastructure for human transplantation does not exist in veterinary medicine.[72]

Future beta cell replacement therapies likely revolve around cellular techniques. Both mesenchymal and induced pluripotent stem cells can be differentiated into beta-cell-like cells in culture.[75] Once again, dogs feature prominently in preclinical development for potential therapies. If these new approaches are clinically successful in human medicine, they have the possibility to be translated to small animal diabetic patients in the future.

SUMMARY

Many novel diabetic therapies are available for human use or are in development that could be applied to veterinary patients with DM. Some, like the smart insulin pens and pen caps, could be directly applied in small animal practice today. Others, including ultra-long-acting insulins, novel GLP-1 analogs, and SGLT-2 inhibitors, could be promising but require further study in veterinary species. Finally, others, such as closed-loop insulin delivery systems and beta cell replacement therapy, are very alluring because of the tight glycemic control and hands-off approach they could potentially offer. However, the implementation of such therapies in dogs and cats would represent a major paradigm shift in the veterinary approach to DM management. Novel diabetic treatments represent an active and rapidly evolving area of research; veterinarians should continue to stay apprised of emerging therapies.

CLINICS CARE POINTS

- DM therapies are a rapidly evolving area of the pharmaceutical industry and veterinarians should be aware of advancements.
- When evaluating a new potential therapy, veterinarians should pay close attention to the quality of evidence supporting its use.
- Ideally, substantial evidence should exist in the target species to support the clinical use a novel DM therapy in a veterinary patient.

DISCLOSURE

The authors have no relevant commercial or financial conflicts of interest to disclose. Dr J.M. Reinhart is currently receiving funding from the University of Illinois, United States, College of Veterinary Medicine, Companion Animal Research Grant Program, which is not in conflict with the topic of this article.

REFERENCES

1. Semlitsch T, Engler J, Siebenhofer A, et al. Ultra-)long-acting insulin analogues versus NPH insulin (human isophane insulin) for adults with type 2 diabetes mellitus. Cochrane Database Syst Rev 2020;(11):CD005613.
2. Jackson B, Grubbs L. Basal-bolus insulin therapy and glycemic control in adult patients with type 2 diabetes mellitus: a review of the literature. J Am Assoc Nurse Pract 2014;26:348–52.
3. Toujeo. Package insert. Sandofi-Aventis U.S. LLC; 2015.
4. Oda H, Mori A, Ishii S, et al. Time-action profiles of insulin degludec in healthy dogs and its effects on glycemic control in diabetic dogs. J Vet Med Sci 2018; 80:1720–3.
5. Salesov E, Zini E, Riederer A, et al. Comparison of the pharmacodynamics of protamine zinc insulin and insulin degludec and validation of the continuous glucose monitoring system iPro2 in healthy cats. Res Vet Sci 2018;118:79–85.
6. Miller M, Pires J, Crakes K, et al. Day-to-day variability of porcine lente, insulin glargine 300 U/mL and insulin degludec in diabetic dogs. J Vet Intern Med 2021;35:2131–9.
7. Saini NK, Wasik B, Pires J, et al. Comparison of pharmacodynamics between insulin glargine 100 U/mL and insulin glargine 300 U/mL in healthy cats. Domest Anim Endocrinol 2021;75:106595.
8. Nishimura E, Pridal L, Glendorf T, et al. Molecular and pharmacological characterization of insulin icodec: a new basal insulin analog designed for once-weekly dosing. BMJ Open Diabetes Res Care 2021;9:e002301.
9. Kjeldsen TB, Hubalek F, Hjorringgaard CU, et al. Molecular engineering of insulin icodec, the first acylated insulin analog for once-weekly administration in humans. J Med Chem 2021;64:8942–50.
10. Wronkowitz N, Hartmann T, Gorgens SW, et al. (LAPS) Insulin115: a novel ultra-long-acting basal insulin with a unique action profile. Diabetes Obes Metab 2017;19:1722–31.
11. Gilor C, Hulsebosch SE, Pires J, et al. An ultra-long-acting recombinant insulin for the treatment of diabetes mellitus in cats. J Vet Intern Med 2021;35:2123–30.

12. Hulsebosch SE, Pires J, Bannasch MJ, et al. Ultra-long-acting recombinant insulin for the treatment of diabetes mellitus in dogs. J Vet Intern Med 2022;36:1211–9.

13. Gilor C, Rudinsky AJ, Hall MJ. New approaches to feline diabetes mellitus: glucagon-like peptide-1 analogs. J Feline Med Surg 2016;18:733–43.

14. Oda H, Mori A, Lee P, et al. Characterization of the use of liraglutide for glycemic control in healthy and Type 1 diabetes mellitus suffering dogs. Res Vet Sci 2013;95:381–8.

15. Lee YS, Jun HS. Anti-diabetic actions of glucagon-like peptide-1 on pancreatic beta-cells. Metabolism 2014;63:9–19.

16. American Diabetes Association. Standards of medical care in diabetes-2022 abridged for primary care providers. Clin Diabetes 2022;40:10–38.

17. Riederer A, Zini E, Salesov E, et al. Effect of the glucagon-like peptide-1 analogue exenatide extended release in cats with newly diagnosed diabetes mellitus. J Vet Intern Med 2016;30:92–100.

18. Scuderi MA, Ribeiro Petito M, Unniappan S, et al. Safety and efficacy assessment of a GLP-1 mimetic: insulin glargine combination for treatment of feline diabetes mellitus. Domest Anim Endocrinol 2018;65:80–9.

19. Gilor C, Graves TK, Gilor S, et al. The GLP-1 mimetic exenatide potentiates insulin secretion in healthy cats. Domest Anim Endocrinol 2011;41(1):42–9.

20. Padrutt I, Lutz TA, Reusch CE, et al. Effects of the glucagon-like peptide-1 (GLP-1) analogues exenatide, exenatide extended-release, and of the dipeptidylpeptidase-4 (DPP-4) inhibitor sitagliptin on glucose metabolism in healthy cats. Res Vet Sci 2015;99:23–9.

21. Seyfert TM, Brunker JD, Maxwell LK, et al. Effects of a glucagon-like peptide-1 mimetic (exenatide) in healthy cats. Intern J Appl Res Vet Med 2012;10:147–56.

22. Blevins T, Pullman J, Malloy J, et al. DURATION-5: exenatide once weekly resulted in greater improvements in glycemic control compared with exenatide twice daily in patients with type 2 diabetes. J Clin Endocrinol Metab 2011;96:1301–10.

23. Rudinsky AJ, Adin CA, Borin-Crivellenti S, et al. Pharmacology of the glucagon-like peptide-1 analog exenatide extended-release in healthy cats. Domest Anim Endocrinol 2015;51:78–85.

24. Hazuchova K, Gostelow RF, Scudder CJ, et al. Effect of monthly injections of GLP-1 analogue exenatide extended release on beta-cell function in newly diagnosed diabetic cats. J Vet Intern Med 2019;33:1042–3. Abstract.

25. Kramer AL, Riederer A, Fracassi F, et al. Glycemic variability in newly diagnosed diabetic cats treated with the glucagon-like peptide-1 analogue exenatide extended release. J Vet Intern Med 2020;34:2287–95.

26. Schneider EL, Reid R, Parkes DG, et al. A once-monthly GLP-1 receptor agonist for treatment of diabetic cats. Domest Anim Endocrinol 2020;70:106373.

27. Gilor C, Klotsman M, Adin C, et al. Safety and tolerability of OKV-119: a novel exenatide long-term drug-delivery-system in cats. J Vet Intern Med 2021;35:3026. Abstract.

28. Knudsen LB, Lau J. The discovery and development of liraglutide and semaglutide. Front Endocrinol 2019;10:155.

29. Hall MJ, Adin CA, Borin-Crivellenti S, et al. Pharmacokinetics and pharmacodynamics of the glucagon-like peptide-1 analog liraglutide in healthy cats. Domest Anim Endocrinol 2015;51:114–21.

30. Werner U, Haschke G, Herling AW, et al. Pharmacological profile of lixisenatide: a new GLP-1 receptor agonist for the treatment of type 2 diabetes. Regul Pept 2010;164:58–64.

31. Moore MC, Werner U, Smith MS, et al. Effect of the glucagon-like peptide-1 receptor agonist lixisenatide on postprandial hepatic glucose metabolism in the conscious dog. Am J Physiol Endocrinol Metab 2013;305:E1473–82.

32. Umpierrez G, Tofe Povedano S, Perez Manghi F, et al. Efficacy and safety of dulaglutide monotherapy versus metformin in type 2 diabetes in a randomized controlled trial (AWARD-3). Diabetes Care 2014;37:2168–76.

33. Pratley RE, Nauck MA, Barnett AH, et al. Once-weekly albiglutide versus once-daily liraglutide in patients with type 2 diabetes inadequately controlled on oral drugs (HARMONY 7): a randomised, open-label, multicentre, non-inferiority phase 3 study. Lancet Diabetes Endocrinol 2014;2:289–97.

34. Rosenstock J, Allison D, Birkenfeld AL, et al. Effect of additional oral semaglutide vs sitagliptin on glycated hemoglobin in adults with type 2 diabetes uncontrolled with metformin alone or with sulfonylurea: the PIONEER 3 randomized clinical trial. J Am Med Assoc 2019;321:1466–80.

35. Rybelsus. Package insert. Novo Nordisk Inc.; 2019.

36. Yin R, Xu Y, Wang X, et al. Role of dipeptidyl peptidase 4 inhibitors in antidiabetic treatment. Molecules 2022;27:3055.

37. Edgerton DS, Johnson KM, Neal DW, et al. Inhibition of dipeptidyl peptidase-4 by vildagliptin during glucagon-like peptide 1 infusion increases liver glucose uptake in the conscious dog. Diabetes 2009;58:243–9.

38. Brown E, Heerspink HJL, Cuthbertson DJ, et al. SGLT2 inhibitors and GLP-1 receptor agonists: established and emerging indications. Lancet 2021;398:262–76.

39. Furrer D, Kaufmann K, Tschuor F, et al. The dipeptidyl peptidase IV inhibitor NVP-DPP728 reduces plasma glucagon concentration in cats. Vet J 2010;183:355–7.

40. Lee B, Shi L, Kassel DB, et al. Pharmacokinetic, pharmacodynamic, and efficacy profiles of alogliptin, a novel inhibitor of dipeptidyl peptidase-4, in rats, dogs, and monkeys. Eur J Pharmacol 2008;589:306–14.

41. Mori A, Ueda K, Lee P, et al. Effect of acarbose, sitagliptin and combination therapy on blood glucose, insulin, and incretin hormone concentrations in experimentally induced postprandial hyperglycemia of healthy cats. Res Vet Sci 2016;106:131–4.

42. Oda H, Mori A, Lee P, et al. Preliminary study characterizing the use of sitagliptin for glycemic control in healthy Beagle dogs with normal gluco-homeostasis. J Vet Med Sci 2014;76(10):1383–7.

43. McTigue KM, Wellman R, Nauman E, et al. Comparing the 5-Year diabetes outcomes of sleeve gastrectomy and gastric bypass: the national patient-centered clinical research network (PCORNet) Bariatric Study. JAMA Surg 2020;155:e200087.

44. Buote NJ, Porter I, Loftus J, et al. Laparoscopic vertical sleeve gastrectomy in felines: a cadaveric feasibility study and experimental case series in two cats. Vet Surg 2022. https://doi.org/10.1111/vsu.13862.

45. Nauck MA, Wefers J, Meier JJ. Treatment of type 2 diabetes: challenges, hopes, and anticipated successes. Lancet Diabetes Endocrinol 2021;9:525–44.

46. Lopaschuk GD, Verma S. Mechanisms of cardiovascular benefits of sodium glucose co-transporter 2 (SGLT2) inhibitors: a state-of-the-art review. JACC Basic Transl Sci 2020;5:632–44.

47. Mamidi RN, Cuyckens F, Chen J, et al. Metabolism and excretion of canagliflozin in mice, rats, dogs, and humans. Drug Metab Dispos 2014;42:903–16.

48. Hoenig M, Clark M, Schaeffer DJ, et al. Effects of the sodium-glucose cotransporter 2 (SGLT2) inhibitor velagliflozin, a new drug with therapeutic potential to treat diabetes in cats. J Vet Pharmacol Ther 2018;41:266–73.

49. Gal A, Burton SE, Weidgraaf K, et al. The effect of the sodium-glucose cotransporter type-2 inhibitor dapagliflozin on glomerular filtration rate in healthy cats. Domest Anim Endocrinol 2020;70:106376.

50. Burchell RK, Preet S, Weidgraaf K, et al. Salt and sugar in your larder make your kidneys work harder. J Vet Intern Med 2019;33:1096. Abstract.

51. Gal A, Burton SE, Weidgraaf K, et al. Isolated renal glycosuria does not lead to polyuria in a feline model. J Vet Intern Med 2018;32:2224–5. Abstract.

52. Benedict SL, Mahony OM, McKee TS, et al. Evaluation of bexagliflozin in cats with poorly regulated diabetes mellitus. Can J Vet Res 2022;86:52–8.

53. Niessen SJM, Voth R, Kroh C, et al. Once-daily oral therapy for feline diabetes mellitus: SGLT-2-inhibitor velagliflozin as standalone therapy compared to insulin injection therapy in diabetic cats September 2022;1-3.

54. Li D, Wang T, Shen S, et al. Urinary tract and genital infections in patients with type 2 diabetes treated with sodium-glucose co-transporter 2 inhibitors: A meta-analysis of randomized controlled trials. Diabetes Obes Metab 2017;19:348–55.

55. E Quality1 Study Group. Quality of life and treatment satisfaction in adults with type 1 diabetes: a comparison between continuous subcutaneous insulin infusion and multiple daily injections. Diabet Med 2008;25:213–20.

56. Niessen SJ, Powney S, Guitian J, et al. Evaluation of a quality-of-life tool for cats with diabetes mellitus. J Vet Intern Med 2010;24:1098–105.

57. Niessen SJM, Powney S, Guitian J, et al. Evaluation of a quality-of-life tool for dogs with diabetes mellitus. J Vet Intern Med 2012;26:953–61.

58. Afrezza. Package insert. MannKind Corporation; 2014.

59. DeClue AE, Leverenz EF, Wiedmeyer CE, et al. Glucose lowering effects of inhaled insulin in healthy cats. J Feline Med Surg 2008;10:519–22.

60. El Maalouf IR, Capoccia K, Priefer R. Non-invasive ways of administering insulin. Diabetes Metab Syndr 2022;16:102478.

61. Halberg IB, Lyby K, Wassermann K, et al. Efficacy and safety of oral basal insulin versus subcutaneous insulin glargine in type 2 diabetes: a randomised, double-blind, phase 2 trial. Lancet Diabetes Endocrinol 2019;7:179–88.

62. Eldor R, Neutel J, Homer K, et al. Efficacy and safety of 28-day treatment with oral insulin (ORMD-0801) in patients with type 2 diabetes: a randomized, placebo-controlled trial. Diabetes Obes Metab 2021;23:2529–38.

63. Eldor R, Kidron M, Greenberg-Shushlav Y, et al. Novel glucagon-like peptide-1 analog delivered orally reduces postprandial glucose excursions in porcine and canine models. J Diabetes Sci Technol 2010;4:1516–23.

64. Jiao X, Shen Y, Chen Y, et al. HbA1c, and less hypoglycemia in closed-loop insulin system in patients with type 1 diabetes: a meta-analysis. BMJ Open Diabetes Res Care 2022;10:e002633.

65. Zhang E, Cao Z. Tissue Response to subcutaneous infusion catheter. J Diabetes Sci Technol 2020;14:226–32.

66. Jarosinski MA, Dhayalan B, Rege N, et al. Smart' insulin-delivery technologies and intrinsic glucose-responsive insulin analogues. Diabetologia 2021;64:1016–29.

67. Masierek M, Nabrdalik K, Janota O, et al. The review of insulin pens-past, present, and look to the future. Front Endocrinol 2022;13:827484.

68. Domingo-Lopez DA, Lattanzi G, Schreiber LHJ, et al. Medical devices, smart drug delivery, wearables and technology for the treatment of diabetes mellitus. Adv Drug Deliv Rev 2022;185:114280.

69. Haidar A, Legault L, Messier V, et al. Comparison of dual-hormone artificial pancreas, single-hormone artificial pancreas, and conventional insulin pump therapy for glycaemic control in patients with type 1 diabetes: an open-label randomised controlled crossover trial. Lancet Diabetes Endocrinol 2015;3:17–26.

70. Taleb N, Emami A, Suppere C, et al. Efficacy of single-hormone and dual-hormone artificial pancreas during continuous and interval exercise in adult patients with type 1 diabetes: randomised controlled crossover trial. Diabetologia 2016;59:2561–71.

71. Jarosinski MA, Chen YS, Varas N, et al. New horizons: next-generation insulin analogues: structural principles and clinical goals. J Clin Endocrinol Metab 2022; 107:909–28.

72. Harrington S, Williams SJ, Otte V, et al. Improved yield of canine islet isolation from deceased donors. BMC Vet Res 2017;13:264.

73. Moshref M, Tangey B, Gilor C, et al. Concise review: canine diabetes mellitus as a translational model for innovative regenerative medicine approaches. Stem Cells Transl Med 2019;8:450–5.

74. Harrington S, Karanu F, Ramachandran K, et al. PEGDA microencapsulated allogeneic islets reverse canine diabetes without immunosuppression. PLoS One 2022;17:e0267814.

75. Wan XX, Zhang DY, Khan MA, et al. Stem cell transplantation in the treatment of type 1 diabetes mellitus: from insulin replacement to beta-cell replacement. Front Endocrinol 2022;13:859638.

Hypersomatotropism and Other Causes of Insulin Resistance in Cats

Stijn J.M. Niessen, DVM, PhD, DECVIM, PGCertVetEd, FHEA, MRCVS[a,b,*]

KEYWORDS

- Hypersomatotropism • Hypercortisolism • Diabetes mellitus • Insulin resistance

KEY POINTS

- Hypersomatotropism is the leading cause of clinically relevant insulin-resistant diabetes mellitus in the cat.
- Hypersomatotropism does not always lead to diabetes mellitus, or to difficult-to-control diabetes mellitus.
- Serum IGF-1 is an effective screening test for hypersomatotropism in the diabetic cat, but false-negative results occur in 10% of cases.
- Hypercortisolism is a seemingly less common yet still relevant cause of insulin resistance and diabetes mellitus in the cat.
- There are currently various treatment options for both hypersomatotropism and hypercortisolism; both surgical and medical options are effective.

INTRODUCTION

The project ALIVE (Agreeing Language in Veterinary Endocrinology) recommendation is to use the term "insulin resistance" to describe the presence of varying degrees of interference of insulin action on target cells. The recommendation further specifies that the term is not defined by the exogenous insulin dose required or by the change of blood glucose following insulin injection. However, when there is concern over the need for a high insulin dose, the presence of insulin resistance should be considered among other potential causes.[1,2]

Overall, the treatment of diabetes mellitus (DM) in the cat is often rewarding, with relatively high owner acceptance of the need for insulin injections and subsequent fast resolution of the DM-associated clinical signs.[1,3,4] Some diabetic cats can even enter a state of diabetic remission.[5] In most diabetic cats, however, clinical control

[a] Royal Veterinary College London, UK; [b] Veterinary Specialist Consultations and VIN Europe, Loosdrechtseweg 56, Hilversum 1215 JX, the Netherlands
* Veterinary Specialist Consultations and VIN Europe, Loosdrechtseweg 56, Hilversum 1215 JX, the Netherlands.
E-mail address: info@veterinaryspecialistconsultations.com

Vet Clin Small Anim 53 (2023) 691–710
https://doi.org/10.1016/j.cvsm.2023.02.005
0195-5616/23/© 2023 Elsevier Inc. All rights reserved.

Table 1
Table depicting the clinical signs displayed by diabetic cats with confirmed hypersomatotropism, compared with a group of cats with primary diabetes mellitus (non-acromegalic)

Clinical Sign	Prevalence in Cats with Hypersomatotropism-Induced Diabetes Mellitus	Prevalence in Cats with Primary Diabetes Mellitus
Polyuria	87%	75%
Polydipsia	87%	85%
Polyphagia	75%, of which extreme: 20%	55%, of which extreme: 0%
Weight loss	42%	60%
Weight gain	17%	0%
Respiratory stridor/"snoring"	38%	10%
CNS signs (excluding lethargy)	1.7%	0%
Lethargy	25%	35%
Stiffness/mobility problems	10%	10%
Abdominal organomegaly (renomegaly and/or hepatomegaly)	40%	25%
Prognathia inferior	18%	10%
Clubbed paw appearance	13%	0%
Broad facial features	37%	0%
Heart murmur	18%	20%
Plantegrade stance	3%	10%

Case 1: Laboratory and Clinical Data of a Diabetic Cat (11-Year-Old MN DSH) with Rising IGF-1; Month 0 Depicts the Initial Presentation and Start of the Exogenous Insulin Treatment. Screening at the Start of Treatment Did Not Exclude Presence of Hypersomatotropism

	Fructosamine (μmol/L)	Exogenous Insulin Dose	Body Weight (kg)	Serum IGF-1 (ng/mL)
Month 0	680	1	3.95	212
Month 1	654	4	3.95	505
Month 2	575	5	4.5	1143

Abbreviation: CNS, central nervous system.
Adapted from Niessen et al.[6]

appears challenging to achieve. Broadly, 4 categories (**Box 1**) could be used to summarize the causes of poor control in these cats. If clinical signs are present despite effective appropriate insulin treatment, clinicians should be on alert for the presence of other diseases that share some of the same clinical signs of DM (eg, polyuria/polydipsia and weight loss with chronic kidney disease and hyperthyroidism, polyphagia with gastrointestinal disease [although inappetence is more common], hyperthyroidism, and hypersomatotropism). If frequent hypoglycemia occurs or periods of good response to insulin are intermixed with periods of poor response, insulin administration technique including type of syringe used (eg, U-40 versus U-100) should be revisited, glucose targets might need to be broadened, remission might be on the horizon, or variable appetite (eg, due to pancreatitis) or gastrointestinal absorption could be the culprit. **Box 2** summarizes the broad categories of factors leading to difficulty in regulating a diabetic cat. This article focuses on "lack of glucose response to insulin" (see **Box 1**) and "cat-associated factors" (see **Box 2**), which can be considered true forms of insulin resistance and therefore should be differentiated from pseudo-insulin resistance (eg, short duration of insulin action, incorrect handling or administration of insulin).

LACK OF GLUCOSE RESPONSE TO INSULIN-TRUE INSULIN RESISTANCE

The most prevalent causes of cat-associated insulin resistance are listed in **Box 3**. It should be pointed out that a host of causes of insulin resistance are presented in this box as well as traditionally in textbooks covering this topic. However, for most of these causes, clinically overt lack of glucose-lowering effect of high-dose exogenous insulin is rare, except for hypersomatotropism (HST), hypercortisolism (HC) (iatrogenic or spontaneous), or, rarely, obesity. All other frequently cited causes are associated with varying degrees of impact on insulin sensitivity, although rarely are they associated with the need to administer more than 1.5 U of insulin per kg body weight on a twice daily basis; as highlighted by the ALIVE definition, insulin resistance is not defined by the exogenous insulin dose required or by the change of blood glucose following insulin injection.[2] The remainder of this article focuses on the most prevalent and important causes of insulin resistance in the cat: HST and HC.

HYPERSOMATOTROPISM

Acromegaly is the clinical syndrome that results from growth hormone (GH) excess. The term HST is preferred, because it does not make assumptions about qualitative and quantitative consequences of GH excess; this is important because recent research has shown that, as in people, GH excess in cats develops months to years before the appearance of external acromegalic features. During that seemingly latent period, DM secondary to GH excess often ensues.

Key general features of HST are summarized in **Box 4**.

Box 1
Management problems in diabetes mellitus

Categories of problems in cats suffering from diabetes mellitus that is difficult to regulate
- Clinical signs despite appropriate insulin treatment
- Lack of glucose response to insulin treatment (insulin resistance)
- Frequent hypoglycemia
- Periods of good control intermixed with periods of poor control

---

Box 2
Factors involved in problem diabetes mellitus

A systematic approach to the insulin-resistant diabetic: assessment of factors associated with the 3 main protagonists involved in diabetes management
- Owner-associated factors
- Veterinarian-associated factors
- Cat-associated factors

PREVALENCE AND CAUSE

Historically, HST was thought to be a rare condition. However, when preconceived ideas about its presentation (eg, all cats suffering from acromegaly have broad facial features and insulin-resistant DM) were set aside, screening studies showed a different picture (**Box 5**). The largest screening study to date evaluated 1221 diabetic cats[6]; 319 (26.1%) demonstrated a serum insulin-like growth factor-1 (IGF-1) greater than 1000 ng/mL (95% confidence interval: 23.6%–28.6%). Of these 319 cats, 63 (20%) underwent pituitary imaging and/or necropsy. Of the 63, 60 cats (95%) had a pituitary mass identified on computed tomography (CT) (56 cats), magnetic resonance imaging (MRI) (3 cats), or necropsy (1 cat). These data suggest a positive predictive value (PPV) of 95% (95% confidence interval: 90%–100%) when serum IGF-1 concentrations are used for screening of HST. However, the true PPV is probably

---

Box 3
Cat-associated conditions frequently linked with decreased insulin sensitivity; italicized are conditions most frequently associated with clinically detectable insulin resistance.

1. Infection
   a. Urinary tract infection
   b. Dental infections
2. Inflammation
   a. Pancreatitis
   b. Inflammatory bowel disease
   c. Gingivostomatitis
   d. *Obesity*
3. Medication
   a. *Corticosteroids (including topical medications)*
   b. *Megestrol acetate*
4. Other hormonal disturbances
   a. Hyperthyroidism
5. Misdiagnosis of the type of diabetes mellitus
   a. *Hypersomatotropism-induced diabetes mellitus (acromegaly)*
   b. *Hyperadrenocorticism-induced diabetes mellitus (Cushing syndrome)*
   c. Pancreatic destruction (eg, neoplasia, abscess, pancreatitis)
6. Other diseases (through known and unknown mechanisms)
   a. Cardiac disease
   b. CKD
   c. Neoplasia
   d. *Obesity (also through inflammation)*

Abbreviations: CKD, chronic kidney disease; IBD, inflammatory bowel disease.

Box 4
Definitions and relevance

1. Hypersomatotropism and acromegaly are related yet different terms

2. Hypersomatotropism is the excess of growth hormone production

3. Acromegaly refers to detectable physical changes and metabolic consequences that occur secondary to GH excess

4. Hypersomatotropism/acromegaly is increasingly being detected among diabetic and nondiabetic cats

5. Hypersomatotropism/acromegaly is the most likely differential diagnosis in the truly insulin-resistant cat

---

higher, because the gold standard in that study was a demonstrable structural pituitary abnormality, whereas it is now known that a CT or MRI can prove false-negative. Regardless, these data suggest that about 25% of diabetic cats in the United Kingdom have HST. However, most cats that were diagnosed with HST in that study did not have the phenotypical acromegaly signs, resulting in only 24% of clinicians indicating a strong pretest suspicion of HST in cases that were confirmed as HST.[6] When similar studies were conducted in the United States, the Netherlands, and Switzerland, a similar prevalence was noted, with approximately 1 in 5 diabetic cats being diagnosed with HST.[7,8] It is also becoming increasingly clear that not all cats have a pituitary acidophil adenoma, with pituitary acidophil hyperplasia being equally commonly.[9] Furthermore, although it is commonly assumed that the DM is more difficult to control in cats with HST than without, this might not be the case in the early phase of HST-associated DM. HST-associated DM can initially undergo remission or be associated with modest insulin requirement, suggesting robust beta cells in these cases, unlike the beta cells in regular DM cases. In addition, a growing number of cats with HST but without DM are being discovered.[10,11]

Further studies regarding the possible cause of somatotroph hyperplasia in cats are warranted such as studies on the ability to transform into a somatotroph adenoma, determination of inhibitory receptor expression, investigation of germline mutations, and the possible association of HST with exposure to endocrine-disrupting chemicals.[12,13]

CLINICAL PRESENTATION

Cats suffering from HST can be of any breed and sex, although they tend to be middle aged and older (**Table 1**). Cats seem to be able to tolerate even large pituitary masses

---

Box 5
Prevalence of hypersomatotropism

1. Prevalence seems the highest among diabetic cats

2. Estimates among diabetic cats range from 1 in 3 to 1 in 5

3. Estimates among non-diabetic cats with HCM-like phenotype currently range from 1 in 20

4. Other non-diabetic presentation types are becoming apparent when the disease is being screened for in the wider population

> **Box 6**
> **Diagnosis**
>
> 1. Serum or plasma IGF-1 is the most useful diagnostic screening test
> 2. Absence of a pituitary tumor on imaging does not exclude hypersomatotropism
> 3. Both CT and MRI are useful in imaging the pituitary
> 4. MRI is slightly more sensitive than CT, but CT can be performed under sedation

without exhibiting central nervous system compromise.[6] The presence of discomfort and dysfunction secondary to a large pituitary tumor (eg, headaches, blindness) cannot, however, be excluded. GH's negative effect on insulin sensitivity can lead to DM and, at times, difficult-to-control DM.[14] The exact mechanisms of decreased insulin sensitivity are not completely understood, although it likely includes a decrease in expression of insulin receptors, as well as competition between GH and insulin for mutually used postreceptor signaling processes. Because cats with HST are different from those with regular DM and, in principle, have healthy pancreatic beta cells, it is likely that increased endogenous insulin production initially compensates for the developing insulin resistance. In many cats, although not all, this compensatory response is not sustained or is insufficient, resulting in a diabetic state.[14]

The effect of both GH and IGF-1 excesses on soft tissue, bone, and cartilage is gradual and could result in illness of various body systems. Cats ultimately share many clinical similarities with people with acromegaly, such as bone growth and cardiovascular and respiratory complications. Visceral organomegaly and cardiac hypertrophy, potentially reversible with treatment, are described in both species[6,14,15] (**Fig. 1**). Inspiratory stridor and snoring are commonly reported in cats.[14]

Importantly, the absence of the acromegaly phenotype in a diabetic cat should not deter the clinician from considering HST as a differential for easy- or difficult-to-control DM in a cat.

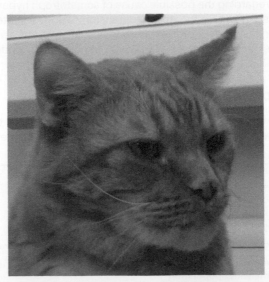

Fig. 1. Broad facial features in a diabetic cat with HST. These features are often not present.

CHARACTERISTICS OF DIABETES MELLITUS SECONDARY TO HYPERSOMATOTROPISM

There are no pathognomonic features that allow discrimination between cats with primary DM and those with DM secondary to early, preacromegaly HST. The diabetic cat with HST might seem to be an unremarkable diabetic and might go into diabetic remission (albeit with high likelihood of relatively quick relapse). Other diabetic cats with HST are extremely challenging to treat, sometimes with seemingly unlimited demand for exogenous insulin. It is expected that with time, most diabetic cats with HST, regardless of the initial level of control, will become difficult to control. This progression presumably relates to increased GH production with increasing tumor size, as well as advancing pancreatic beta cell failure and decreasing endogenous insulin production. A unique, although not universal, feature of DM secondary to HST is increasing body weight despite poor glycemic control. In some cats, the impact of the uncontrolled DM seems to override the anabolic effects of excessive GH and IGF-1 concentrations, and these cats, therefore, tend to lose weight.

DIAGNOSIS
Assessing Serum Insulin-like Growth Factor-1 Concentrations

For most veterinarians, assessing serum total IGF-1 concentrations represents the most feasible and accessible means of screening for HST in diabetic cats (**Box 6**). The PPV of increased IGF-1 (>1000 ng/mL, radioimmunoassay) concentrations is 95% (with a 95% confidence interval: 90%–100%), rendering it very useful clinically.[6] Lower values (600–1000 ng/mL) are also in principle abnormal (although with lower specificity for an HST diagnosis) and should at the very least be followed up when encountered in a patient. Using unvalidated assays is ill advised because clinical data are needed to substantiate the suggested cutoffs. Differences in the performance and expected reference intervals of IGF-1 assays exist.

INSULIN-LIKE GROWTH FACTOR-1 DYNAMICS AND IMPACT ON DIAGNOSIS

The liver is the predominant site of IGF-1 production; this process is insulin dependent. Because some newly diagnosed diabetic cats can be insulin deficient, their IGF-1 concentrations might be decreased, potentially resulting in false-negative results. With insulin therapy, IGF-1 increases in these cats above the diagnostic cutoff for HST within 6 to 8 weeks. In addition, elevation of IGF-1 has been reported in non-HST diabetic cats. As such, at the range of 500 to 1000 ng/mL, the sensitivity and specificity of IGF-1 for the diagnosis of HST is low.[16] Screening for HST could therefore be considered both at the time of diagnosis and after 2 months of insulin therapy.

Serum Growth Hormone, Growth Hormone Suppression, and Other Tests

GH suppression tests are not currently performed because there is no commercially available GH assay despite a radioimmunoassay for GH having been validated for use in cats.[17] GH suppression through glucose administration represents a valuable tool in human medicine, although its value in feline HST has not been established. Administration of glucose intravenously did not suppress GH concentrations in healthy cats in one study.[18] An octreotide suppression test has been described but has only been used for research purposes.[19] Serum type III procollagen propeptide (PIIIP), a peripheral indicator of collagen turnover, was recently shown to provide evidence of active disease or GH bioactivity in the cat.[20] Given that PIIIP is not dependent on portal (hepatic) insulin availability, it might have greater sensitivity than IGF-1 and potentially could be used as part of a panel, to improve diagnosis of feline HST without the explicit need for intracranial imaging. The orexigenic peptide ghrelin is a GH secretagogue and was significantly higher in control cats compared with cats with HST-induced DM.[21] However, the latter group had similar concentrations as those with primary uncomplicated DM, rendering this test not useful for diagnosis. However, after successful radiotherapy, serum ghrelin concentrations increase significantly in cats with HST-induced DM, whereas IGF-1 changes were not significant. This finding suggests a possible role for serum ghrelin as a marker of treatment effect.

IMAGING

After establishing increased IGF-1 concentrations in a cat, imaging (CT or MRI scans of the pituitary area) represents the logical next step in the evaluation of cats suspected of having HST. In most cats with serum IGF-1 concentrations greater than 1000 ng/mL, a protrusion of the pituitary gland beyond the dorsal rim of the sella turcica is identified, indicating enlargement of the pituitary gland (**Fig. 2**). A pituitary height greater than 4 mm is considered to be pituitary enlargement in cats.[6,22] MRI is more sensitive than CT in identifying pituitary enlargement or irregularity.[6] Nevertheless, given the ease and reduced cost of CT in most facilities, contrast-enhanced CT is often chosen.[6] Approximately 95% of cats with HST will demonstrate a pituitary abnormality on CT. This is a high percentage, further implying that overall HST is still diagnosed at a relatively late stage in cats. Because microscopic tumors can have significant systemic endocrine effects, it is questionable whether pituitary enlargement is a necessary criterion for the diagnosis of HST. In the author's opinion, hormonal tests with positive results should usually overrule any negative imaging findings. At the very least, a suspicion of HST should not be discarded.

TREATMENT

Various treatment options are now available (**Box 7, Table 2**). Treating any single consequence of HST alone (such as DM, or in non-DM cats with HST, congestive heart failure [CHF] or arthropathy) is rarely good enough. Nevertheless, insulin treatment can be tried if other options are not possible in a particular diabetic cat. Diabetic cats with HST tend to require higher doses of insulin in the long run, which is

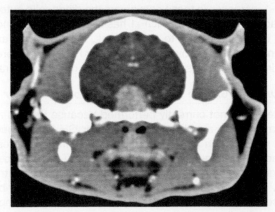

Fig. 2. Postcontrast CT image showing a pituitary enlargement protruding from the sella turcica in a cat with HST. Intracranial imaging can be normal in cats with HST with a microadenoma or pituitary hyperplasia.

Box 7
Treatment options

1. Decreasing/removing the cause of GH excess
   a. Curative
      i. Hypophysectomy
   b. Noncurative
      i. Radiotherapy
      ii. Pasireotide/cabergoline
      iii. Cryotherapy
2. Treating the consequences of the hypersomatotropism only; examples:
   a. Exogenous insulin for diabetes mellitus
   b. Cardiac medications for congestive heart failure
   c. Analgesia for joint pain

---

determined on a case-by-case and temporal basis. No particular insulin type has been shown to be superior, although it could be argued that any insulin type that lacks a pronounced peak effect is preferable, especially when extremely high dosages of insulin are needed. Education of the owner is essential, both in terms of general expectations and in terms of specific complications, particularly with regard to hypoglycemia.

Hypophysectomy is the only treatment able to completely remove the inciting cause, and experience with this procedure has been growing rapidly.[23–25] Most commonly, cats are placed in sternal recumbency in a commercially available surgical head frame (Brainsight, Rogue Research, Montreal, Canada) for rigid immobilization, allowing an approach to the pituitary through opening of the soft palate and drilling a hole transsphenoidally. The entire pituitary gland is removed. Postoperatively cats receive desmopressin (topically applied on the conjunctiva) and are treated with a hydrocortisone infusion until they begin to eat, at which point they transition to long-term oral hydrocortisone as well as levothyroxine. Insulin administration is tapered over the following days based on ongoing glucose monitoring. Desmopressin supplementation can be ceased in most cats following the immediate postoperative period.[23–25] **Box 8** further details postoperative medication. Serum IGF-1 concentrations decrease markedly and consistently within 4 weeks postoperatively and normalize in more than 90% of cases.[23] About 70% of cats undergo diabetic remission.[23] When a cat is in CHF, surgery can still be considered after stabilization of CHF. For these cats, hypophysectomy represents the only treatment option for effective reversal of cardiac pathology. The perioperative and postoperative mortality rate is 15% (and decreasing with experience) and is generally acceptable to most cat owners given the paucity of equally effective alternative treatment modalities.[23]

It is reasonable to consider radiation therapy (RT) a treatment option when hypophysectomy is not available or when dealing with a big pituitary tumor (the definition of "big" is not well established though). However, clinicians and owners should realize that treatment success is less certain than with surgery and that the timing and extent of any success, if it occurs, is unpredictable and could take more than a year. It is worth noting that diabetic remission rates are lower following RT and that RT requires multiple procedures under general anesthesia. For some owners, this may be an unacceptable risk. Success, in some cats, can be followed by remission. From an endocrinological point of view, RT does not reduce GH and IGF-1 concentrations effectively, whereas hypophysectomy does.[26]

In the author's clinic, hypophysectomy has been successfully performed on several cats with disease reoccurrence after RT, which is encouraging; this implies that in

Table 2
Currently available treatment options for hypersomatotropism

Treatment Modality	Advantages	Disadvantages
Hypophysectomy	Highest success rates Treats underlying cause and removes tumor Most cats enter diabetic remission Predictable success Normalizes IGF-1	Availability Cost Morbidity and mortality (<10%) Lifelong supplementation of thyroid hormone, cortisone, and in 20%–50% desmopressin
Radiotherapy	Can reduce the tumor size Little morbidity and mortality A minority of cats enter diabetic remission	Availability Does not normalize hormones—IGF-1 elevations persist GH- and IGF-1-induced pathologic condition progresses Multiple anesthetic procedures required Cost Does not remove tumor, reoccurrence relatively frequent Unpredictability of effect
Pasireotide	Good success rates No anesthetics required Little morbidity and mortality	Costs Does not normalize hormones Leaves tumor in place Some self-limiting gastrointestinal side effects
Cabergoline	Modest success rate (<40%) No anesthetics required Little morbidity and mortality Available and cost-effective	Ineffective in many cats Does not normalize hormones Leaves tumor untreated Some self-limiting gastrointestinal side effects
Treating the consequences of GH excess, not the hypersomatotropism	Available to all A minority (±1 in 5) of cats can have adequate quality of life for a short period	Most cats do not have a good quality of life despite high-dose insulin treatment Hypoglycemia with high-dose insulin, when pulsatile GH secretion is low Leaves tumor untreated GH- and IGF-1-induced pathologic condition progresses
Cryotherapy	Success rate reported in 2 cases	Very limited experience

---

Box 8
Supplementation details posthypophysectomy

1. Glucocorticoid supplementation (eg, hydrocortisone or cortisone acetate 0.5 mg/kg once or twice daily, prednisolone can sometimes be too potent and lead to muscle atrophy and accelerated aging)

2. Thyroid supplementation (eg, levothyroxine 0.1 mg once daily)

3. Conjunctival desmopressin (1 drop three times a day, decreased gradually over 1 month, complete cessation possible in 80% of cases)

4. Insulin injections (as required—70% cease to require insulin)

---

case of large pituitary tumors, and thus with possible increased risk for hypophysectomy complications, RT could be performed first to reduce tumor size, followed by hypophysectomy to enable permanent cure.

Pasireotide (SOM230, Novartis, Basel, Switzerland) is a novel somatostatin receptor (SSTR) analogue with binding affinity for SSTR subtypes 1, 2, 3, and 5; it is the only medical therapy to consistently and markedly improve insulin sensitivity.[27] In cats receiving 8 mg/kg subcutaneous pasireotide long-acting release once monthly for 6 months, significant decreases in IGF-1 concentrations, insulin dose, and fructosamine concentrations were documented.[27]

Decreased dopamine D2 receptor expression in larger feline tumors has been demonstrated. This observation may hint toward a mechanism that allows unchecked adenoma growth, as well as likely confirms the cause behind previous disappointing treatment results with dopamine agonists like cabergoline. Nevertheless, recent reports suggest that in a subpopulation of cats, possibly with smaller tumors, dopamine agonists have improved diabetic control (and even induced diabetic remission) in some cats treated with cabergoline (10 μg/kg every 24 hours, orally), although not in others.[28,29]

Cryotherapy constitutes the damaging of the tumor through local exposure to extremely low temperatures. Only 2 cases of pituitary tumor cryotherapy, although both successful, have been described, and it is therefore difficult to provide strong recommendations in favor or against this treatment option.[30]

PROGNOSIS

A recent study of quality of life (QoL) showed that median QoL score at diagnosis of HST was 2 (range 1–5; 1 poor; 5 excellent) with improvement in all treatment groups. Cabergoline (4; range 1–5), RT (4; range 2–5), and hypophysectomy (5; range 4–5) showed more improvement in median QoL scores compared with insulin therapy alone (3; range 1–5).[31] Overall median survival time (MST) was 24 months (range 0–75 months). Cats treated with insulin alone showed shorter MST (22 months; range 0–69 months) compared with cats receiving other treatments (36 months; range 3–75 months; $P = 0.04$).

HYPERCORTISOLISM

Excess glucocorticoid activity can result in DM and therefore represents another possible cause for the insulin-resistant diabetic cat.[32,33] Glucocorticoids are able to induce DM through a variety of mechanisms, including impairment of insulin-dependent glucose uptake in the periphery and enhanced gluconeogenesis in the liver. In addition, glucocorticoids oppose several other actions of insulin, including its central inhibitory effect on appetite. Finally, steroid-induced inhibition of insulin secretion by pancreatic beta cells has also been shown to occur in a variety of species (although still only suspected and not proven in the cat).[32]

PREVALENCE AND ETIOLOGY

Noniatrogenic (spontaneous) feline HC, with or without subsequently induced DM, seems to be a rare condition with approximately 100 cases reported in the veterinary literature.[32,33] However, in contrast to the situation with feline HST, it is currently unknown what exact proportion of the diabetic cat population is indeed suffering from it. Iatrogenic feline HC is also rare and certainly less common than iatrogenic HC in dogs. Interestingly, 7.5% of diabetic cats included in a study concerning insured diabetic cats in the United Kingdom had a confirmed history of glucocorticoid administration indirectly implicating glucocorticoids in the cause of their (assumed type 2) DM.[34] Just like canine HC, spontaneous feline HC is caused by either a functional pituitary tumor (pituitary-dependent hypercortisolism [PDH]) oversecreting adrenocorticotropic hormone (ACTH) or a functional tumor of the adrenal cortex oversecreting hormones with glucocorticoid activity. PDH is the most prevalent form (75%–80% of cases) and is usually caused by an adenoma of the pars intermedia or pars distalis of the pituitary gland.[32] Pituitary carcinomas have been described rarely. The remaining 20% to 25% of cases suffer from adrenal-dependent HC (ADH). Of the latter group, a benign functional adenoma of the cortex of one of the adrenals is most likely (65%) with a malignant cortical carcinoma affecting a minority of cats with ADH.[32] Interestingly, variations of these causes exist including unilateral and bilateral cortical carcinomas overproducing sex hormones with glucocorticoid effects (eg, progesterone, androstenedione, testosterone), ACTH-independent cortisol production due to the excess alpha-melanocyte stimulating hormone production by a pituitary tumor exerting glucocorticorticotropic effects, and pituitary adenomas overproducing both GH and ACTH resulting in HST and HC.[32,35,36] Finally, rare cases of multiple endocrine neoplasia have been described to include HC.

CLINICAL PRESENTATION AND CHARACTERISTICS OF DIABETES MELLITUS SECONDARY TO HYPERCORTISOLISM

Cats suffering from HC can be of any breed or sex, although most cats are middle aged to older. About 80% of cats with HC present with signs referable to DM (polyuria, polydipsia, polyphagia, and peripheral neuropathy), which, over time, could become less sensitive to insulin. Nevertheless, insulin requirements in those patients tend to be less extreme than those of some cats with HST.[32] Interestingly, weight loss, instead of weight gain, is most common with feline HC (as opposed to HST). A minority of HC cats will present with predominance of dermatologic abnormalities such as skin fragility, or with polyphagia and weight gain, instead of DM-related clinical signs (Fig. 3). The perceived lack of polyuria and polydipsia in the cases without overt DM illustrates the relative inherent resistance cats have (compared with dogs) to the glucocorticoid-induced inhibition of secretion and action of antidiuretic hormone. Polyuria and polydipsia tend to only ensue once DM has arisen.

Clinical signs of HC that cats share with dogs affected by HC include abdominal enlargement or pot-bellied appearance, panting, muscle atrophy, unkempt hair coat, bilateral symmetrical alopecia, and predisposition for infections (urinary tract, skin, abscesses, respiratory tract, toxoplasmosis). More specific to the cat is skin fragility, which is thought to relate to the protein catabolism and can result in tearing of the skin under otherwise innocuous circumstances, such as self-grooming or

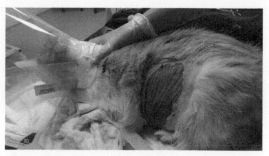

Fig. 3. Fragile skin resulting in an extensive spontaneous wound in a cat with PDH.

minimal restrain. Cats can develop hair coat color changes as well as (perhaps more rarely than in dogs) calcinosis cutis.[32]

Finally, there are rare cases in which blindness (due to a pituitary macroadenoma or induced by hypertension), abnormal behavior, compulsive walking, circling, and continuous vocalization have also been reported. Virilization has been encountered in cases with sex hormone-secreting (androstenedione and testosterone) adrenal carcinomas, which might be manifested as spines on the penis of a castrated male cat.[32] **Box 9** summarizes the clinical differences between diabetic cats with HST and those with HC.

DIAGNOSIS

There are currently no studies demonstrating the accuracy of any test for the diagnosis of HC in cats. Endocrine tests that might be useful in substantiating a diagnosis of feline HC, including their advantages and disadvantages, are shown in **Table 3**. As is the case with many endocrine tests, these tests will demonstrate low PPV when used in cases with a clinical picture that does not strongly support the possible presence of HC (see clinical presentation). Conversely, given the low prevalence of feline HC in general, routine screening in clinically unremarkable diabetic cats is not recommended. Results of differentiating tests should not be interpreted as proof of the presence of the disease in the first place; only screening tests should be used for diagnosis.

IMAGING

In feline HC, pituitary imaging (using CT or MRI) lacks the sensitivity that endocrine testing offers (45% of cats with PDH had normal CT scan results) and is usually more expensive, as well as requiring sedation/anaesthesia.[32] In addition, cases with

---

Box 9
Clinical differences between feline hypersomatotropism and hypercortisolism

1. HC seemingly less prevalent in cats than HST

2. Weight loss more common with HC; weight gain with HST

3. Cases with extreme insulin resistance are more likely to suffer from HST

4. Fragile skin and fur changes are associated with HC

5. Muscle atrophy more associated with HC

Table 3
Overview and characteristics of screening and discriminating tests for feline hypercortisolism[32]

Differentiating Test	Protocol	Interpretation	Advantage	Disadvantage
LDDST (screening and differentiating test)	1. Baseline serum cortisol (t = 0) 2. Intravenous 0.1 mg/kg dexamethasone (or intramuscular) 3. Serum cortisol t = 4 and 8 h	If suppression at t = 8 h, HC unlikely; if no suppression & t = 4 h > 50% of t = 0 h: ADH and PDH possible; if t = 4 h < 50% of t = 0 h: PDH possible	Can be performed in any clinic Can serve as screening test and as discriminating test	1. Long duration of test and need for multiple samples 2. Vulnerable to false-positives
ACTH stimulation test (screening test)	1. Baseline serum cortisol (t = 0) 2. Intravenous 5 μg/kg synthetic ACTH (IM possible) 3. Serum cortisol t = 30 min, 60 min, 90 min, 120 min (all or at least 2 of these advocated)	If overstimulating abovementioned laboratory's reference interval, HC possible	Can be performed in any clinic	1. Unreliable timing of peak stimulation/need for multiple samples 2. Vulnerable to false-negatives
HDDST (differentiating test)	1. Baseline serum cortisol (t = 0) 2. Intravenous 1.0 mg/kg dexamethasone (or intramuscular) 3. Serum cortisol t = 4 and 8 h	If cortisol <50% of t = 0 h: ADH unlikely	Can be performed in any clinic	In-hospital: stress 50% of PDH cats do not show suppression
UCCR with oral dexamethasone suppression (screening & differentiating test)	1. 2 at home collected morning samples for UCCR (sample 1 & 2): calculate average 2. Owner administers 0.5 mg dexamethasone orally at 12 PM, 6 PM, and 12 AM midnight 3. Next morning: home-collected morning sample for UCCR (sample 3)	average baseline samples 1&2 > laboratorys reference interval:H possible; 75% of cats with PDH will show <50% of average UCCR ofsamples 1 & 2 in 3rd sample	At home: less influence of stress Can serve as screening test and as discriminating test	25% of PDH cats do not show suppression

Endogenous ACTH (differentiating test)	1. Usually collected in EDTA collection tube 2. Put immediately on ice 3. Plasma separated and stored at −80°C 4. Transported to laboratory on dry ice. 5. Exact protocol to be verified with laboratory performing the assay	If high or high normal: PDH likely If low or low normal: ADH likely	Only one sample needed	Unstable hormone: false low results (special sampling and transport conditions crucial, contact laboratory)
Adrenal size and morphology on abdominal ultrasonography or CT (differentiating tests)	1. Measurements of adrenal width are taken 2. Structure of adrenals is assessed 3. Includes assessment for vena cava invasion	Bilaterally enlarged adrenals suggestive of PDH One large adrenal and small contralateral adrenal suggestive of ADH Vena cava invasion suggests adrenal carcinoma	Availability Vena cava invasion or evidence of metastases suggest presence of a carcinoma and informs treatment decisions Other causes of insulin-resistant DM can be screened for (eg, pancreatitis)	Equipment and experience needed
Pituitary size and morphology on intracranial imaging (CT, MRI) (differentiating tests)	1. Imaging of the sella turcica 2. Precontrast and postcontrast enhancement	If macroadenoma present (pituitary height > 3 mm) usually definitive	If no macroadenoma present, abdomen can also be imaged using the same modality screening for ADH Essential step for planning of hypophysectomy or radiation therapy Useful for assessment of vena cava invasion in case of ADH and before considering adrenalectomy	Limited availability Costs Need for sedation or anesthesia Microadenoma (50% of PDH cases) could be missed/limited sensitivity Rare immediate contrast side effects (usually only limited to waking up from sedation and vomiting)

Abbreviation: EDTA, Ethylenediaminetetraacetic acid; HC, hypercortisolism; IM, intramuscular; LDDST, low dose dexamethasone suppression test; UCCR, urinary corticoid creatinine ratio.

nonfunctional pituitary tumors or nonfunctional adrenal enlargements might be misdiagnosed if endocrine testing is not performed. Nevertheless, during the discriminatory phase, performing an abdominal ultrasonography in cats suspected of suffering from HC might help. Visualization of adrenal glands in cats is easier to accomplish than in dogs, although it remains operator and equipment dependent.[37] In one study, 34 of 41 cats (83%) were correctly classified as ADH or PDH based on ultrasound findings when the combination of one large adrenal gland (or having an adrenal mass) and one small adrenal gland was considered consistent with ADH, whereas the presence of equal-sized (normal or enlarged) adrenal glands was considered consistent with PDH.[32] Ultrasound-guided biopsy of adrenal masses is possible, although not without risk (especially hemorrhage, and also risk of failure to reach a histologic diagnosis), and one could question the need for this procedure when adrenalectomy represents the gold-standard treatment option for ADH.[38]

Abdominal radiography adds little value to the diagnostic process, especially when abdominal ultrasonography is available, with the exception of large adrenal tumors, which can sometimes be seen on regular radiographs. It is also important to emphasize that adrenal gland calcification can occur in cats as part of the normal aging process and does not indicate presence of an adrenal tumor.[32] Abdominal CT might also prove useful in the assessment if adrenal morphology as well as assessment for vena cava invasion or metastases from an adrenal carcinoma. In the differentiation process, both the pituitary and the adrenal glands could be imaged in one CT session. Finally, a sex hormone-secreting tumor should be suspected in cats with clinical signs of HC when an adrenal mass is observed on ultrasonography or CT but normal or even suppressed cortisol concentrations are found on dynamic tests.[32]

TREATMENT OPTIONS FOR HYPERCORTISOLISM

Comparable to HST, treatment options consist of medical treatment, surgical options, RT, and mere treatment of the consequences of cortisol excess. Similar to feline HST, when treatment is initiated, rapid changes in insulin demands might occur and clinicians and owners need to be vigilant and monitor closely.

MEDICAL TREATMENT (PITUITARY-DEPENDENT HYPERADRENOCORTICISM AND ADRENAL-DEPENDENT HYPERADRENOCORTICISM)

Medical treatment could be considered in the following situations: (1) if a definitive treatment option (hypophysectomy or adrenalectomy) is declined or not feasible; (2) in the preoperative period with the goal of reducing the risk of surgical complications, especially in terms of improving wound healing; (3) pre-RT, peri-RT, and post-RT (PDH); and (4) as a palliative option in case of metastatic disease. At present, using trilostane above all other medical options is recommended, given its superior efficacy, relative lack of side effects, and ease of use.[39] A good QoL can be achieved long term with trilostane in a significant proportion of cats, and some even achieve diabetic remission.[40] Cabergoline also seems effective in some cats with PDH,[41] as is pasireotide (personal communication author, SJM Niessen, 2023).

HYPOPHYSECTOMY (PITUITARY-DEPENDENT HYPERADRENOCORTICISM)

As described above for feline HST, hypophysectomy is the only potentially curative option in human, canine, and feline PDH. The largest case series to date consisted of 7 cats with PDH but likely underestimates the potential of this procedure because experience has been gained since, alongside increased success rates.[42]

UNILATERAL OR BILATERAL ADRENALECTOMY (ADRENAL-DEPENDENT HYPERADRENOCORTICISM OR PITUITARY-DEPENDENT HYPERADRENOCORTICISM)

Bilateral adrenalectomy is another surgical option for PDH, whereas unilateral adrenalectomy might be curative in cases of ADH.[32,43,44] Adrenalectomy requires less expertise than a hypophysectomy, although perioperative and postoperative management are equally important and impaired wound healing secondary to chronic hypercortisolemia can represent an added level of difficulty. In the author's institution, a hydrocortisone infusion is started as soon as the surgeon starts working on the adrenal glands and the infusion is continued until the patient is eating postoperatively. Whenever possible, presurgical treatment with trilostane is advocated by the author, to reduce the risk of impaired wound healing. When impaired wound healing and/or skin fragility is a great concern, a flank incision approach to the adrenal glands is often preferred, because it is associated with decreased tension on the incision compared with a midline incision approach, reducing the risk of incision breakdown.[32,44]

In case of bilateral adrenalectomy, the patient will require lifelong supplementation of mineralocorticoid and glucocorticoid hormones. In case of unilateral adrenalectomy, glucocorticoid treatment is continued in the immediate postoperative period, and then tapered gradually over a period of 6 weeks in order for the remaining adrenal gland to gradually resume glucocorticoid production. Measuring basal serum cortisol concentrations 12 hours after the prednisolone or hydrocortisone was administered can guide the assessment of the activity levels of the remaining adrenal gland during the last part of the tapering period and can inform the ultimate decision to stop treatment completely.[32]

RADIATION THERAPY (PITUITARY-DEPENDENT HYPERADRENOCORTICISM)

RT is also discussed in the feline HST section. In summary, the unreliability in terms of response to treatment is the greatest pitfall of using this modality, as is the case when treating feline HS.

QUALITY OF LIFE AND PROGNOSIS

High-quality research on QoL and prognosis of cats suffering from HC is not available given the paucity of reports in the literature. If adequate, preferably curative, treatment aimed at lowering cortisol concentrations is provided, a good QoL can be achieved in many cats. HC tends to result in more acute complications with seriously debilitating effects compared with feline HST. Therefore, intervention to reduce endogenous cortisol levels is usually more urgently needed, and treating DM without addressing the underlying HC is usually not recommended. Meticulous wound management is indicated in case of wounds caused by fragile skin (wounds will be challenging, though not impossible, to heal), as well as adequate prevention and treatment of opportunistic infections and screening for HC-associated hypertension. A low-carbohydrate canned diet would be advocated, as in other cases of feline DM.

CLINICS CARE POINTS

- Hypersomatotropism is often referred to as acromegaly, despite the fact that most cats do not have external features that fit with acromegaly-any cat with diabetes mellitus, regardless of insulin requirements, could have underlying hypersomatotropism-serum IGF-1 is an effective screening tool for hypersomatotropism-a diabetic cat with extreme insulin resistance is more likely to suffer from hypersomatotropism than Cushing's Syndrome/ hypercortisolism.

- HC cats are more likely to have pathology of the skin and/or fur than those with hypersomatotropism.
- Treatment of the underlying cause is a more successful route to good quality of life than treating any possible resulting diabetes mellitus alone.

DISCLOSURE

Professor S. Niessen provides regular consultation to Boehringer Ingelheim, Dechra, MSD Animal Health, Nestlé Purina, and Hill's. Research on the use of pasireotide was supported by Novartis, its manufacturer.

REFERENCES

1. Niessen SJ, Powney S, Guitian J, et al. Evaluation of a quality-of-life tool for cats with diabetes mellitus. J Vet Intern Med 2010;24:1098–105.
2. Niessen SJM, Bjornvad C, Church DB, et al, ESVE/SCE Membership. Agreeing Language in Veterinary Endocrinology (ALIVE): Diabetes mellitus - a modified Delphi-method-based system to create consensus disease definitions. Vet J 2022;289:105910.
3. O'Neill DG, Gostelow R, Orme C, et al. Epidemiology of diabetes mellitus among 193,435 cats attending primary-care veterinary practices in England. J Vet Intern Med 2016;30(4):964–72.
4. Callegari C, Mercuriali E, Hafner M, et al. Survival time and prognostic factors in cats with newly diagnosed diabetes mellitus: 114 cases (2000-2009). J Am Vet Med Assoc 2013;243:91–5.
5. Gostelow R, Forcada Y, Graves T, et al. Systematic review of feline diabetic remission: separating fact from opinion. Vet J 2014;202(2):208–21.
6. Niessen SJ, Forcada Y, Mantis P, et al. Studying Cat (Felis catus) Diabetes: Beware of the Acromegalic Imposter. PLoS One 2015;10(5):e0127794.
7. Berg RI, Nelson RW, Feldman EC, et al. Serum insulin-like growth factor-I concentration in cats with diabetes mellitus and acromegaly. J Vet Intern Med 2007; 21(5):892–8.
8. Schaefer S, Kooistra HS, Riond B, et al. Evaluation of insulin-like growth factor-1, total thyroxine, feline pancreas-specific lipase and urinary corticoid-to-creatinine ratio in cats with diabetes mellitus in Switzerland and the Netherlands. J Feline Med Surg 2017;19(8):888–96.
9. Scudder CJ, Mirczuk SM, Richardson KM, et al. Pituitary Pathology and Gene Expression in Acromegalic Cats. J Endocr Soc 2018;3(1):181–200.
10. Steele MM, Borgeat K, Payne JR, et al. Increased insulin-like growth factor 1 concentrations in a retrospective population of non-diabetic cats diagnosed with hypertrophic cardiomyopathy. J Feline Med Surg 2021;23(10):952–8.
11. Fletcher JM, Scudder CJ, Kiupel M, et al. Hypersomatotropism in 3 Cats without Concurrent Diabetes Mellitus. J Vet Intern Med 2016;30(4):1216–21.
12. Dirtu AC, Niessen SJ, Jorens PG, et al. Organohalogenated contaminants in domestic cats' plasma in relation to spontaneous acromegaly and type 2 diabetes mellitus: a clue for endocrine disruption in humans? Environ Int 2013;57-58:60–7.
13. Scudder CJ, Niessen SJ, Catchpole B, et al. Feline hypersomatotropism and acromegaly tumorigenesis: a potential role for the AIP gene. Domest Anim Endocrinol 2017;59:134–9.

14. Niessen SJ, Petrie G, Gaudiano F, et al. Feline acromegaly: an underdiagnosed endocrinopathy? J Vet Intern Med 2007;21(5):899–905.

15. Borgeat K, Niessen SJM, Wilkie L, et al. Time spent with cats is never wasted: Lessons learned from feline acromegalic cardiomyopathy, a naturally occurring animal model of the human disease. PLoS One 2018;13(3):e0194342.

16. Woolhead VL, Whee Wen LT, Scudder CJ, et al. Serial changes in insulin-like growth factor 1 and impact on hypersomatotropism-screening in feline diabetes mellitus, research communications of the 27th ECVIM-CA congress. J Vet Intern Med 2018;32:525–609.

17. Niessen SJ, Khalid M, Petrie G. et al. Validation and application of a radioimmunoassay for ovine growth hormone in the diagnosis of acromegaly in cats, Vet Rec, 2007;160(26):902–907.

18. Kokka N, Garcia JF, Morgan M, et al. Immunoassay of plasma growth hormone in cats following fasting and administration of insulin, arginine, 2-deoxyglucose and hypothalamic extract. Endocrinology 1971;88(2):359–66.

19. Slingerland LI, Voorhout G, Rijnberk A, et al. Growth hormone excess and the effect of octreotide in cats with diabetes mellitus. Domest Anim Endocrinol 2008; 35(4):352–61.

20. Keyte SV, Kenny PJ, Forcada Y, et al. Serum N-Terminal Type III procollagen propeptide: an indicator of growth hormone excess and response to treatment in feline hypersomatotropism. J Vet Intern Med 2016;30(4):973–82.

21. Jensen KB, Forcada Y, Chruch DB, et al. Evaluation and diagnostic potential of serum ghrelin in feline hypersomatotropism and diabetes mellitus. J Vet Intern Med 2015;29(1):14–20.

22. Lamb CR, Ciasca TC, Mantis P, et al. Computed tomographic signs of acromegaly in 68 diabetic cats with hypersomatotropism. J Feline Med Surg 2014; 16(2):99–108.

23. Fenn J, Kenny PJ, Scudder CJ, et al. Efficacy of hypophysectomy for the treatment of hypersomatotropism-induced diabetes mellitus in 68 cats. J Vet Intern Med 2021;35(2):823–33.

24. Van Bokhorst KL, Galac S, Kooistra HS, et al. Evaluation of hypophysectomy for treatment of hypersomatotropism in 25 cats. J Vet Intern Med 2021;35(2):834–42.

25. Neilson DM, Viscasillas J, Alibhai HI, et al. Anaesthetic management and complications during hypophysectomy in 37 cats with acromegaly. J Feline Med Surg 2019;21(4):347–52.

26. Watson-Skaggs ML, Gieger TL, Yoshikawa H, et al. Endocrine response and outcome in 14 cats with insulin resistance and acromegaly treated with stereotactic radiosurgery (17 Gy). Am J Vet Res 2021;83(1):64–71.

27. Gostelow R, Scudder C, Keyte S, et al. Pasireotide long-acting release treatment for diabetic cats with underlying hypersomatotropism. J Vet Intern Med 2017; 31(2):355–64.

28. Miceli DD, Vidal PN, Pompili GA, et al. Diabetes mellitus remission in three cats with hypersomatotropism after cabergoline treatment. JFMS Open Rep 2021; 7(1). 20551169211018991.

29. Scudder CJ, Hazuchova K, Gostelow R, et al. Pilot study assessing the use of cabergoline for the treatment of cats with hypersomatotropism and diabetes mellitus. J Feline Med Surg 2021;23(2):131–7.

30. Blois SL, Holmberg DL. Cryohypophysectomy used in the treatment of a case of feline acromegaly. J Small Anim Pract 2008;49(11):596–600.

31. Corsini A, Niessen SJ, Miceli DD, et al. Quality of life and response to treatment in cats with hypersomatotropism: the owners' point of view. J Feline Med Surg 2022; 24(8):e175–82.

32. Niessen SJ, Church DB, Forcada Y. Hypersomatotropism, acromegaly, and hyperadrenocorticism and feline diabetes mellitus. Vet Clin North Am Small Anim Pract 2013;43(2):319–50.

33. Gilor C, Niessen SJ, Furrow E, et al. What's in a Name? Classification of Diabetes Mellitus in Veterinary Medicine and Why It Matters. J Vet Intern Med 2016;30(4): 927–40.

34. McCann TM, Simpson KE, Shaw DJ, et al. Feline diabetes mellitus in the UK: the prevalence within an insured cat population and a questionnaire-based putative risk factor analysis. J Feline Med Surg 2007;9(4):289–99.

35. Harro CC, Refsal KR, Shaw N, et al. Retrospective study of aldosterone and progesterone secreting adrenal tumors in 10 cats. J Vet Intern Med 2021;35(5): 2159–66.

36. Valentin SY, Cortright CC, Nelson RW, et al. Clinical findings, diagnostic test results, and treatment outcome in cats with spontaneous hyperadrenocorticism: 30 cases. J Vet Intern Med 2014;28(2):481–7.

37. Combes A, Pey P, Paepe D, et al. Ultrasonographic appearance of adrenal glands in healthy and sick cats. J Feline Med Surg 2013;15(6):445–57.

38. Bertazzolo W, Didier M, Gelain ME, et al. Accuracy of cytology in distinguishing adrenocortical tumors from pheochromocytoma in companion animals. Vet Clin Pathol 2014;43(3):453–9.

39. Mellett Keith AM, Bruyette D, Stanley S. Trilostane therapy for treatment of spontaneous hyperadrenocorticism in cats: 15 cases (2004-2012). J Vet Intern Med 2013;27(6):1471–7.

40. Muschner AC, Varela FV, Hazuchova K, et al. Diabetes mellitus remission in a cat with pituitary-dependent hyperadrenocorticism after trilostane treatment. JFMS Open Rep 2018;4(1). 2055116918767708.

41. Miceli DD, Zelarayán GS, García JD, et al. Diabetes mellitus remission in a cat with hyperadrenocorticism after cabergoline treatment. JFMS Open Rep 2021; 7(2). 20551169211029896.

42. Meij BP, Voorhout G, Van Den Ingh TS, et al. Transsphenoidal hypophysectomy for treatment of pituitary-dependent hyperadrenocorticism in 7 cats. Vet Surg 2001;30(1):72–86.

43. Duesberg CA, Nelson RW, Feldman EC, et al. Adrenalectomy for treatment of hyperadrenocorticism in cats: 10 cases (1988-1992). J Am Vet Med Assoc 1995; 207(8):1066–70.

44. Daniel G, Mahony OM, Markovich JE, et al. Clinical findings, diagnostics and outcome in 33 cats with adrenal neoplasia (2002-2013). J Feline Med Surg 2016;18(2):77–84.

Cushing's Syndrome and Other Causes of Insulin Resistance in Dogs

Linda Fleeman, BVSc, PhD, MANZCVS*,
Renea Barrett, BSc, DVM, MANZCVS

KEYWORDS

- Dog • Canine • Diabetes mellitus • Insulin resistance • Cushing's syndrome
- Hypercortisolism • Basal-bolus insulin • Diestrus

KEY POINTS

- Cushing syndrome is the most common cause of insulin resistance in diabetic dogs in populations where neutering of young dogs is routine.
- The most pronounced effects of hypercortisolism on glucose metabolism are insulin resistance, perceived short duration of insulin action, excessive postprandial hyperglycemia, and substantial within-day and day-to-day glycemic variability.
- Successful strategies to manage excessive glycemic variability include basal insulin monotherapy and combined basal-bolus insulin treatment.
- Diestrus is the most common cause of insulin resistance in diabetic dogs in populations where neutering of young dogs is not routinely recommended.
- Obesity and other causes of insulin resistance have an additive effect on insulin requirements and the risk of progression to clinical diabetes in dogs.

INSULIN RESISTANCE
Definition of Insulin Resistance

Project ALIVE (Agreeing Language In Veterinary Endocrinology)[1] recommends using the term "insulin resistance" "to describe the presence of varying degrees of interference of insulin action on target cells. The term is not defined by the exogenous insulin dose required or by the change of blood glucose following insulin injection. However, when there is concern over the need for a high insulin dose, the presence of insulin resistance should be considered among other potential causes."[1]

Animal Diabetes Australia, 5 Hood Street, Collingwood, Victoria 3066, Australia
* Corresponding author.
E-mail address: L.Fleeman@AnimalDiabetesAustralia.com.au

[1] Project ALIVE (Agreeing Language In Veterinary Endocrinology) was founded by the European Society of Veterinary Endocrinology in 2016 and endorsed by the Society for Comparative Endocrinology in 2017 and focuses on creating agreement over the definition of common terminology in veterinary endocrinology.

Vet Clin Small Anim 53 (2023) 711–730
https://doi.org/10.1016/j.cvsm.2023.01.009
0195-5616/23/© 2023 Elsevier Inc. All rights reserved.

Causes of Insulin Resistance in Dogs

Causes of insulin resistance in dogs are listed in **Table 1**. The 3 most common causes of insulin resistance in dogs are discussed in the following section.

CUSHING SYNDROME
Definition of Cushing Syndrome

Project ALIVE defines Cushing syndrome as "the umbrella term for a range of *clinical syndromes* that are caused by a chronic excess of glucocorticoid activity, which can be due to a range of endogenous or exogenous steroid hormones."[1]

How Glucocorticoids Cause Impairment of Glucose Metabolism

- Impairment in glucose metabolism caused by glucocorticoids is multifactorial and includes increased glucogenesis, decreased glycogenosis, decreased glucose uptake and oxidation, impaired insulin secretion, and insulin resistance (reduced sensitivity of tissues to insulin). Insulin resistance may be manifested by direct changes in insulin receptor signaling or via indirect mechanisms through changes in lipid, carbohydrate, and protein metabolism.[2] The main organs involved are the liver, skeletal muscle, endocrine pancreas, and adipose tissue. Glucocorticoids cause increased glucogenesis in the liver. Glucocorticoid response elements within the promoter region of genes are activated, and this leads to increased expression of enzymes involved in the glucogenesis pathway. In addition, increased lipolysis and proteolysis augment this effect with increased substrates available for glucogenesis. Glucocorticoids also inhibit the suppressive effects of insulin on this pathway.
- There is interindividual variability in the susceptibility of people to the adverse effects of glucocorticoids and to the degree of insulin resistance they induce. The situation is likely similar in dogs. Dogs that develop unexpectedly pronounced side effects to treatment with systemic or topical glucocorticoids might have concurrent spontaneous hypercortisolism and experience additive effects of exogenous and endogenous glucocorticoids.
- Basal and postprandial insulin resistance occur but in nondiabetic human patients the diabetogenic effects of prednisolone were most prominent in the postprandial, hyperinsulinemic state.[3,4]

Table 1	
Causes of insulin resistance in dogs	
Cause	**Mechanism**
Cushing syndrome (hypercortisolism/glucocorticoid treatment)	Excess cortisol or cortisone
Diestrus/pregnancy/progestogen treatment	Predominantly due to progestogens and growth hormone
Obesity	Via hormonal signals from adipose tissue (eg, leptin)
Hypothyroidism	Excess growth hormone induced by thyrotropin-releasing hormone
Stress hyperglycemia	Increased counterregulatory hormones (cortisol, catecholamines)
Inflammatory, traumatic, and other health conditions	Via increased stress hormones (cortisol, catecholamines)
Pheochromocytoma/paraganglioma	Increased catecholamines

- Within nonhepatic tissues, insulin resistance is associated with impaired glucose metabolism and decreased glucose uptake; this may involve a direct effect on receptor signaling pathways and reduced glucose transporters, but not all of the pathways and molecular mechanisms of insulin resistance are understood.[5]
- Within the acute phase of corticosteroid use, insulin-stimulated glucose uptake is inhibited in skeletal muscle. More chronically, decreased muscle mass and inhibition of capillary recruitment leads to a decreased surface area for exchange and reduced glucose uptake.[6,7]
- Hormones released from adipose tissue are termed adipokines. Glucocorticoids influence the synthesis and release of adipokines, which leads to a more diabetogenic profile (increased leptin and resistin, which then decrease insulin sensitivity). Increased lipolysis also increases the substrates for glucogenesis, although this glucocorticoid-associated dyslipidemia has not been proved to cause insulin resistance on its own.[8]
- In the endocrine pancreas, insulin synthesis and secretion from beta cells is impaired, and this especially affects glucose-stimulated insulin secretion.[9]
- Glucocorticoids potentiate the action of glucagon and cause incomplete suppression of glucagon after meals. High-dose (30 mg) prednisolone treatment in healthy humans leads to an increase in fasting and postprandial glucagon concentrations.[10]

Canine Cushing Syndrome and Insulin Resistance

- Insulin resistance associated with Cushing syndrome in dogs has been recognized for more than 40 years.[11]
- The gold standard for assessment of insulin sensitivity is the euglycemic-hyperinsulinemic glucose clamp. Using this gold standard, dogs with spontaneous Cushing syndrome have severe insulin resistance, even more severe than bitches in diestrus.[12]
- Nondiabetic dogs with Cushing syndrome secrete more insulin from beta cells in response to the insulin resistance.[13] If this compensation fails, diabetes ensues.
- Most dogs with Cushing syndrome remain euglycemic (146/235 [62%] in a prospective study); however, those that developed mild hyperglycemia (100–180 mg/dL; 5.6–10.0 mmol/L) had increased risk for becoming more severely hyperglycemic within a year.[14]

Association of Hypercortisolism and Diabetes Mellitus in Dogs

- For dogs that have both Cushing syndrome and diabetes, it is logical that Cushing usually precedes the onset of diabetes. Clinical signs consistent with Cushing are often reported to have been present for several years before diagnosis of diabetes. However, as the diagnosis of diabetes is much more straightforward than the diagnosis of hypercortisolism in dogs, diabetes will often be diagnosed before Cushing syndrome.
- Clinical experience suggests that in populations where neutering of young dogs is routine, Cushing syndrome is the most common cause of insulin resistance in diabetic dogs.
- A major limitation for reporting data on the prevalence of Cushing syndrome in diabetic dogs is the unreliability of diagnostic tests for hypercortisolism in this population with both false-positive and false-negative results occurring commonly. Nevertheless, a positive association between Cushing syndrome and diabetes is well recognized. Diabetic dogs were 6 times more likely than controls to be diagnosed with hypercortisolism in first-opinion practices[15]; this aligns

with a reported 23% prevalence of hypercortisolism in diabetic dogs[16] and 13.6% prevalence of diabetes in dogs with hypercortisolism.[14]

- Insulin resistance typically causes compensatory increase of beta cell function. Therefore, progression to diabetes mellitus in insulin-resistant individuals always requires concurrent loss of beta cell function. In diabetic dogs with all forms of insulin resistance including Cushing syndrome, the mechanisms of beta cell loss are likely the same as for diabetic dogs without insulin resistance.

- Risk factors associated with the diagnosis of diabetes in dogs with Cushing syndrome included hypercholesterolemia, hypertriglyceridemia, pituitary-dependent hypercortisolism, and nonspayed females.[14] However, significantly increased plasma cholesterol and triglycerides occurred after the onset of diabetes, and not in the euglycemic or mildly hyperglycemic dogs with hypercortisolism, indicating that these factors were likely a consequence rather than a cause of the diabetic state.[14]

Iatrogenic Cushing Syndrome in Diabetic Dogs

- The effect of systemic glucocorticoid treatments on insulin requirement in diabetic dogs is predictable. Such treatments will often increase insulin requirement and protect against insulin-induced hypoglycemia. Conversely, insulin requirement can markedly decrease when glucocorticoid treatment is withdrawn.

- The effect of topical glucocorticoid treatments on insulin requirement in diabetic dogs is less predictable. Twice daily application of prednisolone acetate eye drops to healthy dogs for 2 weeks suppressed the hypothalamic-pituitary-adrenal axis,[17] yet application 4 times daily for 4 weeks to diabetic dogs was associated with no detectable differences in diabetic control compared with topical diclofenac.[18] However, dogs with hypercortisolism and poorly controlled diabetes were excluded from the latter study, and our experience is that patients from those specific populations often seem to have increased insulin requirement when treated with prednisolone acetate eye drops and decreased insulin requirement when the treatment is discontinued. Therefore, although there is no contraindication for treatment of diabetic dogs with prednisolone acetate eye drops, this might affect diabetic control in dogs with poorly controlled diabetes and/or hypercortisolism.

Clinical Presentation of Cushing Syndrome in Diabetic Dogs

- Underlying Cushing syndrome can be difficult to recognize in diabetic dogs because there is overlap of clinical signs, laboratory abnormalities, age of diagnosis, and breed predispositions. An important difference is that diabetes typically causes weight loss whereas Cushing does not. Therefore, once glycemic control is sufficient to arrest weight loss, persistent polyphagia, polyuria, polydipsia, and lethargy might be indicators of Cushing syndrome.

- The Project ALIVE Cushing's Clinical Score[1] will often be difficult to apply in diabetic dogs because of the overlap of clinical signs. It is recommended to instead focus on signs specific to Cushing syndrome.

- As it is presumed that in dogs affected concurrently by Cushing syndrome and diabetes, Cushing typically precedes the onset of diabetes, owners may have become accustomed to the Cushing signs and describe their dog as "normal" once the diabetes is controlled.

- There are marked interindividual and breed differences in the clinical presentation of Cushing syndrome. For example, endocrine alopecia presents differently in short- versus long-haired breeds and in those with curly versus straight hair coats. Similarly, deep-chested breeds are less likely to present with a pot-bellied appearance than those breeds with relatively broad chests. As awareness of canine hypercortisolism has increased over time, more subtle case presentations have been recognized.[19] Specific clinical signs of Cushing syndrome include endocrine alopecia, a pot-bellied appearance and muscle wasting that persist after diabetes is controlled, heat and exercise intolerance, increased anxiety or behavioral changes, and signs reflecting premature aging. Hepatomegaly, hypertriglyceridemia, and an alkaline phosphatase that is much more elevated than alanine transaminase can also be indicators of underlying Cushing syndrome, especially if these persist or increase after diabetes is controlled. Dogs with Cushing syndrome are also at increased risk for cruciate ligament rupture.

- The more clinical abnormalities identified that are specific for Cushing syndrome, the stronger the suspicion that hypercortisolism might be present.[19] However, there is no requirement to identify multiple indicators, and suspicion of underlying Cushing syndrome may be based on the presence of only one specific clinical sign (eg, endocrine alopecia) in addition to diabetes. Caution is advisable considering the overlap of clinical signs of the 2 conditions.
- Suspicion of underlying Cushing syndrome may also be based solely on persistently poor response to high doses of insulin not attributable to another cause.[19]

THE EFFECT OF CUSHING-ASSOCIATED DYSGLYCEMIA IN DIABETIC DOGS

- The ALIVE project states that insulin resistance is not defined by the exogenous insulin dose. Therefore, insulin resistance is not necessarily associated with requirement for a higher exogenous insulin dose than is typical for the general diabetic dog population. It follows that there is no insulin dose "threshold" that defines a state of insulin resistance.
- Diabetes in dogs with hypercortisolism is not necessarily more difficult to manage than in dogs with uncomplicated diabetes; this is because glycemic control depends on the interaction in the individual between residual beta cell function and the degree of insulin resistance. These factors may change over time because of ongoing beta cell loss and/or increased or decreased influence of endogenous glucocorticoids. Therefore, there may be good diabetic control for a variable period with subsequent deterioration.
- Diabetes can be very difficult to manage when substantial Cushing-associated dysglycemia is present. The most pronounced effects are typically
  ○ Excessive postprandial hyperglycemia,
  ○ Perceived short duration of insulin action,
  ○ Substantial within-day and/or day-to-day glycemic variability.
- Glycemic variability is best appreciated using continuous glucose monitoring systems (**Figs. 1–5**).
- Glucocorticoids confer protection against insulin-induced hypoglycemia. However, unexpected neuroglycopenia can occur when there is substantial day-to-day glycemic variability necessitating a more cautious approach to insulin treatment (see **Fig. 3**A).

Insulin Treatment to Manage Cushing-Associated Dysglycemia

- Strategies to manage the excessive glycemic variability can provide immediate clinical benefit for diabetic dogs; this can also minimize the confounding effect of poor diabetic control on the diagnostic investigation for the underlying cause of the insulin resistance.

A

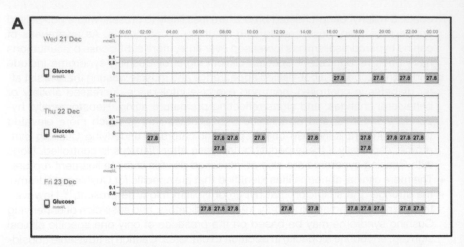

B

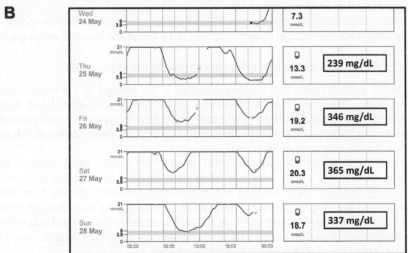

Fig. 1. Example of the effect of Cushing-associated insulin resistance on glycemic control in diabetic dogs: within-day glycemic variability. (*A*) Continuous glucose graph from a diabetic dog soon after commencing treatment with an intermediate-acting insulin formulation at 0.5 U/kg q12 h. All interstitial glucose results were greater than 500 mg/dL (>27.8 mmol/L). (*B*) Continuous glucose graph from the same dog in Fig. 1A 6 months later when treated with the same intermediate-acting insulin formulation at 2.0 U/kg q12 h. Average daily interstitial glucose results are provided in the right panel. Note that there is large within-day glycemic variability and apparent short duration of insulin action.

- The most successful approaches mimic the pattern of endogenous insulin secretion of nondiabetic, insulin-resistant individuals:
  - Basal insulin requirements, and hence basal insulin secretion, typically increase in response to insulin resistance (although this might be either a constant or an intermittent effect).
  - Glucocorticoids additionally increase postprandial insulin requirement by inhibiting the suppressive effects of insulin on glucogenesis, along with incomplete suppression of glucagon after meals.

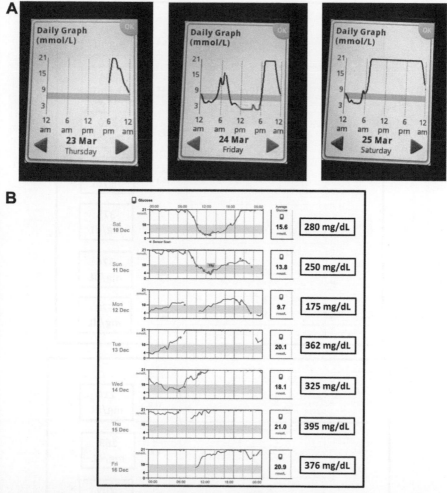

Fig. 2. Examples of the effect of Cushing-associated insulin resistance on glycemic control in diabetic dogs: day-to-day glycemic variability. (*A*) Daily graphs from consecutive days showing marked day-to-day glycemic variability despite a consistent insulin dosing and feeding routine. (*B*) Continuous glucose graph from a different dog showing marked day-to-day glycemic variability despite a consistent insulin dosing and feeding routine. Average daily interstitial glucose results are provided in the right panel.

- *Basal insulin monotherapy* aims to address background insulin resistance without specifically addressing postprandial hyperglycemia. This simple approach provides good-to-excellent control in most of the dogs with Cushing-associated diabetes (**Fig. 6**). Ideally, a basal insulin formulation should have a similar action at every hour of the day and minimal day-to-day variability. There are only 2 options that fulfill these criteria in dogs: insulin glargine U300 and insulin degludec insulin (see Chapter 9, Insulin therapy in dogs).[20,21]
- As there is large variability in the severity of insulin resistance in dogs with Cushing-associated diabetes, there is corresponding large variability of the required dose of basal insulin. Therefore, dose titration is only feasible if response to treatment is monitored using a continuous glucose monitor.[22]

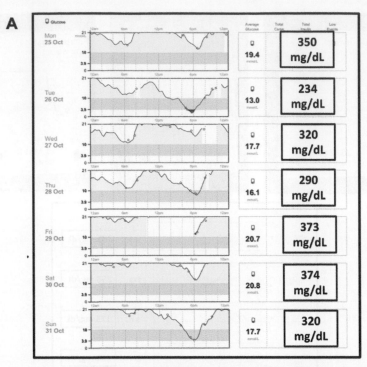

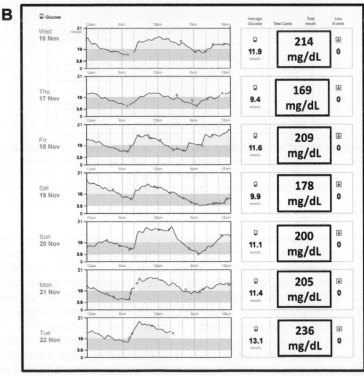

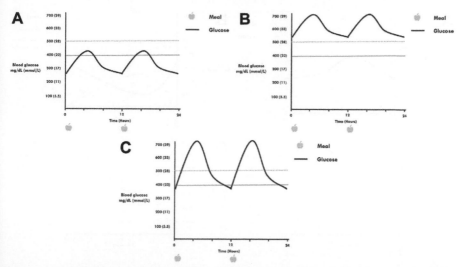

Fig. 4. Graphical illustration of the influence of insulin resistance on glucose control in diabetic dogs. Graphs show examples of 24-hour glucose data. The x-axis shows time, and the y-axis shows blood/interstitial glucose concentrations. The solid gray line denotes the upper limit of the Freestyle Libre graph (400 mg/dL; 22 mmol/L) and the broken gray line the highest glucose concentration measured by that device (500 mg/dL; 27.8 mmol/L). (*A*) Example of a 24-hour glucose graph in a diabetic dog with no underlying insulin resistance. The same meal is consumed every 12 hours, and no insulin treatment is administered. Note that the typical postprandial hyperglycemic period is 6 to 9 hours. (*B*) Example of a 24-hour glucose graph in a diabetic dog with insulin resistance that is relatively constant over the day. The same meal is consumed every 12 hours, and no insulin treatment is administered. (*C*) Example of a 24-hour glucose graph in a diabetic dog with insulin resistance associated with excessive postprandial hyperglycemia, for example, due to Cushing syndrome. The same meal is consumed every 12 hours, and no insulin treatment is administered.

- *Combined basal-bolus insulin treatment* aims to address both background insulin resistance and postprandial hyperglycemia. This approach typically requires that 2 different insulin formulations are administered with a meal twice daily (**Fig. 7**). Intermediate-acting insulin formulations are the most appropriate for bolus insulin treatment of dogs, rather than the short-acting formulations used for this purpose in diabetic people (see Chapter 9, Insulin therapy in dogs).

Fig. 3. Example of the effect of Cushing-associated insulin resistance on glycemic control in diabetic dogs: response to trilostane treatment. (*A*) Continuous glucose graph from a diabetic dog with hypercortisolism 4 months after starting trilostane treatment. There was still marked postprandial hyperglycemia and day-to-day glycemic variability despite good control of hypercortisolism. The low glucose event on Tuesday October 26 was associated with mild signs of neuroglycopenia. Average daily interstitial glucose results are provided in the right panel. (Treatment: insulin glargine U300 at 1 U/kg BID; trilostane at 3 mg/kg BID). (*B*) Continuous glucose graph from the same dog in Fig. 3A 15 months after starting trilostane treatment. Glycemic variability has substantially decreased, so the insulin dose could be safely increased to improve overall glycemic control without associated increased risk of neuroglycopenia. Average daily interstitial glucose results are provided in the right panel. (Treatment: insulin glargine U300 at 2 U/kg BID; trilostane at 3 mg/kg BID).

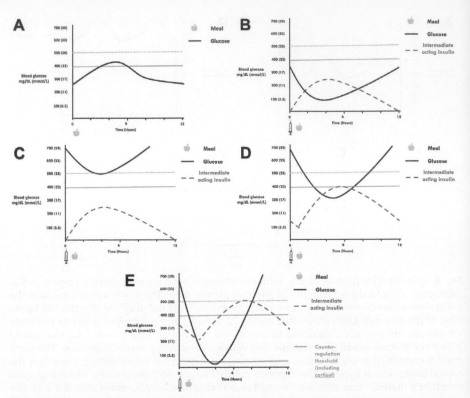

Fig. 5. Graphical illustration of the effect of treatment of a diabetic dog with insulin resistance using an intermediate-acting insulin. Graphs show examples of 12-hour glucose data. The x-axis shows time, and the y-axis shows blood/interstitial glucose concentrations. The solid gray line denotes the upper limit of the Freestyle Libre graph (400 mg/dL; 22 mmol/L) and the broken gray line the highest glucose concentration measured by that device (500 mg/dL; 27.8 mmol/L). The same meal is consumed every 12 hours. (*A*) Example of a 12-hour glucose graph in a diabetic dog with no underlying insulin resistance. No insulin treatment is administered. (*B*) Example of a 12-hour glucose graph in a diabetic dog with no insulin resistance treated with a standard dose of intermediate-acting insulin. Note that the expected (yet not always achieved) graph is U-shaped. (*C*) Example of a 12-hour glucose graph in a diabetic dog with insulin resistance treated with a standard dose of intermediate-acting insulin q12 h. (*D*) Example of a 12-hour glucose graph in a diabetic dog with insulin resistance treated with 1.5 times a standard dose of intermediate-acting insulin q12 h. Note that the duration of action of the insulin increases as the dose increases. (*E*) Example of a 12-hour glucose graph in a diabetic dog with insulin resistance treated with 2 times a standard dose of intermediate-acting insulin q12 h. The insulin decreases the blood glucose to the hypoglycemic range, which triggers a counterregulatory response. Dogs with Cushing syndrome might have excessive cortisol counterregulation.

- When switching to a basal-bolus protocol, it is recommended that the same total insulin dose (per unit) is used every 12 hours by reducing the dose of the intermediate-acting insulin by 50%, and the remainder of the total insulin dose is divided and given by basal insulin twice daily.[23] The doses can then be adjusted based on the dog's response. In this situation, it is crucial that there is very clear communication with owners regarding the dose of each of the insulin preparations. The response to treatment is much more predictable with this

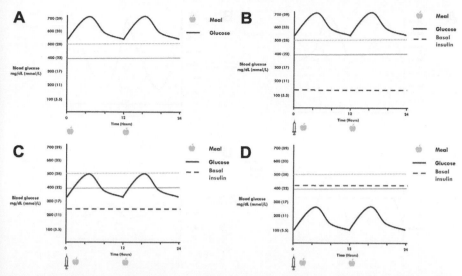

Fig. 6. Graphical illustration of the effect of treatment of a diabetic dog with insulin resistance using a basal insulin. Graphs show examples of 24-hour glucose data. The x-axis shows time, and the y-axis shows blood/interstitial glucose concentrations. The solid gray line denotes the upper limit of the Freestyle Libre graph (400 mg/dL; 22 mmol/L) and the broken gray line the highest glucose concentration measured by that device (500 mg/dL; 27.8 mmol/L). The same meal is consumed every 12 hours. (*A*) Example of a 24-hour glucose graph in a diabetic dog with insulin resistance. No insulin treatment is administered. (*B*) Example of a 24-hour glucose graph in a diabetic dog with insulin resistance treated with a standard dose of basal insulin q24 h. Note the postprandial increase of glucose that causes the graph to be an inverse of the U-shape expected following intermediate-acting insulin. (*C*) Example of a 24-hour glucose graph in a diabetic dog with insulin resistance treated with 1.5 times a standard dose of basal insulin q24 h. (*D*) Example of a 24-hour glucose graph in a diabetic dog with insulin resistance treated with 3 times a standard dose of basal insulin q24 h.

approach compared with basal insulin monotherapy and so it is not necessary to use a continuous glucose monitor during the changeover.

DIAGNOSIS OF CANINE HYPERCORTISOLISM

- Details regarding the diagnosis of hypercortisolism in dogs are available in the Project ALIVE resources.[1] The "General definitions for diagnostic tests for Cushing's and Hypoadrenocorticism" section provides information on the various tests.
- The ALIVE criteria for the diagnosis of naturally occurring Cushing syndrome are as follows:
  - "Identification of a set of clinical features attributable to Cushing's Syndrome including supportive history, physical examination findings, and clinicopathologic test results;
  - AND demonstration of an excess of cortisol through dynamic testing of pituitary-adrenal function; dynamic testing of pituitary-adrenal function can include a dexamethasone suppression test based on blood or urine or an adrenocorticotropic hormone (ACTH) stimulation test."[1]
- Importantly, Project ALIVE provides a definition for "subdiagnostic" Cushing syndrome:

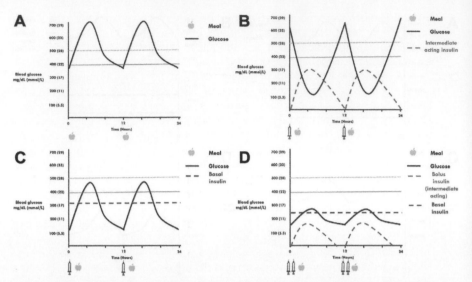

Fig. 7. Graphical illustration of the effect of treatment of a diabetic dog with insulin resistance using basal-bolus insulin. Graphs show examples of 24-hour glucose data. The x-axis shows time, and the y-axis shows blood/interstitial glucose concentrations. The solid gray line denotes the upper limit of the Freestyle Libre graph (400 mg/dL; 22 mmol/L) and the broken gray line the highest glucose concentration measured by that device (500 mg/dL; 27.8 mmol/L). The same meal is consumed every 12 hours. (*A*) Example of a 24-hour glucose graph in a diabetic dog with insulin resistance associated with excessive postprandial hyperglycemia, for example, due to Cushing syndrome. No insulin treatment is administered. (*B*) Example of a 24-hour glucose graph in a diabetic dog with insulin resistance associated with excessive postprandial hyperglycemia treated with an intermediate-acting insulin q12 h. (*C*) Example of a 24-hour glucose graph in a diabetic dog with insulin resistance associated with excessive postprandial hyperglycemia treated with a basal insulin q12 h. The same pattern can be achieved in many dogs with q24 h dosing. (*D*) Example of a 24-hour glucose graph in a diabetic dog with insulin resistance associated with excessive postprandial hyperglycemia treated with basal-bolus insulin treatment q12 h. The same pattern can be achieved in many dogs with q24 h dosing of the basal insulin.

- ○ "A clinical syndrome in which a dog or cat appears to have Cushing's syndrome, yet the results of dynamic testing of pituitary-adrenal function fall into appropriate (normal) reference intervals.
- ○ Testing requires a normal dexamethasone suppression test (based on blood or urine estimates of corticoid activity) and a normal ACTH stimulation test.
- ○ "Subdiagnostic Cushing's syndrome" has previously been referred to as Atypical or Occult Cushing's/Hyperadrenocorticism."[1]
- • "Subdiagnostic Cushing syndrome" therefore defines the relatively common situation when there are false-negative results for both a dexamethasone suppression test and an ACTH stimulation test for an individual case.

Diagnosis of Hypercortisolism in Diabetic Dogs: Specificity, Sensitivity, and the Relationship Between Pretest Probability and the Positive and Negative Predictive Values of Diagnostic Tests

- • Reported sensitivities and specificities for both the low-dose dexamethasone suppression test and the ACTH stimulation test for diagnosis of canine hypercortisolism were mostly determined decades ago with cortisol assays that are no longer used. Nevertheless, although updated and current sensitivity and specificity data are scarce, it is recognized that false-positive and false-negative results still commonly occur with both tests.[24]

- It is recommended that individual features of each case are carefully considered to assist with assessment of the likelihood of false-positive and false-negative results because this will vary from case to case and over time for the one case:
  - False-positive results are typically associated with stress and/or nonadrenal illness, including diabetes; this means that it is necessary to achieve control of the diabetes before testing for hypercortisolism to improve the specificity of the tests and reduce the likelihood of a false-positive result. It is the authors' experience that a practical guideline is to first achieve sufficient control of the diabetes to arrest weight loss before performing diagnostic tests for hypercortisolism. It is also advisable to ensure that there are no signs of malaise or inappetence on the day the test is performed and that the dog is housed in a low-stress environment during the test.
  - Pretest probability is influenced by disease prevalence. There is a positive association between hypercortisolism and diabetes in dogs, which means that a diabetic dog is more likely to have hypercortisolism than a nondiabetic dog. If care is taken to minimize the likelihood of false-positive results as outlined earlier, then this increased prevalence affects the pretest probability in diabetic dogs as follows:
    - The negative predictive value of a diagnostic test for hypercortisolism is decreased compared with nondiabetic dogs.
    - The positive predictive value of a diagnostic test for hypercortisolism is increased compared with nondiabetic dogs.
- Negative (normal) test results cannot exclude a diagnosis of hypercortisolism.
- If it is suspected that the first test returned a false-negative result, then it is recommended that the other alternative test is performed. For example, if the first test was an ACTH stimulation test, then a low-dose dexamethasone suppression test is recommended (and vice versa). If it is suspected that both tests returned false-negative results, then subdiagnostic Cushing syndrome may be present.
- The situation where there is no perfectly reliable test for hypercortisolism and there is a possibility of subdiagnostic Cushing syndrome can result in a frustrating situation where hypercortisolism is strongly suspected but diagnosis cannot be confirmed. An appropriate approach in many cases will be to retest after 3 to 6 months if clinical signs persist. However, if clinical signs are severe and negatively affecting the dog's and/or the owner's quality of life, and there is no other likely reason for the dog's clinical signs, then a carefully monitored trilostane treatment trial should be considered. Improvement in response to treatment can thus be used as a diagnostic test. Dogs with normal adrenal function seem to be more resistant to adverse effects associated with trilostane treatment than dogs with hypercortisolism[25,26]; this means that a carefully monitored trilostane treatment trial might be unlikely to cause problems in dogs that do not have hypercortisolism.

Treatment of Cushing Syndrome in Diabetic Dogs

- Glucocorticoid treatment should ideally be withdrawn if iatrogenic Cushing syndrome is present. However, it is acknowledged that this might not always be possible.

- If the cause of ACTH-dependent or ACTH-independent hypercortisolism cannot be removed, then medical treatment to control excess adrenal hormone secretion is indicated.
- If trilostane treatment is used, a twice-daily administration protocol is typically recommended for diabetic dogs.
- Use of clinical signs to monitor the response to treatment of Cushing syndrome is likely less reliable in diabetic dogs than in nondiabetic dogs. Therefore, direct measurement of cortisol response is recommended, for example, with an ACTH stimulation test.
- Short-acting glucocorticoid tablets should be dispensed when Cushing treatment commences. Administration of these tablets is recommended whenever there is potential for absolute or relative hypocortisolism, for example, when there is inappetence, malaise, a stressful event, or surgery. Administration will also protect diabetic dogs against the potential for hypoglycemia. It is additionally noted that one of the differential diagnoses for owners reporting inappetence in trilostane-treated dogs is resolution of polyphagia.

What Happens to the Insulin Resistance When Cushing Syndrome Is Treated?

- Insulin resistance and associated within-day and/or day-to-day glycemic variability seems to persist for many months after very good control of hypercortisolism is achieved with trilostane treatment (see **Fig. 3**). Resolution of insulin resistance and glycemic variability seems to correlate with resolution of hepatomegaly.
- Therefore, there is no requirement to decrease the insulin dose at the same time as commencing trilostane treatment.
- This is in contrast to treatment methods that eliminate the cause of hypercortisolism, such as surgical removal of a functional adrenal tumor. In those cases, insulin resistance and dysglycemia seem to resolve rapidly after treatment.

DIESTRUS
Why Diestrus Is Associated with Insulin Resistance

- Entire female dogs undergo cyclical changes in insulin sensitivity associated with their estrous cycle. Insulin resistance occurs during diestrus,[12] which, in dogs, is a prolonged, progesterone dominant luteal stage that lasts for 2 to 3 months. Many of the hormonal changes during diestrus mimic those that occur during pregnancy.
- In women, no single hormone or metabolic mechanism has been found to explain insulin resistance during pregnancy.[27] Instead insulin resistance results from the summation of multiple effects and increases as pregnancy progresses.[28] However, unlike people, progesterone-induced growth hormone secretion from the mammary glands is an important hormonal change in dogs.
- Progesterone and growth hormone are 2 diabetogenic hormones that are associated with insulin resistance. Growth hormone and progesterone concentrations are comparable in diestrus and pregnancy in dogs, with reduced insulin sensitivity during both stages. However, pregnant dogs are more insulin resistant and have a 43% reduction in insulin sensitivity in late pregnancy.[12,29]
- Progesterone can stimulate growth hormone production and release from the mammary gland of entire bitches. In some individuals, hypersecretion of growth hormone is induced, causing hypersomatotropism, an acromegalic phenotype, and greater insulin resistance compared with normal diestrus.[30]

- In susceptible dogs, diabetes mellitus develops in association with insulin resistance during diestrus.[31] This subtype of canine diabetes is likely comparable to gestational diabetes in women in that progression from insulin resistance to diabetes requires concurrent loss of beta cell function (because insulin resistance alone does not directly cause beta cell loss). The mechanisms of beta cell loss are likely the same as for diabetic dogs without insulin resistance.
- There is interindividual variability of the diabetogenic effects of diestrus with recognized breed predispositions, including Border Collies and Swedish Elkhounds.[31] The increased risk of Swedish Elkhounds does not seem to be associated with beta cell autoimmunity because all affected dogs were negative for GAD-65-autoantibodies.[32]

The Effect of Routine Neutering of Young Female Dogs on Risk Factors for Diabetes in Dog Populations

- In contrast to the female predisposition for diabetes in populations where neutering of young female dogs is not routinely recommended (eg, 72% female predisposition for diabetes in Swedish dogs),[31] there tends to be a marginal male predisposition for diabetes where neutering is routine.[15,33]
- There is an interaction of neutering status with common causes of insulin resistance in dogs. Compared with intact dogs, neutered dogs have an increased risk of obesity and for developing Cushing syndrome.[34] However, entire female dogs with hypercortisolism have increased risk for diabetes compared with males and neutered females.[14]

Treatment and Remission of Diestrus Diabetes

- Ovariohysterectomy can promptly resolve progesterone-associated insulin resistance. The chance of diabetic remission is likely much higher if neutering is performed as soon as practical after the diagnosis of diabetes. In addition, prompt insulin treatment is important to attempt to preserve pancreatic beta cell function. This approach has been reported to achieve diabetic remission in about 10% of cases.[35] Remission usually occurs within 4 to 39 days after ovariohysterectomy, but the time to resolution of insulin resistance and decreased exogenous insulin requirements is unpredictable.[30]
- Remission may spontaneously occur at the end of diestrus.[31] Ovariohysterectomy should be performed before subsequent estrus cycles to prevent relapse of diabetes and risk of progression to permanent diabetes.

OBESITY
Obesity Results in Compensatory Increase of Insulin Secretion in Dogs

- Obesity causes insulin resistance in dogs as it does in all species, with the degree of insulin resistance positively correlated with the severity of adiposity.[36]
- Spontaneously obese dogs compensate for reduced insulin sensitivity with hyperinsulinemia, with the result that glucose tolerance is maintained. In one study, obese dogs had approximately half the insulin sensitivity of lean dogs, with a 4-fold increase in insulin concentrations, while maintaining euglycemia.[37]
- Adipose tissue is an active endocrine organ that secretes adipokines that modify insulin sensitivity. In spontaneously obese dogs, leptin seems to be the main adipokine associated with obesity-associated changes in insulin sensitivity and compensatory hyperinsulinemia. Glucagon-like peptide 1 also likely has a role in compensatory hyperinsulinemia.[38]

- Similar to other species, obesity is associated with hypertriglyceridemia in dogs, but, unlike other species, obesity-associated hypertriglyceridemia might not contribute to insulin resistance in dogs.[39]

Obesity and Canine Diabetes Mellitus

- Type 2 diabetes mellitus, a condition strongly associated with obesity in people, is not recognized in dogs.
- Disease processes that cause progressive loss of beta cells, such as immune-mediated destruction or chronic pancreatitis, will limit the capacity of obese dogs to compensate for obesity-associated insulin resistance; this might result in earlier presentation with diabetes than if the dog was lean.
- Insulin is an anabolic hormone and so treatment with exogenous insulin promotes weight gain. If an insulin-treated diabetic dog becomes obese, the resulting insulin resistance will increase basal insulin requirement; this can lead to a cycle of increasing insulin doses and increasing adiposity. Conversely, if an obese diabetic dog loses weight, insulin sensitivity will improve and exogenous insulin requirement will decrease.
- Obesity and other causes of insulin resistance have an additive effect on insulin requirements and the risk of progression to clinical diabetes in dogs. Dogs with Cushing syndrome had greater risk for developing diabetes if they were entire females and/or were overweight or obese on initial presentation.[14] The same cumulative insulin resistance occurs in obese female dogs in diestrus.[40]

SUMMARY

- CUSHING SYNDROME is the most common cause of insulin resistance in diabetic dogs in populations where neutering of young dogs is routine.
- Suspicion of underlying Cushing syndrome may be based solely on persistently poor response to high insulin doses not attributable to another cause. There is no requirement to identify multiple indicators; although, the more abnormalities identified, the stronger the suspicion for hypercortisolism.
- The most pronounced effects of Cushing syndrome on glucose metabolism are insulin resistance, excessive postprandial hyperglycemia, perceived short duration of insulin action, and/or substantial within-day and/or day-to-day glycemic variability.
- Strategies to manage excessive glycemic variability can provide immediate clinical benefit for diabetic dogs and minimize the confounding effect of poor diabetic control on the diagnostic investigation for the underlying cause of the insulin resistance.
- Successful strategies include basal insulin monotherapy and combined basal-bolus insulin treatment.
- False-positive and false-negative results commonly occur with diagnostic tests for hypercortisolism in dogs.
- False-positive results are typically associated with stress and/or nonadrenal illness, including diabetes. A practical guideline before testing for hypercortisolism to reduce the likelihood of a false-positive result is to first achieve sufficient control of the diabetes to arrest weight loss.
- Diabetic dogs are more likely to have hypercortisolism than nondiabetic dogs. Therefore, if care is taken to minimize the likelihood of false-positive results as outlined above:
  - The negative predictive value of a diagnostic test for hypercortisolism is decreased compared with nondiabetic dogs.

- ○ The positive predictive value of a diagnostic test for hypercortisolism is increased compared with nondiabetic dogs.
- The situation where there is no perfectly reliable test for hypercortisolism and there is a possibility of subdiagnostic Cushing syndrome can result in a frustrating situation where hypercortisolism is strongly suspected but diagnosis cannot be confirmed. If clinical signs are severe and negatively affecting the dog's and/or the owner's quality of life, and there is no other likely reason for the dog's clinical signs, then a carefully monitored trilostane treatment trial may be considered.
- DIESTRUS is the most common cause of insulin resistance in diabetic dogs in populations where neutering of young dogs is not routinely recommended.
- Ovariohysterectomy and insulin treatment can achieve diabetic remission in about 10% of cases of diestrus diabetes.
- OBESITY: spontaneously obese dogs compensate for reduced insulin sensitivity with hyperinsulinemia, with the result that glucose tolerance is maintained. There is no evidence that obesity is associated with type 2 diabetes mellitus in dogs.
- Obesity and other causes of insulin resistance have an additive effect on insulin requirements and the risk of progression to clinical diabetes in dogs.

CLINICS CARE POINTS

- Suspicion of underlying Cushing syndrome may be based solely on persistently poor response to high insulin doses not attributable to another cause. There is no requirement to identify multiple indicators, although, the more abnormalities identified, the stronger the suspicion for hypercortisolism.

- Strategies to manage excessive glycemic variability can provide immediate clinical benefit for diabetic dogs and minimize the confounding effect of poor diabetic control on the diagnostic investigation for the underlying cause of the insulin resistance.

- Successful strategies include basal insulin monotherapy and combined basal-bolus insulin treatment.

- False positive and false negative results commonly occur with diagnostic tests for hypercortisolism in dogs.

- The situation where there is no perfectly reliable test for hypercortisolism and there is a possibility of subdiagnostic Cushing syndrome can result in a frustrating situation where hypercortisolism is strongly suspected but diagnosis cannot be confirmed. If clinical signs are severe and negatively affecting the dog's and/or the owner's quality of life, and there is no other likely reason for the dog's clinical signs, then a carefully monitored trilostane treatment trial may be considered.

- Ovariohysterectomy and insulin treatment can achieve diabetic remission in about 10% of cases of diestrus diabetes.

DISCLOSURE

L. Fleeman has received honoraria for educational seminars for MSD Animal Health, Zoetis, Royal Canin, Nestle Purina, and consulting fees from Dechra.

REFERENCES

1. European Society of Veterinary Endocrinology. Project ALIVE. Available at: https://www.esve.org/alive/search.aspx. Accessed Dec 5, 2022.

2. Pivonello R, De Leo M, Vitale P, et al. Pathophysiology of diabetes mellitus in Cushing's syndrome. Neuroendocrinology 2010;92(Suppl 1):77–81.

3. van Raalte DH, Diamant M. Steroid diabetes: from mechanism to treatment? Neth J Med 2014;72(2):62–72.

4. van Raalte DH, Brands M, van der Zijl NJ, et al. Low-dose glucocorticoid treatment affects multiple aspects of intermediary metabolism in healthy humans: a randomised controlled trial. Diabetologia 2011;54(8):2103–12.

5. Rizza RA, Mandarino LJ, Gerich JE. Cortisol-induced insulin resistance in man: impaired suppression of glucose production and stimulation of glucose utilization due to a postreceptor detect of insulin action. J Clin Endocrinol Metab 1982; 54(1):131–8.

6. DeFronzo RA, Jacot E, Jequier E, et al. The effect of insulin on the disposal of intravenous glucose. Results from indirect calorimetry and hepatic and femoral venous catheterization. Diabetes 1981;30(12):1000–7.

7. Khaleeli AA, Edwards RH, Gohil K, et al. Corticosteroid myopathy: a clinical and pathological study. Clin Endocrinol 1983;18(2):155–66.

8. Ouchi N, Parker JL, Lugus JJ, et al. Adipokines in inflammation and metabolic disease. Nat Rev Immunol 2011;11(2):85–97.

9. van Raalte DH, Ouwens DM, Diamant M. Novel insights into glucocorticoid-mediated diabetogenic effects: towards expansion of therapeutic options? Eur J Clin Invest 2009;39(2):81–93.

10. van Raalte DH, Kwa KA, van Genugten RE, et al. Islet-cell dysfunction induced by glucocorticoid treatment: potential role for altered sympathovagal balance? Metabolism: Clinical and Experimental 2013;62(4):568–77.

11. Peterson ME, Nesbitt GH, Schaer M. Diagnosis and management of concurrent diabetes mellitus and hyperadrenocorticism in thirty dogs. Journal of the American Veterinary Medical Association 1981;178(1):66–9.

12. Fukuta H, Mori A, Urumuhan N, et al. Characterization and comparison of insulin resistance induced by Cushing Syndrome or diestrus against healthy control dogs as determined by euglycemic- hyperinsulinemic glucose clamp profile glucose infusion rate using an artificial pancreas apparatus. J Vet Med Sci 2012;74(11):1527–30.

13. Montgomery TM, Nelson RW, Feldman EC, et al. Basal and glucagon-stimulated plasma C-peptide concentrations in healthy dogs, dogs with diabetes mellitus, and dogs with hyperadrenocorticism. J Vet Intern Med 1996;10(3):116–22.

14. Miceli DD, Pignataro OP, Castillo VA. Concurrent hyperadrenocorticism and diabetes mellitus in dogs. Res Vet Sci 2017;115:425–31.

15. Yoon S, Fleeman LM, Wilson BJ, et al. Epidemiological study of dogs with diabetes mellitus attending primary care veterinary clinics in Australia. Vet Rec 2020;187(3):e22.

16. Hess RS, Saunders M, van Winkle TJ, et al. Concurrent disorders in dogs with diabetes mellitus: 221 cases (1993-1998). Journal of the American Veterinary Medical Association 2000;217(8):1166–73.

17. Kline KE, Walton SA, Specht AJ, et al. Comparison of ophthalmic loteprednol etabonate and prednisolone acetate effects on adrenocortical response to ACTH in dogs. Vet Ophthalmol 2022;25(6):468–75.

18. Rankin AJ, KuKanich KS, Schermerhorn T, et al. Evaluation of diabetes mellitus regulation in dogs treated with ophthalmic preparations of prednisolone acetate versus diclofenac sodium. American Journal of Veterinary Research 2019;80(12): 1129–35.

19. Behrend EN, Kooistra HS, Nelson R, et al. Diagnosis of spontaneous canine hyperadrenocorticism: 2012 ACVIM consensus statement (small animal). J Vet Intern Med 2013;27(6):1292–304.

20. Fink H, Herbert C, Gilor C. Pharmacodynamics and pharmacokinetics of insulin detemir and insulin glargine 300 U/mL in healthy dogs. Domest Anim Endocrinol 2018;64:17–30.

21. Oda H, Mori A, Ishii S, et al. Time-action profiles of insulin degludec in healthy dogs and its effects on glycemic control in diabetic dogs. J Vet Med Sci 2018; 80(11):1720–3.

22. Gilor C, Fleeman LM, Fracassi F. Insulin glargine U300 in dogs: Clinical experience and simple guidelines. Paper presented at: ACVIM Forum; virtual presentation available Sept 22 to Nov 30 2022.

23. Gilor C, Fleeman LM. One hundred years of insulin: Is it time for smart? Journal of Small Animal Practice 2022;63(9):645–60.

24. Bennaim M, Shiel RE, Mooney CT. Diagnosis of spontaneous hyperadrenocorticism in dogs. Part 2: Adrenal function testing and differentiating tests. Vet J (London, England 1997) 2019;252:105343.

25. Teshima T, Hara Y, Takekoshi S, et al. Trilostane-induced inhibition of cortisol secretion results in reduced negative feedback at the hypothalamic-pituitary axis. Domest Anim Endocrinol 2009;36(1):32–44.

26. de Gier J, Wolthers CH, Galac S, et al. Effects of the 3β-hydroxysteroid dehydrogenase inhibitor trilostane on luteal progesterone production in the dog. Theriogenology 2011;75(7):1271–9.

27. Plows JF, Stanley JL, Baker PN, et al. The Pathophysiology of Gestational Diabetes Mellitus. Int J Mol Sci 2018;19(11):3342.

28. Kampmann U, Knorr S, Fuglsang J, et al. Determinants of Maternal Insulin Resistance during Pregnancy: An Updated Overview. J Diabetes Res 2019;2019: 5320156.

29. Johnson CA. Glucose homeostasis during canine pregnancy: Insulin resistance, ketosis, and hypoglycemia. Theriogenology 2008;70(9):1418–23.

30. Eigenmann JE, Eigenmann RY, Rijnberk A, et al. Progesterone-controlled growth hormone overproduction and naturally occurring canine diabetes and acromegaly. Acta Endocrinol 1983;104(2):167–76.

31. Fall T, Hamlin HH, Hedhammar A, et al. Diabetes mellitus in a population of 180,000 insured dogs: incidence, survival, and breed distribution. J Vet Intern Med 2007;21(6):1209–16.

32. Fall T, Hedhammar A, Wallberg A, et al. Diabetes mellitus in elkhounds is associated with diestrus and pregnancy. J Vet Intern Med 2010;24(6):1322–8.

33. Heeley AM, O'Neill DG, Davison LJ, et al. Diabetes mellitus in dogs attending UK primary-care practices: frequency, risk factors and survival. Canine Medicine and Genetics 2020;7(1):6.

34. Carotenuto G, Malerba E, Dolfini C, et al. Cushing's syndrome-an epidemiological study based on a canine population of 21,281 dogs. Open Vet J 2019;9(1):27–32.

35. Pöppl AG, Mottin TS, González FH. Diabetes mellitus remission after resolution of inflammatory and progesterone-related conditions in bitches. Res Vet Sci 2013; 94(3):471–3.

36. German AJ, Hervera M, Hunter L, et al. Improvement in insulin resistance and reduction in plasma inflammatory adipokines after weight loss in obese dogs. Domest Anim Endocrinol 2009;37(4):214–26.

37. Verkest KR, Fleeman LM, Rand JS, et al. Evaluation of beta-cell sensitivity to glucose and first-phase insulin secretion in obese dogs. American Journal of Veterinary Research 2011;72(3):357–66.

38. Verkest KR, Fleeman LM, Morton JM, et al. Compensation for obesity-induced insulin resistance in dogs: assessment of the effects of leptin, adiponectin, and glucagon-like peptide-1 using path analysis. Domest Anim Endocrinol 2011; 41(1):24–34.

39. Verkest KR, Rand JS, Fleeman LM, et al. Spontaneously obese dogs exhibit greater postprandial glucose, triglyceride, and insulin concentrations than lean dogs. Domest Anim Endocrinol 2012;42(2):103–12.

40. Mattheeuws D, Rottiers R, Kaneko JJ, et al. Diabetes mellitus in dogs: Relationship of obesity to glucose tolerance and insulin response. American Journal of Veterinary Research 1984;45(1):98–103.

Moving?

Make sure your subscription moves with you!

To notify us of your new address, find your **Clinics Account Number** (located on your mailing label above your name), and contact customer service at:

Email: journalscustomerservice-usa@elsevier.com

800-654-2452 (subscribers in the U.S. & Canada)
314-447-8871 (subscribers outside of the U.S. & Canada)

Fax number: 314-447-8029

Elsevier Health Sciences Division
Subscription Customer Service
3251 Riverport Lane
Maryland Heights, MO 63043

*To ensure uninterrupted delivery of your subscription, please notify us at least 4 weeks in advance of move.

Printed and bound by CPI Group (UK) Ltd, Croydon, CR0 4YY

03/10/2024

01040471-0005